OXFORD STATISTICAL SCIENCE SERIES

SERIES EDITORS

OXFORD STATISTICAL SCIENCE SERIES

The Statistical Evaluation
of Medical Tests
for Classification and Prediction

Margaret Sullivan Pepe

*Professor of Biostatistics, University of Washington
and Fred Hutchinson Cancer Research Center*

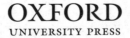

OXFORD
UNIVERSITY PRESS

OXFORD

UNIVERSITY PRESS

Great Clarendon Street, Oxford OX2 6DP

Oxford University Press is a department of the University of Oxford.
It furthers the University's objective of excellence in research, scholarship,
and education by publishing worldwide in

Oxford New York

Auckland Bangkok Buenos Aires Cape Town Chennai
Dar es Salaam Delhi Hong Kong Istanbul Karachi Kolkata
Kuala Lumpur Madrid Melbourne Mexico City Mumbai Nairobi
São Paulo Shanghai Tokyo Toronto

Oxford is a registered trade mark of Oxford University Press
in the UK and in certain other countries

Published in the United States
by Oxford University Press Inc., New York

© Oxford University Press, 2003

The moral rights of the author have been asserted

Database right Oxford University Press (maker)

First published 2003
Reprinted 2003, 2004

British Library Cataloguing in Publication Data
Data available

Library of Congress Cataloging in Publication Data

ISBN 0 19 850984 7

10 9 8 7 6 5 4 3

Typeset using the author's L^AT_EX files by Julie Harris

Printed in Great Britain
on acid-free paper by
Biddles Ltd, King's Lynn, Norfolk

PREFACE

The purpose of this book is to provide a systematic framework for the statistical theory and practice of research studies that seek to evaluate clinical tests used in the practice of medicine. My hope is that it will be found useful by both practicing biostatisticians and more academic research biostatisticians. In addition, it could be used as a textbook for a graduate level course in medical statistics.

While my background is set in mainstream biostatistical research (survival analysis, clinical trials, measurement error, missing data and so forth), I was first introduced to the problem of diagnostic test evaluation in 1995 when collaborating on a hearing screening study. To my surprise, the statistical concepts that the audiology researchers were using were only vaguely familiar to me. They were not part of standard biostatistical training. Moreover, the methods available were fairly rudimentary, lacking, for example, flexibility to adjust for covariates or to handle clustered data. Since then my involvement with several other projects has led me to conclude that these statistical concepts should be applied more widely. At the same time, a more rigorous and expansive development of statistical methodology in this field has been taking place. This book should serve as both a reference for the statistician applying these techniques in practice and as a survey of the current state of statistical research for the academic interested in developing new methodology in this field.

There is a growing need for the rigorous scientific evaluation of tests that purport to identify disease or other conditions. The pace at which new medical technologies are being developed to detect disease, to predict its course and to evaluate response to therapy, is truly amazing. Proteomics, genomics, cell flow cytometry and imaging modalities are among the array of new tools available. In addition, improvements to existing technologies are continually being made. My recent experience with the National Cancer Institute-sponsored Early Detection Research Network (EDRN), which seeks to develop biomarkers for cancer, has greatly reinforced the perspective that rigorous scientific studies must be conducted to determine the accuracy and value of these biotechnologies. The statistical methods described in this book should be useful for the design and evaluation of such studies.

Much of the literature on evaluating biomedical tests appears in substantive journals, particularly in radiology journals. Methods have not been developed to the same extent or with the same rigor as they have for therapeutic research and for epidemiologic research. There is a recent trend towards articles appearing in mainstream biostatistical journals. I hope that this book will serve in some capacity to stimulate further development of statistical methods and to place them firmly within the realm of mainstream biostatistical research. Although most of the book is written with the practicing statistician as the intended audience,

v

some sections are written specifically for the academic research biostatistician. In particular, the comments on needed research that appear in the remarks at the end of each chapter may be of interest.

My challenge and delight in writing has been to give a coherent structure to the existing statistical methodology for evaluating tests and biomarkers. The book of course reflects my understanding and perspectives on the field. Although I have tried hard to provide a broad, balanced exposition, it is colored by my experience with applications and by my research interests. Others would see the field somewhat differently and provide more or less emphasis to various topics. I hope that the book will provide a point of departure for productive discourse in the field.

Writing this book has been both an enormously satisfying and exhausting process. I could not have done it without a great deal of help. First, those who typed the manuscript at various stages, especially Noelle Noble, who took on the task with no prior knowledge of LaTeX and amazed us with her skills obtained over a short period of time. Others who worked on the book are Sandy Walbrek, Pete Mesling and Molly Jackson. I have been fortunate to work with such a talented and efficient group of people over the years.

Gary Longton, a superb statistician and colleague, not only produced analyses and figures for the book, but in doing so helped clarify my thinking on numerous points. Our datasets and programs, written in STATA, are posted at the website http://www.fhcrc.org/labs/pepe/book.

My initial work on the book was supported by the University of Washington Genentech Professorship (1999–2001). I am grateful to the faculty at the UW, especially Tom Fleming and Patrick Heagerty, who encouraged me to undertake the project and who provided space and funding. Later work was supported by the EDRN. I admire the foresight of our funding agency who saw the need for statistical development in this field. I appreciate input from colleagues at the EDRN and at the General Clinical Research Center at the University of Washington.

Graduate students at the University of Washington were key to my completing the book. They provided detailed critical feedback on the chapters, worked through illustrations and ran simulation studies. Equally important, their interest in the topic and high expectations of me fueled my work to the end. I thank especially Todd Alonzo (now at the University of Southern California), Chaya Moskowitz (now at Memorial Sloan Kettering), Lori Dodd (now at the National Cancer Institute), San-San Ou, Zheng Zhang, Elizabeth Rosenthal, Yingye Zheng and Kyeong Kim. A number of people that I consider experts in the field were kind enough to review the book for me. Although remaining weaknesses are entirely my doing, I want to thank Ziding Feng, Les Irwig, Larry Kessler, Charles Metz, Carolyn Rutter, David Shapiro, Jeremy Taylor, Gerald van Belle, Stephen Walter, Noel Weiss, Stuart Baker and Ray Carroll for providing me with valuable feedback.

I am grateful for the educational and professional opportunities afforded me that provided me with the background to write this book. I cannot thank all of my teachers and mentors by name here, but I do want to thank Ross Prentice in particular, my boss at the Fred Hutchinson Cancer Research Center. His support at the early stages of my career was very important. I thank my parents, of course. Their personal support remains as important as ever.

Finally, I want to thank my husband Mike who, while extremely supportive of this endeavor, has always helped me maintain it in a healthy perspective. His love, his companionship, his sense of fun and his educated interest in the book lead me to dedicate it to him.

University of Washington and   M. S. P.
Fred Hutchinson Cancer Research Center
July 2002

The author is donating royalties from the sale of this book to the charity

Doctors Without Borders

CONTENTS

CONTENTS xi

NOTATION

D — disease status = $\begin{cases} 1 & \text{diseased} \\ 0 & \text{non-diseased} \end{cases}$

$D, \bar{D}$ — subscripts for diseased and non-diseased populations

ρ — disease prevalence = $P[D = 1]$

Y — result of medical test

$n_D, n_{\bar{D}}$ — number of diseased and non-diseased study subjects

N — $n_D + n_{\bar{D}}$ in a cohort study

Z — covariate

X — covariables, numerical variables that quantify Z

V — indicates if D has been ascertained or not

$\mathcal{LR}(y)$ — likelihood ratio function = $P[Y = y|D = 1]/P[Y = y|D = 0]$

$\mathrm{RS}(y)$ — risk score function = $P[D = 1|Y = y]$

Binary tests

τ — probability of a positive test = $P[Y = 1]$

FPF — false positive fraction = $P[Y = 1|D = 0]$

TPF — true positive fraction = $P[Y = 1|D = 1]$

PPV — positive predictive value = $P[D = 1|Y = 1]$

NPV — negative predictive value = $P[D = 0|Y = 0]$

DLR^+ — positive diagnostic likelihood ratio = $\mathcal{LR}(1)$

DLR^- — negative diagnostic likelihood ratio = $\mathcal{LR}(0)$

DP — detection probability in a cohort = $P[Y = 1 \text{ and } D = 1]$

FP — false referral probability in a cohort = $P[Y = 1 \text{ and } D = 0]$

$(\mathrm{rFPF}, \mathrm{rTPF})$ — relative classification probabilities

$(\mathrm{rPPV}, \mathrm{rNPV})$ — relative predictive values

$(\mathrm{rDLR}^+, \mathrm{rDLR}^-)$ — relative diagnostic likelihood ratios

$(\mathrm{rDP}, \mathrm{rFP})$ — relative detection and false referral probabilities

Continuous tests

$S(y)$	–	$\mathrm{P}[Y \geqslant y] =$ survivor function for Y
$S_D(y)$	–	$\mathrm{P}[Y_D \geqslant y] = \mathrm{P}[Y \geqslant y | D = 1]$
$S_{\bar{D}}(y)$	–	$\mathrm{P}[Y_{\bar{D}} \geqslant y] = \mathrm{P}[Y \geqslant y | D = 0]$
$q_{\bar{D}}(1 - t)$	–	$1 - t$ quantile of $Y_{\bar{D}} = S_{\bar{D}}^{-1}(t)$
t	–	false positive fraction variable, $t \in (0, 1)$

$\mathrm{ROC}(t)$	–	receiver operating characteristic curve at $t = S_D(S_{\bar{D}}^{-1}(t))$
AUC	–	area under the ROC curve $= \int_0^1 \mathrm{ROC}(t)\, \mathrm{d}t$
$\mathrm{pAUC}(t_0)$	–	partial AUC $= \int_0^{t_0} \mathrm{ROC}(t)\, \mathrm{d}t$

Mathematical symbols

Φ	–	cumulative normal distribution function
ϕ	–	standard normal density function
$\mathrm{N}(\mu, \sigma^2)$	–	normal distribution with mean μ and variance σ^2

1

INTRODUCTION

1.1 The medical test

1.1.1 *Tests, classification and the broader context*

Accurate diagnosis of a medical condition is often the first step towards its control. Appropriate treatment generally depends on knowing what the condition is. Diagnosis is a familiar part of everyday life. I diagnose a runny nose and sore throat as a cold, that I then treat with chicken soup, orange juice and rest. More formal, familiar medical diagnostic tests include, for example, bacterial cultures, radiographic images and biochemical tests. Consider bacterial culture of a throat swab for streptococcal infection (strep throat), of urine for urinary tract infection, of blood for sepsis and of spinal fluid for meningitis. Diagnostic imaging technologies include X-rays for bone fractures, prenatal ultrasound for diagnosing congenital anomalies, CT scans for evaluating brain injury and MRI of the spine for evaluating herniated discs. Biochemical tests are standard for detecting conditions such as liver dysfunction with serum bilirubin, kidney dysfunction with serum creatinine and pregnancy by measurement of human chorionic gonadotropin in urine.

These are examples of medical diagnostic tests in the classic sense. However, we can consider medical diagnosis in a much broader context and will do so here because statistical methodology pertinent to diagnosing disease also applies to other important classification problems in medicine. In particular, prognosis can be considered as a special type of diagnosis, where the condition to be detected is not disease, *per se*, but is a clinical outcome of interest. For example, we might wish to use clinical or laboratory data on a patient to predict (or 'diagnose') hospitalization within a specified time period. A clinical outcome, hospitalization in this case, is the condition to be diagnosed. Screening for disease is also an important special case of the general medical diagnosis problem as we discuss below.

The test for the condition can be relatively simple, as in the case of bacterial culture for infection, or much more complex. For example, it might be the genetic expression profile of a tissue sample measured using micro-array technology, or a clinical score derived from a multicomponent questionnaire, or it might involve a sequence of procedures specified according to a protocol. Although the statistical methods discussed in this book relate to classifiers used for classification or prediction in general (hence the book title), for discussion purposes we use the simple terminology, 'disease' for the condition to be identified and 'diagnostic test' for the information available to identify the condition, and focus

1

on such applications.

1.1.2 *Disease screening versus diagnosis*

Screening healthy populations for occult disease is attractive because disease is often most successfully treated if it is detected early. Breast cancer screening with mammography and cervical cancer screening with the Pap smear are both well established in developed countries. So too is screening for cardiovascular disease with serum cholesterol and blood pressure monitoring. Programs to screen for infectious diseases have a long history, and this is one approach in the efforts to control the spread of diseases such as AIDS. Newborn babies are routinely screened for conditions such as PKU (phenylketonuria), cystic fibrosis and physical impairments.

From a statistical point of view, screening tests are diagnostic tests. That is, they are procedures geared towards detecting a condition. Their evaluation through research studies is basically the same as that for other diagnostic tests. The context in which they are applied in practice is what sets them apart from other diagnostic tests. First, they are applied to 'healthy' individuals and on a large scale. Thus, they must be non-invasive and inexpensive. Second, a positive screening test is usually followed, not directly with treatment, but with further, more definitive diagnostic procedures. Thus their accuracy can be somewhat less than perfect. Finally, diseases screened are often progressive (cancer, cardiovascular disease) and their evolution over time introduces interesting complications into their evaluation, as will be discussed in Chapter 9. In this book we will use the terms 'screening tests' and 'diagnostic tests' interchangeably, and refer to both as 'medical tests' in a generic sense.

1.1.3 *Criteria for a useful medical test*

The development of a test is useful only if there is some benefit to be gained from diagnosing disease. Table 1.1 displays some key criteria that should be considered before implementing a test.

These criteria are adapted from Wilson and Jungner (1968), Cole and Morrison (1980) and Obuchowski *et al.* (2001), who discussed criteria for useful screening programs, but similar considerations apply to diagnostic tests in general. See also Barratt *et al.* (1999) for practical guidance on selecting a screening test.

The criteria pertain to the disease, its treatment and to the test itself. If

Table 1.1 *Criteria for a useful diagnostic/screening test*

---

(1) Disease should be serious or potentially so
(2) Disease should be relatively prevalent in the target population
(3) Disease should be treatable
(4) Treatment should be available to those who test positive
(5) The test should not harm the individual
(6) The test should accurately classify diseased and non-diseased individuals

---

the disease has no serious consequences in terms of longevity or quality of life, then there is no benefit to be gained from diagnosing it, hence criterion (1). Second, if very few subjects have disease, then the disease has little impact on the population as a whole and the potential benefit from testing subjects is minimal. Third, the purpose of diagnosing disease is so that it can be cured or its progression can be slowed down. Effective treatment (criterion (3)) must exist in order to realize this benefit. Sometimes treatment exists but is not accessible to patients because of the unavailability of financial or other resources. Diagnosing disease in such settings will clearly not be beneficial. Therefore, criterion (4) is a reasonable requirement.

Finally, we come to criteria for the medical test itself. The test procedure ideally should cause no harm whatsoever. However, all tests have some negative impact. They cost money, require trips to the clinic, cause physical or emotional discomfort and sometimes are dangerous to the physical well being of the patient. The overriding principle is that these costs should be reasonable in the context of the population being tested and the potential benefits to be gained by accurately diagnosing disease. Accuracy of the test is the final criterion. This will be quantified in various ways in Chapter 2, but basically an accurate test is one that classifies subjects correctly according to their disease status. Inaccurate tests cause diseased subjects to be misclassified as non-diseased, and conversely they cause non-diseased subjects to be classified as diseased. These misclassifications are termed false negative and false positive errors, respectively. False negatives leave diseased subjects untreated. False positives result in people being subjected to unnecessary procedures, often invasive and costly work-up or treatment, and emotional stress. Clearly such errors need to be kept to a minimum. Therefore, before a test can be recommended for use in practice, its diagnostic accuracy must be rigorously assessed. This book is devoted to statistical methods for the design and evaluation of research studies to assess the accuracy of a diagnostic test.

1.2 Elements of study design

To set up the context, let us first consider how studies are basically designed to evaluate the accuracy of a test. We summarize some of the key elements of study design in this section (Table 1.2). In the next section, examples of real studies are described that illustrate variations on the design elements.

Table 1.2 *Some variations on elements of study design*

Element	Possible variations
Type of test result	Binary, ordinal, continuous
Subject selection	Case-control, cohort, cohort with selection
Comparative design	Paired, unpaired
Integrity of test and disease	Inherent, blinding

1.2.1 *Scale for the test result*

The diagnostic test is used to classify subjects as diseased or not diseased. Some tests yield dichotomous results, such as a test for the presence or absence of a specific methylated DNA sequence in serum. The classification rule is then straightforward: positive if present and negative if absent. For tests that yield results on non-binary scales, the classification rule is usually set by a threshold, with results above it classified as positive for disease and results below classified as negative (or vice versa, if appropriate). Tests that yield quantitative measures on an essentially continuous scale include, for example, biochemical tests such as serum levels of creatinine, bilirubin or PSA. Tests that involve subjective assessments are often measured on ordinal scales. For example, diagnostic radiologic images are often rated by an expert according to the degree of suspicion she/he has that disease is present. The BIRADS scale for mammograms (American College of Radiology, 1995) is an example of a 5-point ordinal scale.

In Chapters 2 and 3 we will define and describe the evaluation of diagnostic accuracy for tests that yield binary results. The methodology for tests with results on ordinal or continuous scales will be discussed in Chapters 4, 5 and 6. Such methodology adapts the framework for binary tests by using the notion of a threshold value to dichotomize the test, which is appropriate given the ultimate purpose of the test for classifying subjects as diseased or not.

1.2.2 *Selection of study subjects*

Enrolment into a study of a diagnostic test usually proceeds in one of two ways. Subjects can be selected on the basis of known true disease status. That is, a fixed number of diseased subjects (cases) are selected and a fixed number of non-diseased subjects (controls) are selected. The diagnostic test is then applied to the subjects or perhaps to stored specimens from those subjects. We call this design a *case-control* study. Although it differs from the classic epidemiologic case-control study in that the diagnostic test result, rather than an exposure, is determined, the case-control terminology seems appropriate because case or control status is the basis for selection into the study.

Alternatively, the diagnostic test can be applied to a set of study subjects from the population of interest. In addition, true disease status, as measured by a *gold standard definitive test*, is also determined for them. We call this design a *cohort* study, because membership in the cohort is the basis for selection into the study.

A variation on this design is where ascertainment of true disease status depends on the result of the diagnostic test. If ascertainment of disease status involves expensive or invasive procedures then, for ethical reasons, some of those with a negative diagnostic test result may forego assessment of true disease status. Such two-stage designs will be discussed in Chapter 7, while the simple cohort and case-control designs will be discussed in the preceding chapters. The relative merits of case-control versus cohort studies will be discussed in Section 2.2.5.

1.2.3 *Comparing tests*

When two diagnostic tests are to be compared, it is sometimes possible to apply both tests to study subjects. For example, a comparative study of two biomarkers assayed on serum could apply both assays to an individual's blood sample. We call this a *paired* design because each individual gives rise to a pair of test results. Correlations between test results must be considered in evaluating a study that employs a paired design. An *unpaired* design is one in which each subject receives only one of the diagnostic tests. If the tests involve responding to two different questionnaires, for example, one test could interfere with the subject's performance on the other and a valid comparison would require an unpaired design. Even when multiple tests are involved, we still use the terms paired and unpaired designs to distinguish studies that apply multiple tests to each subject from those that apply one test to each subject. A discussion of principles for conducting studies with paired and unpaired designs is provided in Section 3.1.

1.2.4 *Test integrity*

The valid evaluation of the accuracy of the diagnostic test requires that knowledge of the true disease status of the individual does not influence the assessment of the diagnostic test, and vice versa. If there is a subjective element to either, then one must take precautions in the design of the study. For example, if a radiologist knows that a mammogram is from a woman with breast cancer, she/he might view and assess the mammogram with more suspicion for its showing cancer. The persons administrating and assessing the results of the diagnostic test should be *blinded* to the study subject's true disease status. This will often include the study subject himself.

Similarly, persons involved in procedures for the assessment of true disease status should be blinded to the results of the diagnostic test. For example, if the condition to be diagnosed is a personality disorder whose presence is definitively assessed by an expert (and probably expensive) psychiatrist, and an inexpensive simple questionnaire is to be considered as an alternative diagnostic test, then blinding of the psychiatrist to results of the simple questionnaire should be employed.

Note that in many settings the procedures employed are objective, and assessments cannot interfere with one another. Examples are biochemical tests or bacterial culturing tests. We say that the integrity of such a test is *inherent* to its operation. Even if tests are objective, one must be aware that interference can enter in some subtle ways and take precautions accordingly. For example, if there is a time delay between the experimental diagnostic test and assessment of disease status, altering patient management on the basis of the test might interfere with disease and lead to biased results. As another example, knowledge of true disease status can sometimes influence the care with which the experimental diagnostic test is done, possibly affecting results.

1.2.5 *Sources of bias*

It is well recognized that studies of diagnostic tests are subject to an array
of biases (Table 1.3). Some of these, notably verification bias and imperfect
reference test bias, will be discussed in detail in Chapter 7. Begg (1987) reviews
a variety of other biases in studies of diagnostic tests. See also Begg and McNeil
(1988) and Metz (1989) for an extended discussion concerning radiology studies.

Spectrum bias occurs when diseased subjects in the study are not representative of diseased subjects in the population, or conversely if controls selected for
the study are different from population controls. A common mistake is to select
cases that have severe or chronic disease and controls that are more healthy on
average than non-diseased subjects in the population. Such selection can enhance
the apparent accuracy of the diagnostic test. As with epidemiologic studies, cases
and controls in a diagnostic study should be randomly selected from the diseased
and non-diseased target populations.

We have already mentioned problems that arise when the interpretation of
the test or the assessment of the true disease status interfere with each other.

Table 1.3 *Common sources of bias in study design*

Type of bias	Description
Verification bias	Non-random selection for definitive assessment for disease with the gold standard reference test
Errors in the reference	True disease status is subject to misclassification because the gold standard is imperfect
Spectrum bias	Types of cases and controls included are not representative of the population
Test interpretation bias	Information is available that can distort the diagnostic test
Unsatisfactory tests	Tests that are uninterpretable or incomplete do not yield a test result
Extrapolation bias	The conditions or characteristics of populations in the study are different from those in which the test will be applied
Lead time bias*	Earlier detection by screening may erroneously appear to indicate beneficial effects on the outcome of a progressive disease
Length bias*	Slowly progressing disease is over-represented in screened subjects relative to all cases of disease that arise in the population
Overdiagnosis bias*	Subclinical disease may regress and never become a clinical problem in the absence of screening, but is detected by screening

*Apply only to screening for preclinical states of a progressive disease

Test interpretation bias can also arise if extraneous information, such as clinical symptoms or the result of another test, are allowed to influence the test procedure or its interpretation in a way that is different from how the test will be applied in practice. For example, the results of a mammogram might influence the interpretation of a lump from a clinical breast exam. If a clinical breast exam is to be applied in practice without concurrent mammographic readings available, then assessments in the research study should reflect this.

Unsatisfactory or inadequate test results arise in practice and it is not always clear how these should be handled in the evaluation of a research study. For example, a passive audiology test that requires a child to be quiet will not be completed if the child starts to fuss. An inadequate clinical sample or broken slide cannot be assessed for pathology. If the results of these tests are omitted from analysis, this can make the test appear better than it is. In particular, disease not detected because of unsatisfactory results does not count against the test. On the other hand, the inclusion of unsatisfactory tests can be problematic too. For example, if those tests are counted as negative, but lead to a recommendation for repeat testing, then the test is not given credit for disease that is detected on repeat. We refer the reader to Begg *et al.* (1986) for a good discussion of the issues involved.

Many factors can affect the performance of a test for detecting disease. These include patient-related factors (demographics, health habits, compliance, truthfulness), tester-related factors (experience, training), the environment in which the testing is done (institution, available resources and treatment options, population disease prevalence) and so forth. The analysis of covariate effects on test accuracy is discussed in Chapters 3 and 6. We note here that extrapolation of study results to other populations may not be appropriate if they differ from the study population with regard to factors that influence test accuracy (see Irwig *et al.*, 2002). This, we call, *extrapolation bias*. One point made by Irwig *et al.* (2002) is that the implicit or explicit criterion for defining a positive versus negative test result can differ with the tester or the environment in which the test is done. This has long been a concern, particularly in radiology, and we discuss it further in Chapter 4.

Three additional sources of bias are often of concern in screening studies for progressive diseases like cancer and cardiovascular disease (Cole and Morrison, 1980). The first, *lead time bias*, arises from the fact that by detecting disease earlier in its course, the time from diagnosis to death is increased even if early treatment is totally ineffective. A simple comparison of post-diagnosis survival in screened versus unscreened subjects will be biased in general because of the apparent time gained by earlier detection (Lilienfeld, 1974). The time from early detection by screening to diagnosis in the absence of screening is called the lead time. It must be properly accounted for in evaluating the benefits of screening. A second source of bias, referred to as *length time bias* (Zelen, 1976), acknowledges that disease progresses at different rates in individuals. Subjects with slowly progressing disease will be more prevalent in the population than will subjects who get disease that progresses quickly. A screening program might detect a large fraction of the prevalent cases in the population at any one time but a small proportion of the population that develops disease, if it misses the quickly progressing cases. This would happen if screening was too infrequent, say. Moreover, as noted by Weiss (1996, Chapter 3), survival will usually be better for subjects with slowly progressing disease and therefore screen detected cases may exhibit better survival than non-screen detected cases, even when screening itself does not affect the course of the disease.

Finally, subclinical disease sometimes regresses spontaneously without ever reaching a clinical state. Neuroblastoma is one example. Similarly, in an elderly man, prostate cancer is sometimes sufficiently slow growing that it never becomes a clinical problem in the man's lifetime. A screening test that detects such subclinical disease is not beneficial to the patient. It *overdiagnoses* disease in the sense of leading to unnecessary, often invasive, medical procedures. Considering simply the numbers of cases detected in the subclinical state therefore can mislead one to overestimate the potential benefits of screening tests. This is called overdiagnosis bias.

1.3 Examples and datasets

1.3.1 *Overview*

We will use a variety of datasets in this book to illustrate methodology for evaluating diagnostic tests. All of the datasets can be downloaded from the website http://www.fhcrc.org/labs/pepe/book. These studies employ a variety of different types of designs and we provide brief descriptions of some of them here (see Table 1.4). Others will be described later, when we use them for illustrating statistical methodology.

1.3.2 *The CASS dataset*

As part of the coronary artery surgery study (CASS), Weiner *et al.* (1979) described the results of an exercise stress test (EST) and of a determination of chest pain history (CPH) among 1465 men undergoing coronary arteriography for suspected or probable coronary heart disease. This was a huge study involving fifteen clinical centers in the USA and Canada. Consider now the study design elements listed in Table 1.2. Both diagnostic tests, EST and CPH, are coded dichotomously and are available for all study subjects. The determination of coronary artery disease is with arteriography, the gold standard measure, which is also coded dichotomously as present or absent. This is a simple cohort study, with details of the cohorts, i.e. inclusion/exclusion criteria, given in Weiner *et al.* (1979). The version of the data we use was published in Leisenring *et al.* (2000). Our interest is in comparing the two diagnostic tests. A paired design has been employed for this purpose. All three determinations, EST, CPH and the gold standard, are made in a blinded fashion, in that the results of one does not effect the operation or results of another.

Table 1.4 *Datasets and their source designs*

Study	Reference	Test scale	Subject selection	Comparative design	Comments	Size
CASS	Leisenring *et al.* (2000)	Binary	Cohort	Paired	Compares two tests	1465 men
Pancreatic cancer biomarkers	Wieand *et al.* (1989)	Continuous	Case-control	Paired	Compares two biomarkers	90 cases, 51 controls
Ultrasound for hepatic metastasis	Tostesan and Begg (1988)	Ordinal	Case-control	Unpaired	Compares test performance for two types of tumor	31 cases, 60 controls
CARET PSA	Etzioni *et al.* (1999b)	Continuous	Case-control	Paired	Longitudinal data for two biomarkers	71 cases, 70 controls
Gene expression array study	Pepe *et al.* (2003)	Continuous	Case-control	Paired	Enormous number of tests: how to select and combine tests?	30 cases, 23 controls
Neonatal audiology study	Leisenring *et al.* (1997)	Binary	Cohort	Paired	Clustered incomplete data; evaluation of covariate effects and comparison of tests	973 subjects, 3152 tests
St Louis prostate study	Smith *et al.* (1997)	Binary	Cohort	Paired	Reference test done only for screen positives	20 000 men

1.3.3   Pancreatic cancer serum biomarkers study

This dataset has been used by various statisticians to illustrate statistical techniques for diagnostic tests. First published by Wieand *et al.* (1989), it is a case-control study including 90 cases with pancreatic cancer and 51 controls that did not have cancer but who had pancreatitis. Serum samples from each patient were assayed for CA-125, a cancer antigen, and CA-19-9, a carbohydrate antigen, both of which are measured on a continuous positive scale. The ascertainment of biomarker values and the pathologic determination of disease status are inherently not influenced by each other. A primary question in this study is to determine which of the two biomarkers best distinguishes cases from controls. The design can be summarized as a paired case-control study of continuous tests with the integrity of disease and test being inherent to their measurement.

1.3.4   Hepatitis metastasis ultrasound study

Data from this study were reported in a paper by Tosteson and Begg (1988). It concerns the use of ultrasound to determine hepatic metastasis in cancer patients. The diagnostic test result is the radiologist's assessment of the ultrasound indicating presence of disease, rated on an ordinal scale from 1 to 5, with a rating of 5 indicating 'metastasis definitely present'. Of the 91 patients studied, 31 had hepatic metastasis and 60 did not. There were two groups of cancer patients studied: those with primary cancer of the breast or colon. A primary question was to determine if the diagnostic accuracy of ultrasound is affected by primary tumor type. Although not a comparative study of different diagnostic tests, for the purposes of comparing the performance of the ultrasound test in the two tumor types, it is an unpaired case-control study with ordinal test results.

1.3.5   CARET PSA biomarker study

The beta-carotene and retinol trial (CARET) enrolled over 12 000 men, aged 50 to 65 and at high risk of lung cancer, for randomization to chemoprevention or placebo. A substudy, reported by Etzioni *et al.* (1999b), analyzed serum levels of prostate specific antigen (PSA) for 71 cases of prostate cancer that occurred during the study using serum samples stored prior to their diagnosis. Controls, i.e. subjects not diagnosed with prostate cancer by the time of analysis, matched to cases on date of birth and number of serum samples available for analysis, were included. Two different measures of PSA were considered, namely total serum PSA and the ratio of free to total PSA.

This study is a nested case-control study, nested within the CARET cohort. The data are serial longitudinal measurements of PSA over time. One question to be addressed by the study is how the diagnostic value of PSA varies relative to the onset of clinically diagnosed prostate cancer. That is, how long before the onset of clinical disease can PSA detect cancer? The comparative aspect, comparing the total and ratio PSA measures, is paired since both measures are analyzed for each subject.

1.3.6 *Ovarian cancer gene expression study*

A gene-expression experiment using glass arrays for 1536 cDNA clones was kindly made available to us by Dr Michel Schummer (Institute for Systems Biology, Seattle). We selected data from the 30 cases of ovarian cancer and the 23 subjects with healthy ovary tissues. This is a case-control study with an enormous number (1536) of potential diagnostic tests. Because of the proprietary nature of these data, we will examine data only for some specific genes to illustrate statistical methodology for evaluating and comparing diagnostic potential.

1.3.7 *Neonatal audiology data*

In preparation for the analysis of a study of hearing screening in newborn babies, we generated hypothetical data that followed the key elements of the design of that study (Leisenring *et al.*, 1997). Babies for the study were tested in each ear with three passive hearing tests labeled as A, B and C. Incomplete testing was common since testing is impossible when babies start to fuss. The gold standard behavioral test, the visual reinforcement audiometry (VRA) test, was performed at 9–12 months of age. We generated dichotomous test results and true hearing status for each ear. Incompleteness in the testing protocol was also incorporated into our simulations. Covariates included in the simulation were: a measure of severity of hearing impairment for deaf ears, age of the baby and location (hospital room or sound booth) where the test was performed.

Questions to be addressed by the project were (i) an evaluation of how covariates affected test performance and (ii) a comparison of the three screening tests.

1.3.8 *St Louis prostate cancer screening study*

A study reported by Smith *et al.* (1997) used PSA testing and digital rectal exams (DRE) to screen almost 20 000 healthy men for prostate cancer. If serum PSA was elevated to greater than 4.0 ng/ml or the DRE was considered suspicious for cancer, subjects were referred for biopsy to determine if prostate cancer was present. The results of both screening tests were dichotomized in the reported data.

This is a paired data cohort study to compare DRE and PSA as screening tests. An interesting feature of the data is that true disease status is missing for subjects that screen negative on both tests. This is a common occurrence in prospective screening studies when the definitive test, biopsy in this case, is invasive. Investigators were also interested in racial differences in test performance and the dataset includes information on race.

1.4 Topics and organization

The book is organized into nine chapters, with the basic concepts and methodology contained in Chapters 2 through 6. The first two of these chapters deal with tests that have dichotomous results, because these are simpler than non-binary tests. Indeed, the basis for evaluating non-binary tests is to dichotomize them (in many different ways), so this sets the stage for continuous and ordinal tests too. Various measures for quantifying diagnostic accuracy are described in Chapter 2, along with procedures to estimate them. In Chapter 3 we describe methods to compare diagnostic tests and to evaluate factors influencing the diagnostic accuracy of tests. In particular, we describe several regression modeling frameworks that can be used.

We start over in Chapter 4 with non-binary tests, where measures to quantify diagnostic accuracy are considered. The conceptual basis for the most popular measure, the ROC curve, is described. Methods for estimating the ROC curve are considered in Chapter 5, along with traditional approaches for comparing ROC curves. Next, methods for evaluating covariate effects on the diagnostic accuracy of a non-binary test are described in Chapter 6.

In diagnostic testing, practical and/or ethical issues make incomplete data a frequent occurrence. Consider, for example, the St Louis prostate study. In Chapter 7 we describe methods for statistical analysis that accommodate incompleteness in the data. Another common issue is that the reference test for gold standard assessment of true disease status may itself be subject to error. We discuss the impact of such error and statistical methods that have been proposed for dealing with it.

We return to the design of studies to evaluate diagnostic tests in Chapter 8. The development of a test will usually involve a series of studies, and it is important to specify where in the development process one is, in order to design a study appropriately. One paradigm for the phases of development is defined in Chapter 8. We then proceed to discuss sample size calculations along with other phase-specific considerations for study design.

In Chapter 9 we proceed to describe further extensions and applications of the statistical methodology. We address the analysis of event time data, with application to the CARET PSA biomarker study. The question of how to combine results of several tests to define a better composite test is discussed. In addition, meta-analysis procedures to combine the results of several studies of a diagnostic test are presented. We close Chapter 9, and the book, with some thoughts for the future of diagnostic and prognostic classification in medicine, for broader applications beyond the classification problem and on directions for statistical research in this field. The exercises at the end of each chapter also contain some open-ended questions that may warrant research.

1.5   Exercises

1. New classification systems for cancer may be based on molecular biology measures (gene expression profiles, say) and may even replace current histological classifications. Sub-type classifications are sought for prognostic purposes and for selecting optimal treatment regimens. In this context, what criteria should a classification test satisfy in order to be useful?

2. Consider a progressive disease like cancer. Lead time bias and length bias invalidate observational studies that compare screened and unscreened sub-

jects with regards to disease diagnosis, stage at diagnosis and post-diagnosis survival. These considerations are used to argue for randomized studies of screening versus no screening, with mortality as the primary outcome measure. Discuss how disease incidence, stage and mortality might vary over time in the two arms of a randomized study if:

(a) the diagnostic test is accurate but early treatment does not impact survival;

(b) the diagnostic test is inaccurate but early treatment is beneficial; and

(c) the test is accurate and early treatment is beneficial.

3. The mammography quality improvement program (MQIP) was a study to evaluate an educational intervention for rural radiologists reading screening mammograms. Mammograms were read at baseline and again after the educational program had taken place. Discuss the following issues:

(a) Should each radiologist read the same mammograms at the two reading sessions?

(b) Should the radiologist be told that about half of the images are from subjects known to have cancer? In their usual practice a very small fraction of screening images are from women with cancer because the prevalence of cancer is very low in the screened population.

(c) The BIRADS classification for mammograms is made on an ordinal scale from 1 to 5 and includes a category '3' that allows the radiologist to decline making a recommendation for biopsy and to recommend that a repeat mammogram be performed. Should this be allowed in the research study?

(d) The educational program specifically provides instruction on reading borderline or difficult cases and controls. Should the study include a preponderance of such images in the test sets used for evaluating the intervention?

2

MEASURES OF ACCURACY FOR BINARY TESTS

2.1 Measures of accuracy

The accuracy of a diagnostic test can be defined in various ways. In this chapter we consider only diagnostic tests that yield a binary result. Some tests, by their nature, are dichotomous. A respondent answers 'yes' or 'no' to a question, for example. Others are ordinal or continuous but are dichotomized in practice using a threshold value.

2.1.1 *Notation*

We use the binary variable, D, to denote true disease status:

$$D = \begin{cases} 1 & \text{for disease}; \\ 0 & \text{for non-disease}. \end{cases}$$

The variable Y is the result of the diagnostic test. By convention, larger values of Y are considered more indicative of disease. We write

$$Y = \begin{cases} 1 & \text{positive for disease}; \\ 0 & \text{negative for disease}. \end{cases}$$

Subscripts D and $\bar{D}$ are used occasionally. They index quantities pertinent to disease and non-disease, respectively. Thus, for example, Y_D denotes a test result for a diseased subject.

2.1.2 *Disease-specific classification probabilities*

The result of the test can be classified as a true positive, a true negative, a false positive or a false negative, as shown in Table 2.1. As the names suggest, a true positive result occurs when a diseased subject is correctly classified with a positive test result, and a false negative result occurs when a diseased subject tests negative. Similarly, a true negative or a false positive occurs when a non-diseased subject has a negative or a positive result, respectively.

Table 2.1 *Classification of test results by disease status*

	$D = 0$	$D = 1$
$Y = 0$	True negative	False negative
$Y = 1$	False positive	True positive

The test can have two types of errors, false positive errors and false negative errors. An ideal test has no false positives and no false negatives. We define the *true and false positive fractions* as follows:

$$\text{false positive fraction} = \text{FPF} = P[Y = 1|D = 0], \qquad (2.1)$$

$$\text{true positive fraction} = \text{TPF} = P[Y = 1|D = 1]. \qquad (2.2)$$

Since $1 - \text{TPF}$ is equal to the false negative fraction, the pair (FPF, TPF) defines the probabilities with which errors occur when using the test. Although often called false positive *rate* and true positive *rate*, FPF and TPF are not in fact rates. They are probabilities or fractions. To alleviate the potential for confusion, particularly in epidemiology research where rates have a very specific meaning, we use the more appropriate terms false positive *fraction* and true positive *fraction* in this text. An ideal test has $\text{FPF} = 0$ and $\text{TPF} = 1$. For a useless test on the other hand, disease has no relation to the test outcome and $\text{TPF} = \text{FPF}$.

The TPF and FPF are known by several other terms. In biomedical research, the sensitivity (TPF) and specificity $(1 - \text{FPF})$ are often used to describe test performance. In engineering applications and in audiology, the terms 'hit rate' (TPF) and 'false alarm rate' (FPF) are used. Statisticians using a hypothesis test can be thought of as diagnosticians. In the context of statistical hypothesis testing of a null hypothesis $(D = 0)$ versus an alternative hypothesis $(D = 1)$, the terms significance level (FPF) and statistical power (TPF) are used.

Observe that the overall probability of misclassification, or overall error probability, can be written in terms of (FPF, TPF) and the population prevalence of disease, $\rho = P[D = 1]$. The misclassification probability is

$$P[Y \neq D] = \rho(1 - \text{TPF}) + (1 - \rho)\text{FPF}. \qquad (2.3)$$

This overall misclassification probability is commonly used in engineering and computer science applications but is not considered to be an adequate summary of the diagnostic accuracy of a medical test. Rather, both components of the misclassification probability, $1 - \text{TPF}$ and FPF, should be reported to describe accuracy. The first reason is that the costs and consequences of the two types of errors are usually quite different. False negative errors, i.e. missing disease that is present, can result in people foregoing needed treatment for their disease. The consequence can be as serious as death. False positive errors tend to be less serious. People without disease are subjected to unnecessary work-up procedures or even treatment. The negative impacts include personal inconvenience and stress but the long-term consequences are usually relatively minor. The second reason for preferring the pair of classification probabilities, (FPF, TPF), to the overall misclassification probability for summarizing diagnostic accuracy is that the magnitude of the latter depends on disease prevalence. To illustrate the problem with this, consider a totally uninformative test that classifies all subjects as negative. If the prevalence of disease is low, such a test will have a low overall error probability but clearly is a useless test.

2.1.3 *Predictive values*

As an alternative to considering the frequency of misclassification for each disease state, accuracy can be quantified by how well the test result predicts true disease status. The predictive values are:

$$\text{positive predictive value} = \text{PPV} = P[D = 1 | Y = 1], \qquad (2.4)$$
$$\text{negative predictive value} = \text{NPV} = P[D = 0 | Y = 0]. \qquad (2.5)$$

Observe that the roles of D and Y are reversed in the predictive values relative to their roles in the classification probabilities.

A perfect test will predict disease perfectly, with PPV = 1 and NPV = 1. On the other hand, a useless test has no information about true disease status, so that $P[D = 1 | Y = 1] = P[D = 1]$ and $P[D = 0 | Y = 0] = P[D = 0]$. That is, PPV = ρ and NPV = $1 - \rho$.

We see that the predictive values depend not only on the performance of the test in diseased and non-diseased subjects, but also on the prevalence of disease. A low PPV may simply be a result of low prevalence of disease or it may be due to a test that does not reflect the true disease status of the subject very well. Predictive values are not used to quantify the inherent accuracy of the test. The classification probabilities, TPF and FPF, are considered more relevant to that task because they quantify how well the test reflects true disease status. Rather, predictive values quantify the clinical value of the test. The patient and care-giver are most interested in how likely it is that disease is present given the test result. See Zweig and Campbell (1993) for an in depth discussion of the concepts of accuracy versus usefulness. In many research studies, both the disease-specific classification probabilities and the predictive values are reported.

There is a direct relationship between predictive values and the classification probabilities, although knowledge of prevalence is also required in order to calculate one from the other. Indeed, the complete joint distribution of (D, Y) requires three parameters. One natural parameterization is $(\text{TPF}, \text{FPF}, \rho)$. Another natural parameterization is $(\text{PPV}, \text{NPV}, \tau)$, where $\tau = P[Y = 1]$ is the probability of a positive test. The next result shows the relationship between these parameterizations. The proof is a straightforward application of Bayes' theorem, and is not detailed here.

Result 2.1

(a) We can write $(\text{PPV}, \text{NPV}, \tau)$ in terms of $(\text{TPF}, \text{FPF}, \rho)$:

$$\text{PPV} = \rho\text{TPF} / \{\rho\text{TPF} + (1 - \rho)\text{FPF}\},$$
$$\text{NPV} = (1 - \rho)(1 - \text{FPF}) / \{(1 - \rho)(1 - \text{FPF}) + \rho(1 - \text{TPF})\},$$
$$\tau = \rho\text{TPF} + (1 - \rho)\text{FPF}.$$

(b) We can write $(\mathrm{TPF}, \mathrm{FPF}, \rho)$ in terms of $(\mathrm{PPV}, \mathrm{NPV}, \tau)$:

$$\mathrm{TPF} = \tau\mathrm{PPV}/\{\tau\mathrm{PPV} + (1 - \tau)(1 - \mathrm{NPV})\},$$
$$\mathrm{FPF} = \tau(1 - \mathrm{PPV})/\{\tau(1 - \mathrm{PPV}) + (1 - \tau)\mathrm{NPV}\},$$
$$\rho = \tau\mathrm{PPV} + (1 - \tau)(1 - \mathrm{NPV}).$$ ∎

Example 2.1

In the CASS population, consider the exercise stress test (EST) for the diagnosis of coronary artery disease (CAD). Suppose that probabilities of test result and disease status are as follows:

		CAD $D = 0$	$D = 1$	
EST	$Y = 0$	22.3%	14.2%	36.5%
	$Y - 1$	7.8%	55.6%	63.4%
		30.1%	69.8%	100%

We calculate:

$$\mathrm{TPF} = 0.797, \quad \mathrm{FPF} = 0.259, \quad \rho = 0.698,$$
$$\mathrm{PPV} = 0.877, \quad \mathrm{NPV} = 0.611, \quad \tau = 0.634.$$

The prevalence of disease in patients eligible for this study is very high, almost 70%. The sensitivity of the EST is approximately 80%, while its specificity (i.e. $1 - \mathrm{FPF}$) is 74%. It misses 20% of the truly diseased subjects and incorrectly identifies 26% of the non-diseased subjects as suspicious for CAD. The decision to use the EST as a test for CAD would need to take account of the risks and benefits of the additional diagnostic procedures or treatments that would be recommended following a positive result as well as the consequences of missing disease that is present.

About 63% of the CASS population test positive on EST. Among subjects that test positive, the vast majority, about 88%, do have disease. However, 39% of subjects that test negative also have disease. A negative test does not rule out disease. It might be prudent to seek further non-invasive testing in subjects that test negative on the EST in order to identify the 39% that are truly diseased. However, those that test positive are likely to seek definitive testing immediately, since they have a very high likelihood of being diseased.   ∎

2.1.4 *Diagnostic likelihood ratios*

Likelihood ratios are yet another way of describing the prognostic or diagnostic value of a test. They have gained in popularity during the last decade and we refer the reader to Sackett *et al.* (1985), Boyko (1994) and Boyd (1997) for extensive discussions in favor of their adoption for diagnostic test evaluation. See also Giard and Hermans (1993) and Kerlikowske *et al.* (1996) for examples of their application in substantive research. These parameters are likelihood ratios in the true statistical sense, although we call them diagnostic likelihood ratios (DLR) to distinguish the context. We define them as:

$$\text{positive DLR} = \text{DLR}^+ = \frac{P[Y = 1|D = 1]}{P[Y = 1|D = 0]}, \tag{2.6}$$

$$\text{negative DLR} = \text{DLR}^- = \frac{P[Y = 0|D = 1]}{P[Y = 0|D = 0]}. \tag{2.7}$$

They are, literally, the ratios of the likelihood of the observed test result in the diseased versus non-diseased populations. As before, there are two dimensions to accuracy, the DLR for a positive test, DLR^+, and the DLR for a negative test, DLR^-.

The scale for DLRs is $(0, \infty)$. An uninformative test having no relation to disease status has DLRs of unity. On the other hand, a perfect test, for which $Y = D$ with probability 1, has DLR parameters of $\text{DLR}^+ = \infty$ and $\text{DLR}^- = 0$. A $\text{DLR}^+ > 1$ indicates that a positive test is more likely in a diseased subject than in a non-diseased subject, which is a sensible requirement given our convention about the interpretation of a positive test as indicating presence of disease. Similarly, a sensible test will have $\text{DLR}^- \leqslant 1$.

An attractive feature of the DLRs is that they quantify the increase in knowledge about presence of disease that is gained through the diagnostic test. Consider the odds that a subject has disease before the test is performed, i.e. in the absence of the test result:

$$\text{pre-test odds } = P[D = 1]/P[D = 0].$$

After the test is performed, i.e. with knowledge of the test result, the odds of disease are:

$$\text{post-test odds } (Y) = P[D = 1|Y]/P[D = 0|Y].$$

The DLRs relate these two odds.

Result 2.2

The following results hold:

$$\text{post-test odds } (Y = 1) = \text{DLR}^+ \times (\text{pre-test odds}),$$
$$\text{post-test odds } (Y = 0) = \text{DLR}^- \times (\text{pre-test odds}).$$

Proof   We prove the result for the case of a positive test. The other proof is similar.

$$\begin{aligned}
\text{Post-test odds } (Y = 1) &= \frac{P[D = 1|Y = 1]}{P[D = 0|Y = 1]} \\
&= \frac{P[D = 1, Y = 1]/P[Y = 1]}{P[D = 0, Y = 1]/P[Y = 1]} \\
&= \frac{P[Y = 1|D = 1]P[D = 1]}{P[Y = 1|D = 0]P[D = 0]}
\end{aligned}$$

$$= \text{DLR}^+ \times P[D = 1]/P[D = 0]$$
$$= \text{DLR}^+ \times (\text{pre-test odds}). \qquad \blacksquare$$

Thus, the $(\text{DLR}^+, \text{DLR}^-)$ parameters quantify the change in the odds of disease obtained by knowledge of the result of the diagnostic test. They are also called Bayes factors. If one considers $P[D = 1]$ as the prior probability of disease and $P[D = 1|Y]$ as the posterior probability in a Bayesian sense, then the DLR is the Bayesian multiplication factor relating the prior and posterior distributions.

Observe that the DLRs are motivated by the concept of predicting disease status from the test result. This they share with the predictive value parameters. Indeed, we see that the post-test odds can be written in terms of the predictive values:

$$\frac{\text{PPV}}{1 - \text{PPV}} = \text{post-test odds } (Y = 1), \qquad (2.8)$$

$$\frac{1 - \text{NPV}}{\text{NPV}} = \text{post-test odds } (Y = 0). \qquad (2.9)$$

However, unlike the predictive values, the DLRs do not depend on the prevalence of disease in the population. They are, in fact, simple functions of the classification probabilities. We state this as a result, but it is really a straightforward interpretation of their definitions.

Result 2.3

The following results hold:

$$\text{DLR}^+ = \frac{\text{TPF}}{\text{FPF}},$$

$$\text{DLR}^- = \frac{1 - \text{TPF}}{1 - \text{FPF}}. \qquad \blacksquare$$

In the sense that they relate to prediction but do not depend on population prevalence, they can be considered as a compromise between classification probabilities and predictive values.

Table 2.2 summarizes some of the attributes of the three approaches to quantifying the accuracy of a binary test that we have described. Boyko (1994) and Dujardin *et al.* (1994) provide further discussion of DLRs and contrast them with classification probabilities and predictive values.

Example 2.1 (continued)

By either directly using the proportions in the cross-classification of EST with CAD or by using the previously calculated (FPF, TPF) values and the expression in Result 2.3, we find that

$$\text{DLR}^+ = 3.08 \quad \text{and} \quad \text{DLR}^- = 0.27.$$

Table 2.2 *Three measures of diagnostic accuracy for binary tests and their attributes*

	Classification probabilities	Predictive values	Diagnostic likelihood ratios
Parameter definitions	$\text{FPF} = P[Y = 1\|D = 0]$ $\text{TPF} = P[Y = 1\|D = 1]$	$\text{PPV} = P[D = 1\|Y = 1]$ $\text{NPV} = P[D = 0\|Y = 0]$	$\text{DLR}^+ = \mathcal{L}R(Y = 1)^*$ $\text{DLR}^- = \mathcal{L}R(Y = 0)^*$
Scale	$(0, 1)$	$(0, 1)$	$(0, \infty)$
Perfect test	$\text{FPF} = 0,\ \text{TPF} = 1$	$\text{PPV} = 1,\ \text{NPV} = 1$	$\text{DLR}^+ = \infty,\ \text{DLR}^- = 0$
Useless test	$\text{FPF} = \tau = \text{TPF}$	$\text{PPV} = \rho,\ \text{NPV} = 1 - \rho$	$\text{DLR}^+ = 1 = \text{DLR}^-$
Context for use	Accuracy	Clinical prediction	Test informativeness
Question addressed	To what degree does the test reflect the true disease state?	How likely is disease given the test result?	By how much does the test change knowledge of disease status?
Affected by disease prevalence?	No	Yes	No

$^*\mathcal{L}R(y) = P[Y = y\|D = 1]/P[Y = y\|D = 0]$

The pre-test odds of disease, $0.698/0.302 = 2.31$, are increased to $3.08 \times 2.31 = 7.12$ by a positive test. This is decreased to 0.62 by a negative test. ∎

Example 2.2

The DLRs can be used directly with the prevalence of disease in order to calculate the probability of disease given the result of the test. Consider a population with disease prevalence of 5% and a diagnostic test with DLR values of $\text{DLR}^+ = 5.0$ and $\text{DLR}^- = 0.02$. The odds of disease among those that test positive are $5 \times 0.05/0.95 = 0.263$ and they are $0.02 \times 0.05/0.95 = 0.001$ among those that test negative. That is, the probabilities of disease are 21% and 0.1% following positive and negative tests, respectively, in this population. ∎

Similar to the above example, Fagan (1975) presents a nomogram that maps prevalence and DLRs to predictive values. It is tempting to use this device for inferring the predictive values of the test in populations with different prevalences of disease. One must be careful, however, about assuming that the DLRs of a test will be the same in two different populations. Characteristics of subjects, testers or the environment may differ from population to population, all of which may affect the statistical properties of the test, and hence also the test DLR parameters. We discuss this further in Chapter 3.

2.2 Estimating accuracy with data

We now turn to the estimation of the parameters that quantify accuracy.

2.2.1 Data from a cohort study

We begin our discussion with data derived from a cohort study. Let N denote the number of study subjects or test units in the study, which are assumed to be randomly selected from the population. We represent the data as $\{(D_i, Y_i); i = 1, \dots, N\}$. For the purposes of variance calculations and confidence interval construction we assume that the observations (D_i, Y_i) are independent for now. Later we will discuss modifications for settings when the data are correlated. Suppose that n_D of the observations are diseased and $n_{\bar{D}}$ are truly non-diseased. Also let n^+ and n^- denote the numbers of observations with positive and negative test results.

Data from the cohort study can be tabulated as in Table 2.3.

Table 2.3 *Notation for cross-classified test results and disease status*

	$D = 0$	$D = 1$	
$Y = 0$	$n_{\bar{D}}^-$	n_D^-	n^-
$Y = 1$	$n_{\bar{D}}^+$	n_D^+	n^+
	$n_{\bar{D}}$	n_D	

2.2.2 *Proportions:* (FPF, TPF) *and* (PPV, NPV)

The empirical estimators of the classification probabilities and predictive values are proportions with binomial distributions:

$$\hat{\text{TPF}} = n_D^+/n_D, \quad \hat{\text{FPF}} = n_{\bar{D}}^+/n_{\bar{D}},$$
$$\hat{\text{PPV}} = n_D^+/n^+, \quad \hat{\text{NPV}} = n_{\bar{D}}^-/n^-.$$

If observations are independent, confidence intervals can be calculated using exact binomial or asymptotic methods. For good tests the parameters will be close to the edges of the interval $(0, 1)$, so that the simple normal approximation to a binomial is unlikely to perform well because symmetric confidence intervals may extend outside $(0, 1)$. Rather, exact methods, or asymptotic methods based on a logistic transform, may be preferred in such settings. See Agresti and Caffo (2000) for an alternative method. In the next example all of the approaches yielded the same confidence intervals.

Example 2.3

Data from the CASS study yielded the following estimates and 95% confidence intervals (shown in parentheses):

		CAD			
		$D = 0$	$D = 1$		
EST	$Y = 0$	327	208	535	$\hat{\text{NPV}} = 0.61$ $(0.57, 0.65)$
	$Y = 1$	115	815	930	$\hat{\text{PPV}} = 0.88$ $(0.85, 0.90)$
		442	1023	1465	

$$\hat{\text{FPF}} = 0.26 \quad \hat{\text{TPF}} = 0.80$$
$$(0.22, 0.30) \quad (0.77, 0.82)$$ ∎

It is generally more appropriate to report a joint $1 - \alpha$ confidence region for the pair (FPF, TPF) than to report two univariate confidence intervals. (Similar considerations apply to the pair of predictive values.) After all, accuracy is described by considering both parameters together. There are several ways of generating joint confidence regions. Elliptical regions based on joint asymptotic normality could be used. We can also use rectangular regions constructed from the cross-product of $1 - \alpha^*$ confidence intervals for TPF and FPF, where α^* is defined in the next result.

Result 2.4

If $(\text{FPF}_L, \text{FPF}_U)$ and $(\text{TPF}_L, \text{TPF}_U)$ are $1 - \alpha^*$ univariate confidence intervals for FPF and TPF, where $\alpha^* = 1 - (1 - \alpha)^{1/2}$, then the rectangle $R \equiv (\text{FPF}_L, \text{FPF}_U) \times (\text{TPF}_L, \text{TPF}_U)$ is a $1 - \alpha$ rectangular confidence region for (FPF, TPF).

Proof We use the fact that, statistically, data from diseased and non-diseased subjects are independent. For binary data, the FPF confidence interval is therefore independent of that for the TPF. To prove the result, observe that

$$P[(FPF, TPF) \in R] = P[FPF \in (FPF_L, FPF_U), TPF \in (TPF_L, TPF_U)]$$
$$= P[FPF \in (FPF_L, FPF_U)] \, P[TPF \in (TPF_L, TPF_U)]$$
$$= (1 - \alpha^*)^2 = 1 - \alpha. \qquad \blacksquare$$

Example 2.3 (continued)

The 95% confidence intervals for TPF and FPF yield a rectangular region $(0.22, 0.30) \times (0.77, 0.82)$ that contains both population parameters, (FPF, TPF), with confidence level 90% $(= 95\% \times 95\%)$. A 95% confidence region for (FPF, TPF) is constructed from the $\sqrt{95\%} = 97.5\%$ univariate intervals, $(0.22, 0.31) \times (0.77, 0.82)$, which in this example are only slightly wider. We can say that with 95% confidence the FPF is between 0.22 and 0.31 and the TPF is between 0.77 and 0.82 (see Fig. 2.1). *0.975 for individual test confidence interval*

One advantage of rectangular confidence regions over elliptical regions is that they are easily described by the constituent univariate intervals. A graphical representation is not necessary for rectangular regions. On the other hand, elliptical regions require a plot in order to communicate them to a clinically-oriented audience. When journal space is at a premium, rectangular regions may be preferred.

Joint confidence regions for the predictive values can be calculated using methods analogous to those above for the classification probabilities. Again this

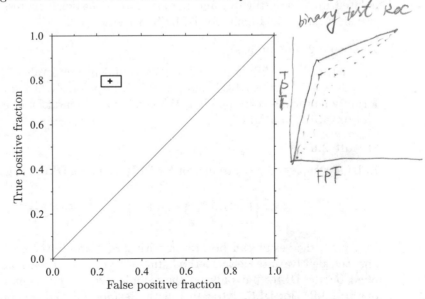

FIG. 2.1. Joint 95% rectangular confidence region for (FPF, TPF) of the exercise stress test based on the CASS data *for 2 dimension*

follows from the statistical independence of the n^+ test positive subjects from the n^- test negative subjects in a cohort study.

2.2.3 Ratios of proportions: DLRs

Empirical estimators of the diagnostic likelihood ratios are

$$\hat{\mathrm{DLR}}^+ = \hat{\mathrm{TPF}}/\hat{\mathrm{FPF}},$$
$$\hat{\mathrm{DLR}}^- = (1 - \hat{\mathrm{TPF}})/(1 - \hat{\mathrm{FPF}}).$$

Because they are written as ratios of statistically independent proportions, asymptotic distribution theory is derived using a logarithmic transform and the delta method (Barndorff-Nielsen and Cox, 1989, Theorem 2.6). The large sample variances are given in the next result, where log denotes the natural logarithm.

Result 2.5

The following results hold:

$$\mathrm{var}\left\{\log \hat{\mathrm{DLR}}^+\right\} = \frac{1 - \mathrm{TPF}}{n_D \mathrm{TPF}} + \frac{1 - \mathrm{FPF}}{n_{\bar{D}} \mathrm{FPF}},$$

$$\mathrm{var}\left\{\log \hat{\mathrm{DLR}}^-\right\} = \frac{\mathrm{TPF}}{n_D(1 - \mathrm{TPF})} + \frac{\mathrm{FPF}}{n_{\bar{D}}(1 - \mathrm{FPF})}. \qquad \blacksquare$$

Confidence limits for $\log \mathrm{DLR}$, based on asymptotic normality, can be calculated from the estimates and the asymptotic variance expressions. These are transformed to yield limits for DLR (Simel *et al.*, 1991).

Example 2.3 (continued)

Applied to the CASS data, we find 95% confidence intervals of $(0.96, 1.28)$ and $(-1.43, -1.17)$ for $\log \mathrm{DLR}^+$ and $\log \mathrm{DLR}^-$, respectively. An exponential transformation provides corresponding 95% confidence intervals of $(2.6, 3.6)$ for DLR^+ and $(0.24, 0.31)$ for DLR^-. $\qquad \blacksquare$

Result 2.6

In large samples, the covariance of $\log \hat{\mathrm{DLR}}^+$ and $\log \hat{\mathrm{DLR}}^-$ is given by

$$\mathrm{cov}\left\{\log \hat{\mathrm{DLR}}^+, \log \hat{\mathrm{DLR}}^-\right\} = -\left(\frac{1}{n_D} + \frac{1}{n_{\bar{D}}}\right). \qquad \blacksquare$$

Again, the result can be proven with large sample theory for $(\hat{\mathrm{FPF}}, \hat{\mathrm{TPF}})$ and the multivariate delta method. Interestingly, the covariance does not depend on the DLRs but only on the sample sizes. Joint asymptotic normality of $(\log \hat{\mathrm{DLR}}^+, \log \hat{\mathrm{DLR}}^-)$ together with Results 2.5 and 2.6 provide elliptical confidence regions for $(\log \mathrm{DLR}^+, \log \mathrm{DLR}^-)$, which can be transformed to confidence regions for $(\mathrm{DLR}^+, \mathrm{DLR}^-)$. Rectangular regions cannot be constructed here in the same way that they were in Section 2.2.2 because of the dependence between $\hat{\text{DLR}}^+$ and $\hat{\text{DLR}}^-$. Another approach is to calculate a rectangular confidence region for (FPF, TPF) and then to map the region to a joint region for $(\hat{\text{DLR}}^+, \hat{\text{DLR}}^-)$ with the transform $g(\text{FPF}, \text{TPF}) = (\text{TPF}/\text{FPF}, (1-\text{TPF})/(1-\text{FPF}))$. Confidence regions calculated with the CASS data are shown in Fig. 2.2.

2.2.4 *Estimation from a case-control study*

In a case-control study pre-determined numbers of diseased and non-diseased subjects are selected for testing. We use the same notation as in Table 2.3, but note that n_D and $n_{\bar{D}}$ are now fixed by design. The relative frequency of diseased subjects is usually much higher in a case-control study than in the population from which the cases and controls are drawn, at least if disease prevalence is relatively low.

Inference for the classification probabilities is exactly the same in a case-control study as in a cohort study because the (FPF, TPF) parameters condition on disease status. The same is true for the DLRs. Inference for predictive values, however, is more difficult in a case-control study. The naive sample proportion, n_D^+/n^+, for example, will overestimate the PPV when cases are oversampled from the population. Formally, oversampling cases in a case-control study causes

$$P[D = 1|Y = 1, \text{ sampled}] > P[D = 1|Y = 1] = \text{PPV}.$$

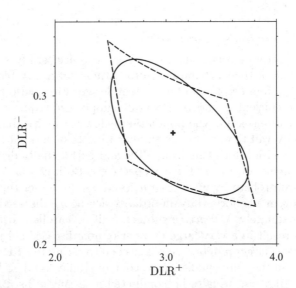

FIG. 2.2. 95% confidence regions for $(\text{DLR}^+, \text{DLR}^-)$ of the EST test based on the CASS data. A region based on asymptotic normality of $(\log \text{DLR}^+, \log \text{DLR}^-)$ is shown by the solid line. A region based on a rectangular region for (FPF, TPF) is shown by the dashed line

In order to estimate $(\mathrm{PPV}, \mathrm{NPV})$ one needs to know the population prevalence, ρ, or at least an estimate of it. Estimates of $(\mathrm{FPF}, \mathrm{TPF})$ from the case-control study can then be substituted into the expressions of Result 2.1(a) to yield estimates of $(\mathrm{PPV}, \mathrm{NPV})$. Equivalently, the formulae of Result 2.2 can be used, along with the estimated DLR values. Indeed, we see from Result 2.2 and eqns (2.8) and (2.9) that

$$\mathrm{logit}\,\mathrm{PPV} = \log(\mathrm{PPV}/(1-\mathrm{PPV})) \quad = \mathrm{logit}\,\rho + \log\mathrm{DLR}^{+}\,,$$
$$\mathrm{logit}\,\mathrm{NPV} = -\log((1-\mathrm{NPV})/\mathrm{NPV}) = -\mathrm{logit}\,\rho - \log\mathrm{DLR}^{-}\,,$$

where we define the function $\mathrm{logit}\,x = \log(x/(1-x))$.

Moreover, confidence intervals for $(\log\mathrm{DLR}^{+}, \log\mathrm{DLR}^{-})$ based on $(\hat{\mathrm{DLR}}^{+}, \hat{\mathrm{DLR}}^{-})$, either univariate or joint, when shifted by $\mathrm{logit}\,\rho$, yield confidence intervals for $(\mathrm{logit}\,\mathrm{PPV}, \mathrm{logit}\,\mathrm{NPV})$, which can in turn be transformed to confidence intervals for $(\mathrm{PPV}, \mathrm{NPV})$.

Example 2.4

Suppose that the 95% confidence interval for $\log\mathrm{DLR}^{+}$ is calculated as $(1.5, 2.5)$ in a population based case-control study and that the disease prevalence is 2%. Then a 95% confidence interval for the $\mathrm{logit}\,\mathrm{PPV}$ of the test, when it is applied in the population, is $\log(0.02/0.98) + (1.5, 2.5) = (-2.39, -1.39)$. This yields a confidence interval of $(0.08, 0.20)$ for the PPV based on the inverse logit transform, $\mathrm{logit}^{-1}\,x = \mathrm{e}^{x}/(1+\mathrm{e}^{x})$. ∎

2.2.5   *Merits of case-control versus cohort studies*

Should a case-control or cohort design be used to select study subjects? Table 2.4 contrasts some of their attributes. Initial studies of a new biomarker or diagnostic test will often employ a case-control design. First, case-control designs tend to be more efficient in terms of overall sample size requirements. That is, if the prevalence of disease in the population is low (or high), the total size of a case-control study will tend to be far smaller than that of a cohort study. This is because the precision for estimating TPF and FPF usually drives the design through requirements on n_D and $n_{\bar{D}}$, respectively. Both can be kept to a minimum in a case-control study, since both n_D and $n_{\bar{D}}$ are under the investigator's control. However, in a cohort study, in order to accrue n_D diseased subjects, say, a total of approximately $N = n_D/\rho$ subjects will be enrolled. If the prevalence is low, this will result in a very large number of non-diseased subjects being enrolled, sometimes a larger number than is needed to estimate FPF with adequate precision. Because they are smaller, case-control studies tend to be less expensive. Moreover, they can usually be conducted at a single institution, whereas a cohort study for a rare disease may need to involve multiple institutions and impose a heavier administrative burden.

Second, case-control studies allow for the exploration of subject-related characteristics on the test. One can deliberately select subjects with different types

Table 2.4 *Attributes of case-control versus cohort studies*

Case-control	Cohort
Small, inexpensive	Large, expensive
Cases already otherwise identified, may exclude mild disease forms	Disease and non-disease representative of population
Deliberate selection of some specific types of cases and controls possible	Can exclude rare subgroups or disease types because of sampling variability
Cannot estimate predictive values directly	Can estimate all measures of diagnostic accuracy
Exploratory	Confirmatory

or manifestations of disease. One can select non-diseased subjects with rare conditions that might potentially be confused with disease by the diagnostic test (Guyatt *et al.*, 1986). These are important issues to be explored at the early phases of test development before embarking on larger cohort studies.

Ironically, a key disadvantage of a case-control study is that the spectrum of disease (and non-disease) may not be representative of the population. The cases have already been diagnosed by some other means. Hence, milder cases that exist in the population but that have not been diagnosed will not be included in the case sample. On the other hand, by its nature a cohort study will include, on average, representative samples of subjects with and without disease.

Cohort studies are often conducted in settings closer to the eventual intended application (see Chapter 8). Moreover, in contrast to case-control studies, in a cohort study disease prevalence can be determined and the clinical value of the test can be assessed with predictive values. Evaluating the true costs and consequences of applying a diagnostic test in practice also requires a cohort study. Thus, a cohort study should ideally be performed before a test enters into routine clinical practice. These confirmatory studies are usually preceded by case-control studies that we consider to be more exploratory in nature. Chapter 8 provides a more thorough discussion of the progressive phases of diagnostic test development, so we will return to this topic again there.

2.3 Quantifying the relative accuracy of tests

We now turn to the comparison of diagnostic tests, considering in particular the comparison of two tests that we label as test A and test B. We use subscripts A and B to index test-specific parameters. Since there are two dimensions to each of the accuracy measures we have discussed, we note that comparisons must also be made in a two-dimensional space.

2.3.1 *Comparing classification probabilities*

Various metrics might be used to compare $(\text{FPF}_A, \text{TPF}_A)$ with $(\text{FPF}_B, \text{TPF}_B)$. In Table 2.5 we define three: absolute differences, odds ratios and relative probabilities.

Our preference is for the latter, which we will denote by $(\text{rFPF}(A, B), \text{rTPF}(A, B))$. First, their interpretations are straightforward. If $\text{rFPF}(A, B) = 2.0$ and $\text{rTPF}(A, B) = 0.8$, the interpretation is that the false positive fraction for test A is twice that of test B, while its true positive fraction is only 80% of that for test B. Interpretations for odds ratios on the other hand are not quite so natural. Moreover, in contrast to traditional epidemiologic studies of disease risk, where odds ratios approximate relative risks, in diagnostic studies relative classification probabilities are usually very different in magnitude from odds ratios (because positive tests are not rare events).

Example 2.5

Consider the classification probabilities of the EST and CPH tests conducted in the CASS study. We see that the classification odds ratios of the CPH test relative to the EST test are much larger than the relative classification probabilities.

	FPF	TPF
EST	26%	80%
CPH	55%	95%
(rFPF, rTPF)	2.12	1.19
(oFPF, oTPF)	3.48	4.75

One drawback associated with absolute differences is that statistical inference on this scale is difficult. The logistic scale, i.e. the odds ratio, is better suited to

Table 2.5 *Three comparative measures for classification probabilities*

	Absolute differences	Odds ratios	Relative probabilities
Definition	$\text{TPF}_A - \text{TPF}_B$	$\frac{\text{TPF}_A(1-\text{TPF}_B)}{\text{TPF}_B(1-\text{TPF}_A)}$	$\text{TPF}_A/\text{TPF}_B$
	$\text{FPF}_A - \text{FPF}_B$	$\frac{\text{FPF}_A(1-\text{FPF}_B)}{\text{FPF}_B(1-\text{FPF}_A)}$	$\text{FPF}_A/\text{FPF}_B$
Notation	$\Delta\text{TPF}(A, B)$	$\text{oTPF}(A, B)$	$\text{rTPF}(A, B)$
	$\Delta\text{FPF}(A, B)$	$\text{oFPF}(A, B)$	$\text{rFPF}(A, B)$
Interpretation	Easy	Awkward	Easy
Statistical inference	Limited	Standard	Easy
Flexible designs accommodated	No	No	Yes

sophisticated statistical inference. Logistic regression can be used, for example, to evaluate odds ratios while controlling for covariate effects. Regression models for classification probabilities are almost never formulated as linear on the original scale. Statistical inference for relative probabilities or fractions is straightforward, though admittedly non-standard. Relative probabilities, being defined on $(0, \infty)$, can be analyzed on a log scale. Generalized linear regression models with a log link, for example, are discussed in Chapter 3 for making inferences about relative probabilities as an alternative to logistic models that make inferences about odds ratios.

Finally, in Chapter 7 we will discuss some common study designs that, unfortunately, do not allow for the estimation of absolute $(\mathrm{FPF}, \mathrm{TPF})$ or for inference about the comparative measures $(\Delta\mathrm{FPF}, \Delta\mathrm{TPF})$ and $(\mathrm{oFPF}, \mathrm{oTPF})$. Inference about relative classification probabilities is, however, possible. The quantification of relative accuracy in terms of relative probabilities applies across a broader range of study designs, and in this sense is more robust.

2.3.2 *Comparing predictive values*

Predictive values can be compared on various scales, such as multiplicative (i.e. relative) or logistic (i.e. odds ratio) scales. Indeed, when the prevalence of disease is low, the relative positive predictive values and odds ratios are approximately equal. This is a standard result used in epidemiology, which we now state formally for our context of diagnostic testing. First we define the following notation:

$$\mathrm{rPPV}(A, B) \equiv \mathrm{PPV}_A/\mathrm{PPV}_B \,, \tag{2.10}$$

$$\mathrm{oPPV}(A, B) \equiv \mathrm{PPV}_A(1 - \mathrm{PPV}_B)/\mathrm{PPV}_B(1 - \mathrm{PPV}_A) \,, \tag{2.11}$$

$$\mathrm{rNPV}(A, B) \equiv \mathrm{NPV}_A/\mathrm{NPV}_B \,, \tag{2.12}$$

$$\mathrm{oNPV}(A, B) \equiv \mathrm{NPV}_A(1 - \mathrm{NPV}_B)/\mathrm{NPV}_B(1 - \mathrm{NPV}_A) \,, \tag{2.13}$$

$$\overline{\mathrm{rNPV}}(A, B) \equiv (1 - \mathrm{NPV}_A)/(1 - \mathrm{NPV}_B) \,. \tag{2.14}$$

Result 2.7

If the prevalence of disease is low, then the following equalities hold approximately: *rare*

$$\mathrm{rPPV}(A, B) = \mathrm{oPPV}(A, B) \,, \qquad RR \doteq OR$$
$$\mathrm{rNPV}(A, B) = 1 \,,$$
$$\overline{\mathrm{rNPV}}(A, B) = 1/\mathrm{oNPV}(B, A) \,. \qquad\blacksquare$$

The result follows from the fact that both PPV_A and PPV_B are approximately 0 for a low prevalence disease. When prevalence is not low, we prefer the relative predictive values, $(\mathrm{rPPV}, \mathrm{rNPV})$, over the odds ratio measures, again for reasons similar to those for preferring relative classification probabilities over classification odds ratios. Their interpretation is more straightforward. As an example, if $\mathrm{rPPV}(A, B) = 2.0$, then a positive result on test A is twice as indicative of disease risk than is a positive result on test B. Note that subjects might be tested with both tests, but that the predictive values involved in rPPV(A, B) are marginal probabilities. That is, PPV$_A$ and PPV$_B$ pertain, respectively, to the risk of disease associated with test A in the absence of knowledge about the result of test B and the risk associated only with knowledge of a positive result on test B.

Although odds ratios in and of themselves are less appealing than relative predictive values, in the next section we provide another interpretation for them in terms of DLRs that is somewhat appealing.

2.3.3 *Comparing diagnostic likelihood ratios*

The relative DLRs are defined as

$$\mathrm{rDLR}^+(A, B) = \mathrm{DLR}_A^+/\mathrm{DLR}_B^+, \tag{2.15}$$
$$\mathrm{rDLR}^-(A, B) = \mathrm{DLR}_A^-/\mathrm{DLR}_B^-. \tag{2.16}$$

Note that odds ratios are not appropriate here because DLRs are not probabilities. The relative DLRs are defined on $(0, \infty)$, with test A being a better test on the DLR$^+$ scale if rDLR$^+(A, B) > 1$ and a better test on the DLR$^-$ scale if rDLR$^-(A, B) < 1$.

Example 2.5 (continued)

Observe that the DLRs of the EST and CPH tests in the CASS population are

$$\mathrm{DLR}_{\mathrm{EST}}^+ = 3.06, \quad \mathrm{DLR}_{\mathrm{CPH}}^+ = 1.71,$$
$$\mathrm{DLR}_{\mathrm{EST}}^- = 0.28, \quad \mathrm{DLR}_{\mathrm{CPH}}^- = 0.12.$$

Therefore, rDLR$^+$(CPH, EST) $= 0.56$ and rDLR$^-$(CPH, EST) $= 0.43$, indicating that a positive result on EST is more indicative of disease than is a positive result on CPH. However, a negative result on EST is not as convincing for indicating the absence of disease as a negative CPH result. ∎

Result 2.8

The following results hold:

$$\mathrm{rDLR}^+(A, B) = \mathrm{oPPV}(A, B),$$
$$\mathrm{rDLR}^-(A, B) = 1/\mathrm{oNPV}(A, B). ∎$$

This result follows from the relationship between DLRs and predictive values described in Result 2.2 and eqns (2.8) and (2.9). It provides an alternative interpretation for the odds ratios of predictive values. In particular, they can be interpreted as ratios of diagnostic likelihood ratios. We will use this fact later in Chapter 3 to make inferences about relative DLRs.

2.3.4 *Which test is better?*

An overall conclusion about the relative performance of one test compared to another is easy if one test outperforms the other on both dimensions of the accuracy scale under consideration. For example, on the classification probability scale, if $rTPF(A, B) > 1$ and $rFPF(A, B) < 1$, then we can say that test A is the more accurate test on this scale. As one would expect, a test that is better than another on both dimensions of the classification probability scale is also better on both dimensions of the other scales that we have mentioned, namely predictive values and diagnostic likelihood ratios. There is a reciprocal relationship with the predictive value scale, but interestingly not with the likelihood ratio scale (Exercise 6).

Result 2.9

The following are equivalent statements:

(i) $\qquad\qquad\qquad$ $rTPF(A, B) > 1$ $\quad$ and $\quad$ $rFPF(A, B) < 1$;

(ii) $\qquad\qquad\qquad$ $rPPV(A, B) > 1$ $\quad$ and $\quad$ $rNPV(A, B) > 1$.

Moreover, (i) implies, but is not implied by the following statement:

(iii) $\qquad\qquad\qquad$ $rDLR^+(A, B) > 1$ $\quad$ and $\quad$ $rDLR^-(A, B) < 1$. $\qquad$ ∎

If test A is more accurate than test B on one dimension, but less accurate on the other dimension, then an overall conclusion about which test is better is more difficult. For example, if a new sample collection method increases the TPF of the Pap smear, but also increases the FPF, what can we conclude about the new test? One approach is to define a single measure that incorporates both dimensions of accuracy and to base a conclusion on the composite single measure. Cost is one composite measure that is often used (Boyko, 1994). Others have been proposed. Chock *et al.* (1997) motivate $(TPF_A - TPF_B)/(FPF_A - FPF_B)$ as a composite measure. A composite measure must balance the two dimensions of accuracy in an appropriate way. Agreement as to what constitutes a valid composite measure is rarely an easy task.

We will consider cost as a composite measure here, simply to give a taste of this aspect in evaluating a test. A broader discussion of cost and cost-effectiveness in healthcare can be found in Weinstein and Fineberg (1980) and Gold *et al.* (1996). Costs can include non-monetary components as well as financial costs. Suppose that a new test for a disease is to be offered to subjects in a certain population. The key components of cost pertinent to the test and the disease in this population include:

(i) C, the cost associated with performing the test itself;

(ii) C_D^+ and C_D^-, the costs of treatment and disease morbidity for diseased subjects that test positive and test negative, respectively. Usually C_D^- will be much larger than C_D^+ because undetected disease will ultimately be harder to treat successfully;

(iii) $C_{\bar{D}}^+$, the cost of work-up, stress and possibly unnecessary treatment for non-diseased subjects that test positive.

The overall cost of disease per subject in the population in the presence of testing can then be written as

$$\text{Cost(testing)} = C + C_D^+ \text{TPF}\rho + C_D^-(1 - \text{TPF})\rho + C_{\bar{D}}^+ \text{FPF}(1 - \rho). \qquad (2.17)$$

In the absence of testing, each diseased subject contributes C_D^-. Hence, the overall cost per subject in the population is

$$\text{Cost(no testing)} = \rho C_D^-.$$

A comparison of Cost(testing) with Cost(no testing) can be used to determine whether a testing program will reduce the overall cost of the disease to the population. A comparison of two different tests can be based on their calculated values for Cost(testing).

Example 2.6

We refer to a report on cervical cancer screening in the United States (AHCPR, 1999). The risk of cervical cancer is estimated to be about 0.8% and therefore $\rho = 0.008$. The Pap smear is estimated to have true and false positive fractions of 0.51 and 0.02, respectively. We consider here monetary costs pertaining only to diagnosis and treatment. Anxiety, reduced work productivity and morbidity are costs that are not considered. The cost of a Pap smear is about $40. Suppose that diseased subjects detected with the Pap screening test average $1730 for work-up and treatment of their disease, while those not detected with the Pap ultimately require more extensive treatment, costing on average $17 500. Subjects with false positive screens require colposcopy and biopsy, costing about $170.

The cost of cervical cancer to the population as a whole in the absence of testing with the Pap, is then calculated as

$$\text{Cost(no testing)} = 0.008 \times \$17\,500 = \$140.$$

This is the cost per person in the general population. The corresponding cost in the presence of screening is

$$\begin{aligned}
\text{Cost(testing)} &= \$40 + \$1730 \times 0.51 \times 0.008 + \$17\,500 \times 0.49 \times 0.008 \\
&\qquad\qquad\qquad\qquad\qquad + \$170 \times 0.02 \times 0.992 \\
&= \$40 + \$7.06 + \$68.60 + \$3.37 \\
&= \$119.
\end{aligned}$$

Thus testing appears to be worthwhile, even when measured in monetary terms.

Would a more sensitive, but less specific, test be better on this cost dimension? Suppose that a new test that costs the same as the Pap to administer has a true positive rate of 0.70 but unfortunately doubles the false positive rate relative to the Pap, i.e. FPF = 0.04. Then,

$$\text{Cost(testing)} = \$40 + \$1730 \times 0.70 \times 0.008 + \$17\,500 \times 0.30 \times 0.008$$
$$+ \$170 \times 0.04 \times 0.992$$
$$= \$40.00 + \$9.69 + \$42.00 + \$6.75$$
$$= \$98.44\,.$$

Cost savings provided by this test relative to the Pap are substantial. Thus it would be preferred over the Pap test on this cost scale. However, other factors, especially the stress and physical morbidity associated with false positive results, would need to be considered by healthcare providers before adopting the new test for widespread use.   ∎

2.4   Concluding remarks

The concept of diagnostic accuracy has several definitions. Three methods for quantifying diagnostic accuracy of binary tests have been described in this chapter, each consisting of two components: the classification probabilities (FPF, TPF), the predictive values (PPV, NPV) and the diagnostic likelihood ratios (DLR$^+$, DLR$^-$). Attributes of the measures were summarized in Table 2.2. The classification probabilities and predictive values are most commonly used in practice, the former being the key parameters derived from case-control studies, while predictive values, which relate to test usefulness, can be estimated from cohort studies. In my opinion, the natural role for the DLRs is to supplement the (FPF, TPF) estimates from a case-control study. They quantify the change in the odds of disease conferred by knowledge of the test result, thereby suggesting the information content in the test when it is used in a prospective fashion. However, the predictive values themselves will be the key quantities of interest from the cohort studies that follow case-control studies.

Simple statistical techniques to make inferences about each of the accuracy measures from data were described in Section 2.2. This material is intended to be accessible to the applied researcher with standard statistical training. The focus here and elsewhere in the book is on estimation and construction of confidence intervals. Hypothesis testing procedures that relate directly to the methods described here are discussed in Chapter 8, where they are used to plan sample sizes for studies. For joint estimation of the two parameters (FPF, TPF) (or (PPV, NPV)), rectangular confidence regions are suggested. These simplify the construction of the regions, their presentation and the sample size calculations in comparison to more traditional elliptical regions. It would be interesting to make some comparisons of the sizes of the rectangular and corresponding elliptical regions.

The relative merits of cohort and case-control studies were summarized in Table 2.4. In fact, for most diagnostic tests the process of their development and evaluation entails a series of research studies, with early studies likely to be of the case-control design while later ones are cohort studies. This is addressed more fully in Chapter 8.

The last section of this chapter concerned the comparison of tests. There are many ways to quantify the relative performance of tests. Indeed, even when one has settled on one of the three measures for quantifying accuracy, classification probabilities, say, there are many scales on which to quantify the comparative accuracy. The multiplicative scale is favored here because of its easy interpretation and inference (see also Chapter 7). However, others may prefer to use the logistic scale or the absolute difference scale.

Comparing tests with a one-dimensional composite measure, such as cost, was discussed in Section 2.3.4. This is an important and relatively well-developed area, which is only touched on briefly here in a much simplified example. The reader is referred to the health economics literature for proper, more sophisticated treatments of the techniques for evaluating and comparing costs.

2.5 Exercises

1. Prove the equalities of Result 2.1. Demonstrate them empirically for the EST test using the CASS study data.

2. The positive DLR can be interpreted as a benefit to cost ratio.

   (a) Provide such an interpretation using the DLR^+ of the EST test as a context.

   (b) Consider the composite comparative measure of test performance, $(TPF_A - TPF_B)/(FPF_A - FPF_B)$, which was proposed by Chock *et al.* (1997). Discuss its interpretation and your opinion of its value in practice. Compare the EST and CPH tests using this measure.

3. Using the neonatal audiology testing data described in Section 1.3.7, compare test C with test A. Write up your analysis and conclusions for a clinical colleague, providing simple relevant interpretations for parameters that you choose to report. Ignore sampling variability in estimates of comparative measures of test performance.

4. Explain intuitively why $\hat{DLR}^+$ and $\hat{DLR}^-$ are negatively correlated.

5. A computationally simple but conservative joint confidence region for (DLR^+, DLR^-) is formed by the rectangle

$$\left(\frac{TPF_L}{FPF_U}, \frac{TPF_U}{FPF_L}\right) \times \left(\frac{1 - TPF_U}{1 - FPF_L}, \frac{1 - TPF_L}{1 - FPF_U}\right),$$

where FPF_L, FPF_U, TPF_L and TPF_U denote the limits of the $\sqrt{1 - \alpha}$ confidence intervals for FPF and TPF. Calculate this for the EST test using the CASS data and contrast it with regions displayed in Fig. 2.2.

6. Prove algebraically the equivalences stated in Result 2.9. Also, construct an example where $rDLR^+(A, B) > 1$ and $rDLR^-(A, B) < 1$, while one of the conditions $rTPF(A, B) > 1$ or $rFPF(A, B) < 1$ fails.

3

COMPARING BINARY TESTS AND REGRESSION ANALYSIS

Various factors can influence the performance of a medical test. The environment in which it is performed, characteristics of testers, characteristics of test subjects and operating parameters for the test are some such factors. It is important to identify and understand the influence of such factors in order to optimize conditions for using a test. Statistical regression analysis can be used to make inferences about such factors, as will be described in this chapter. We also consider the related problem of comparing different tests.

3.1 Study designs for comparing tests

Decisions about which tests to recommend for widespread use and which to abandon are made, in part, on the basis of research studies that compare the accuracies of tests. Before detailing statistical methods for evaluating data from such studies, we first briefly consider options for designing comparative studies.

3.1.1 Unpaired designs

In studies to compare multiple tests, each study subject can be tested with all tests or each subject can undergo a single test. We call the former a paired design and the latter an unpaired design, even when more than two tests are under consideration (see Section 1.2.3).

Unpaired designs are used if tests are invasive, cause the patient discomfort, are time consuming or have significant risk associated with them. Ethical considerations usually require that unpaired comparisons be made to minimize the burden on the subject. Alternatively, the performance of one test might interfere with the implementation or results of another. Two different surgical procedures cannot be done without interfering with each other, for example. Since the objectives are to evaluate each test as a single entity, such interference would invalidate the study. Finally, in observational studies of medical tests, patients will be unlikely to have more than one experimental test performed. Thus, again, the data will be unpaired. Table 3.1 shows the typical layout of data for an unpaired comparison of two binary tests.

An unpaired comparative study for multiple tests should follow the same design principles as those for a parallel-arm randomized clinical trial: well-defined entry criteria should be in place for the study; rigorous definitions for disease and test results are necessary; a detailed protocol should be in place for all study procedures; subjects should be randomized to the different tests and the randomization should ensure that the study arms (subjects receiving test A, test B, etc.) are balanced with regards to factors affecting test performance;

Table 3.1 *Notation and layout of data from an unpaired study design*

	$D=1$			$D=0$		
	$Y=0$	$Y=1$		$Y=0$	$Y=1$	
Test A	$n_D^-(A)$	$n_D^+(A)$	$n_D(A)$	$n_{\bar D}^-(A)$	$n_{\bar D}^+(A)$	$n_{\bar D}(A)$
Test B	$n_D^-(B)$	$n_D^+(B)$	$n_D(B)$	$n_{\bar D}^-(B)$	$n_{\bar D}^+(B)$	$n_{\bar D}(B)$

blinding may be necessary to maintain the integrity of disease and diagnostic test assessments, as mentioned in Chapter 1; a data analysis plan must be in place prior to conducting the study to ensure the integrity of statistical analyses; finally, the sample sizes chosen should be sufficiently large, so that a scientific conclusion can be made with confidence at the end of the study.

3.1.2 *Paired designs*

Comparative studies, where subjects are tested with each test, are valid if tests do not interfere with each other. Interference can be subtle. For example, if some tests are time consuming, the care with which a test is performed or the cooperation of the patient may be less when multiple tests are on the agenda.

When feasible, however, paired designs have several advantages over unpaired designs. Most importantly, the impact of between-subject variability is minimized, thus yielding statistically more efficient studies. On an intuitive basis also, studies that compare performances of several tests in the *same* patients yield stronger conclusions about relative performance. Possibilities for confounding are completely eliminated. Moreover, one can examine characteristics of subjects where tests yield different results. This can lead to insights about test performance and sometimes strategies for improving tests. When multiple tests are performed on individuals, one can assess the value of applying combinations of tests compared with single tests. This, however, will not be discussed further here (see Chapter 9).

Data for a paired study to compare two tests can be summarized in the format of Table 3.2. This table shows the joint classification of the tests. Thus it shows correlations between them as well. Note, however, that comparisons between tests are made on the basis of their singular performances. That is, until we

Table 3.2 *Layout of data for a paired study design*

		$D=1$			$D=0$		
		Test A			Test A		
		$Y_A=0$	$Y_A=1$		$Y_A=0$	$Y_A=1$	
Test B	$Y_B=0$	a	b	$n_D^-(B)$	e	f	$n_{\bar D}^-(B)$
	$Y_B=1$	c	d	$n_D^+(B)$	g	h	$n_{\bar D}^+(B)$
		$n_D^-(A)$	$n_D^+(A)$	n_D	$n_{\bar D}^-(A)$	$n_{\bar D}^+(A)$	$n_{\bar D}$

(b.c) (e.f) are discordant cell

discuss how to combine tests in Chapter 9, we will not be directly interested in their correlations.

Observe that the layout shown in Table 3.1 for unpaired data can be used for a paired study too, and is appropriate when we neglect the correlations between tests. The marginal frequencies for a paired design in Table 3.2 correspond to the entries given in Table 3.1 for an unpaired study. Since subjects tested with test A and test B are the same, in the notation of Table 3.1 we have $n_D(A) = n_D(B) = n_D$ and $n_{\bar{D}}(A) = n_{\bar{D}}(B) = n_{\bar{D}}$. It is important to note that the parameters of interest (such as (rFPF, rTPF), etc.) can be estimated from the marginal frequencies, and hence in essentially the same way from paired and unpaired studies.

A study that yields paired test data will usually be experimental and deliberately designed rather than observational. Well-established principles for cross-over clinical trials should be adhered to in a paired comparative study. Many of the considerations have been mentioned already for unpaired studies. In addition, the order in which tests are performed may need to be randomized.

3.2   Comparing accuracy with unpaired data

3.2.1   *Empirical estimators of comparative measures*

Measures that quantify the relative accuracy of two tests were discussed in Chapter 2. All of these measures can be estimated empirically from cohort data. Empirical estimates of $(\mathrm{rFPF}(A, B), \mathrm{rTPF}(A, B))$ and $(\mathrm{rDLR}^+(A, B), \mathrm{rDLR}^-(A, B))$ are also valid for case-control study data. However, estimates of $(\mathrm{rPPV}(A, B), \mathrm{rNPV}(A, B))$ are not because they, like the predictive values themselves, involve disease prevalence. Thus, we consider inference for (rPPV, rNPV) only for cohort studies. Using the notation of Table 3.1 we formally define the empirical estimators as follows:

$$\mathrm{r\hat{T}PF}(A, B) = \left\{ \frac{n_D^+(A)}{n_D(A)} \right\} \bigg/ \left\{ \frac{n_D^+(B)}{n_D(B)} \right\}, \tag{3.1}$$

$$\mathrm{r\hat{F}PF}(A, B) = \left\{ \frac{n_{\bar{D}}^+(A)}{n_{\bar{D}}(A)} \right\} \bigg/ \left\{ \frac{n_{\bar{D}}^+(B)}{n_{\bar{D}}(B)} \right\}, \tag{3.2}$$

$$\mathrm{r\hat{P}PV}(A, B) = \left\{ \frac{n_D^+(A)}{n_D^+(A) + n_{\bar{D}}^+(A)} \right\} \bigg/ \left\{ \frac{n_D^+(B)}{n_D^+(B) + n_{\bar{D}}^+(B)} \right\}, \tag{3.3}$$

$$\mathrm{r\hat{N}PV}(A, B) = \left\{ \frac{n_{\bar{D}}^-(A)}{n_D^-(A) + n_{\bar{D}}^-(A)} \right\} \bigg/ \left\{ \frac{n_{\bar{D}}^-(B)}{n_D^-(B) + n_{\bar{D}}^-(B)} \right\}, \tag{3.4}$$

$$\mathrm{r\hat{D}LR}^+(A, B) = \left\{ \frac{n_D^+(A)\, n_{\bar{D}}(A)}{n_D(A)\, n_{\bar{D}}^+(A)} \right\} \bigg/ \left\{ \frac{n_D^+(B)\, n_{\bar{D}}(B)}{n_D(B)\, n_{\bar{D}}^+(B)} \right\}, \tag{3.5}$$

$$\mathrm{r\hat{D}LR}^-(A, B) = \left\{ \frac{n_D^-(A)\, n_{\bar{D}}(A)}{n_D(A)\, n_{\bar{D}}^-(A)} \right\} \bigg/ \left\{ \frac{n_D^-(B)\, n_{\bar{D}}(B)}{n_D(B)\, n_{\bar{D}}^-(B)} \right\}. \tag{3.6}$$

3.2.2 *Large sample inference*

Although the empirical estimators are valid in a wider context, our asymptotic distribution theory relies on an assumption of statistical independence between observations. Inference with clustered data will be discussed later. The large sample results technically relate to the condition that $\min(n_D(A), n_D(B), n_{\bar{D}}(A),$ $n_{\bar{D}}(B))$ converges to ∞. In words, all four sample sizes involved are large.

Result 3.1

In large samples, $(\log r\hat{\mathrm{F}}\mathrm{PF}(A, B), \log r\hat{\mathrm{T}}\mathrm{PF}(A, B))$ are independent and normally distributed with mean $(\log r\mathrm{FPF}(A, B), \log r\mathrm{TPF}(A, B))$ and variances approximated by

$$\mathrm{var}(\log r\hat{\mathrm{T}}\mathrm{PF}(A, B)) = \frac{1 - \mathrm{TPF}_A}{n_D(A)\mathrm{TPF}_A} + \frac{1 - \mathrm{TPF}_B}{n_D(B)\mathrm{TPF}_B},$$

$$\mathrm{var}(\log r\hat{\mathrm{F}}\mathrm{PF}(A, B)) = \frac{1 - \mathrm{FPF}_A}{n_{\bar{D}}(A)\mathrm{FPF}_A} + \frac{1 - \mathrm{FPF}_B}{n_{\bar{D}}(B)\mathrm{FPF}_B}.$$

Proof   The result follows from the delta methods as applied by Simel *et al.* (1991) for the ratio of two independent binomial proportions.   ∎

Example 3.1

Let us use the result to construct a joint confidence interval for the $(r\mathrm{FPF}, r\mathrm{TPF})$ of two tests. The (hypothetical) data in Table 3.3 relate to the diagnosis of fetal chromosomal abnormalities during the first trimester of pregnancy in women who are at high risk of fetal chromosomal or genetic disorders. Chorionic villus sampling (CVS) is an invasive procedure that involves removing a sample of placental cells during the first trimester and analyzing them for fetal karyotypes. Amniocentesis, also an invasive procedure, involves removing a sample of amniotic fluid to obtain fetal karyotypes. While amniocentesis is a relatively safe and accurate procedure when it is performed mid-trimester, as is commonly done, early amniocentesis (EA) is done during the first trimester and is still the subject of many questions and concerns. Women were randomized to receive either EA or CVS.

Similar to the approach used in Section 2.2.2, we construct a $1 - \alpha$ rectangular confidence region for $(r\mathrm{FPF}(\mathrm{EA}, \mathrm{CVS}), r\mathrm{TPF}(\mathrm{EA}, \mathrm{CVS}))$ by constructing $1 - \alpha^*$

Table 3.3 *Data from a randomized unpaired study of chorionic villus sampling (CVS) versus early amniocentesis (EA) for fetal abnormality*

	$D = 1$			$D = 0$		
	$Y = 0$	$Y = 1$		$Y = 0$	$Y = 1$	
EA	6	116	122	4844	34	4878
CVS	13	111	124	4765	111	4876

[Handwritten annotations:]

TPF = Sensitivity : EA: 116/122 = 95%

CVS = 111/124 = 90%

FPF = EA: 34/4878 = 0.7%

CVS = 111/4876 = 2.3%

→ EA is a better test

benefit from simultaneous test

confidence intervals for its components, where $\alpha^* = 1 - \sqrt{1 - \alpha}$. The confidence interval for $\log \mathrm{rFPF}$ is

$$(L, H) = \log \mathrm{r\hat{F}PF} \pm \Phi^{-1}\left(1 - \frac{\alpha^*}{2}\right)\sqrt{\mathrm{v\hat{a}r}(\log \mathrm{r\hat{F}PF})},$$

which is exponentiated to yield a confidence interval (e^L, e^H) for rFPF. Similarly for rTPF.

Applying this strategy to the data in Table 3.3 with $\alpha = 0.05$, the joint 95% confidence region for $(\mathrm{rFPF}, \mathrm{rTPF})$ is a rectangle with sides (0.20, 0.47) and (0.98, 1.15). The FPF associated with the EA test is between 20% and 50% of that for the CVS test, while their TPFs are similar, the $\mathrm{rTPF(EA, CVS)}$ being between 98% and 115%. ∎

Result 3.2

In a large cohort study $\log \mathrm{r\hat{P}PV}$ and $\log \mathrm{r\hat{N}PV}$ are approximately normal and independent with variances

$$\mathrm{var}\left(\log \mathrm{r\hat{P}PV}(A, B)\right) = \frac{(1 - \mathrm{PPV}_A)/\mathrm{PPV}_A}{n_D^+(A) + n_{\bar{D}}^+(A)} + \frac{(1 - \mathrm{PPV}_B)/\mathrm{PPV}_B}{n_D^+(B) + n_{\bar{D}}^+(B)},$$

$$\mathrm{var}\left(\log \mathrm{r\hat{N}PV}(A, B)\right) = \frac{(1 - \mathrm{NPV}_A)/\mathrm{NPV}_A}{n_D^-(A) + n_{\bar{D}}^-(A)} + \frac{(1 - \mathrm{NPV}_B)/\mathrm{NPV}_B}{n_D^-(B) + n_{\bar{D}}^-(B)}. \qquad ∎$$

This result is entirely analogous to that in Result 3.1 after interchanging the roles of disease and test result. A joint 90% confidence interval for $(\mathrm{rNPV(EA, CVS)}, \mathrm{rPPV(EA, CVS)})$, calculated using methods similar to those in Example 3.1, is a rectangle with sides (0.999, 1.003) and (1.32, 1.81).

Next we consider large sample inference for the third set of parameters, namely the relative DLRs.

Result 3.3

In large samples, $(\log \mathrm{r\hat{DLR}}^+(A, B), \log \mathrm{r\hat{DLR}}^-(A, B))$ are normally distributed with

$$\mathrm{var}(\log \mathrm{r\hat{DLR}}^+(A, B))$$
$$= \frac{1 - \mathrm{TPF}_A}{n_D(A)\mathrm{TPF}_A} + \frac{1 - \mathrm{FPF}_A}{n_{\bar{D}}(A)\mathrm{FPF}_A} + \frac{1 - \mathrm{TPF}_B}{n_D(B)\mathrm{TPF}_B} + \frac{1 - \mathrm{FPF}_B}{n_{\bar{D}}(B)\mathrm{FPF}_B}, \tag{3.7}$$

$$\mathrm{var}(\log \mathrm{r\hat{DLR}}^-(A, B))$$
$$= \frac{\mathrm{TPF}_A}{n_D(A)(1 - \mathrm{TPF}_A)} + \frac{\mathrm{FPF}_A}{n_{\bar{D}}(A)(1 - \mathrm{FPF}_A)}$$
$$+ \frac{\mathrm{TPF}_B}{n_D(B)(1 - \mathrm{TPF}_B)} + \frac{\mathrm{FPF}_B}{n_{\bar{D}}(B)(1 - \mathrm{FPF}_B)}, \tag{3.8}$$

$$\text{cov}(\log \text{rD}\hat{\text{L}}\text{R}^+(A, B), \log \text{D}\hat{\text{L}}\text{R}^-(A, B))$$

$$= -\left(\frac{1}{n_D(A)} + \frac{1}{n_{\bar{D}}(A)} + \frac{1}{n_D(B)} + \frac{1}{n_{\bar{D}}(B)}\right).$$

(3.9)

Proof This follows from the statistical independence of subjects receiving tests A and B and the large sample results for DLRs given in Results 2.5 and 2.6. ∎

Example 3.1 (continued)

Using the asymptotic normality result we have that a 95% joint confidence region for $\log \text{rDLR}^+(\text{EA}, \text{CVS})$ and $\log \text{rDLR}^-(\text{EA}, \text{CVS})$ is given by the ellipse in Fig. 3.1. Recall from Result 2.8 that, because of the correspondence between rDLRs and predictive value odds ratios, this can also be interpreted as a joint confidence region for the log odds ratios $(\log \text{oPPV}(\text{EA}, \text{CVS}), \log \text{oNPV}(\text{EA}, \text{CVS}))$. ∎

Hypothesis testing is considered in some detail in Chapter 8. We base hypothesis testing procedures on confidence intervals for the parameters of interest, because a wide range of hypotheses can be tested in this framework. Nevertheless, we note that standard statistical tests can be applied to test some simple hypotheses about comparative parameters. For the hypothesis $H_0 : \text{rTPF}(A, B) = 1$, for example, a Pearson chi-squared test can be used with unpaired data.

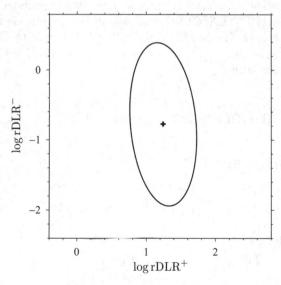

FIG. 3.1. 95% elliptical confidence region for $\log \text{rDLR}^+(\text{EA}, \text{CVS})$ and $\log \text{rDLR}^-(\text{EA}, \text{CVS})$

3.3 Comparing accuracy with paired data

3.3.1 *Sources of correlation*

When multiple tests are applied to each study subject, the test results are likely to be correlated. It is important to be cognizant of this when interpreting data from a comparative study. At the design stage, too, it is important to consider factors giving rise to correlation and to take advantage of these while not allowing them to dominate. Finally, some popular statistical techniques for comparing diagnostic tests require that tests are statistically independent conditional on disease status (see Chapter 7), and this assumption must be carefully considered.

What then are some sources of correlation between tests? Any factor that influences the performance of the tests and that varies across subjects will give rise to correlation (unless properly accounted for as covariates in analyses). Consider, for example, patient-related characteristics such as breast tissue density that will affect the outcomes of both the clinical breast exam and mammography for detecting breast cancer. Alternatively, consider ambient room noise that affects the performance of hearing tests. If the auditory brain-stem response test and the distortion product emissions test are performed in a busy neonatal unit, they will probably both be less accurate than if they are performed in a sound booth. A detailed discussion of factors that influence test performance appears in Section 3.4.

Later in this chapter we will discuss how to adjust for covariates that affect test results. These techniques reduce effects of correlation in data analysis. However, non-measurable factors that influence test results cannot be adjusted for as covariates. For example, if alliquots of a single specimen are used to assay several tests for detecting bacteria, the tests will all depend on the density of viable bacteria in the sample, an unmeasurable entity. Misconceptions of one's behavior can lead to the same errors in responding to several different test questionnaires. Adjustments cannot be made for such unmeasurable entities. Analyses will simply need to acknowledge that correlations exist.

Recall that diagnostic tests themselves can influence each other, either directly or indirectly. Such influences not only give rise to correlation, but, of more concern, they give rise to biases that invalidate the paired study design (see Section 3.1.2). Thus we do not allow this sort of interdependence between tests in a comparative study, and we assume henceforth that it does not exist in the data.

3.3.2 *Estimation of comparative measures*

To estimate relative performance measures with a paired study design, consider first as an example the relative TPF. Recall that the constituent classification probabilities TPF_A and TPF_B are defined as marginal probabilities. The TPF_A is a probability that depends only on the result of test A and disease status. It does not involve test B at all. When data only pertaining to test A is considered for diseased subjects, the empirical probability $n_D^+(A)/n_D$ is a valid estimate of TPF_A. Similarly for test B, and hence the ratio of the empirical values $(n_D^+(A)/n_D)/(n_D^+(B)/n_D)$ is an estimator of $\text{rTPF}(A,B)$. This logic holds true for all of the relative performance measures. Hence the empirical estimators defined in Section 3.2.1 are also valid for paired designs. The notation simplifies with paired data because subjects that receive test A are the same as those that receive test B. Thus, $n_D(A) = n_D(B) = n_D$ and $n_{\bar{D}}(A) = n_{\bar{D}}(B) = n_{\bar{D}}$. We can therefore write

$$\mathrm{r\hat{T}PF}(A, B) = n_D^+(A)/n_D^+(B),$$

$$\mathrm{r\hat{F}PF}(A, B) = n_{\bar{D}}^+(A)/n_{\bar{D}}^+(B),$$

$$\mathrm{r\hat{D}LR^+}(A, B) = \frac{n_D^+(A)n_{\bar{D}}^+(B)}{n_D^+(B)n_{\bar{D}}^+(A)},$$

$$\mathrm{r\hat{D}LR^-}(A, B) = \frac{n_D^-(A)n_{\bar{D}}^-(B)}{n_D^-(B)n_{\bar{D}}^-(A)},$$

while the notation for $\mathrm{r\hat{P}PV}(A, B)$ and $\mathrm{r\hat{N}PV}(A, B)$ remains the same.

3.3.3 Wide or long data representations

Data on two tests for n_D diseased subjects and for $n_{\bar{D}}$ non-diseased subjects can be represented in two ways. In 'wide' format, we write each subject's data as (I, D, Y_A, Y_B), where I is a subject identifier and as before D is disease status, while Y_A and Y_B are the results of tests A and B, respectively. Typically, data are in this format to produce the cross-classification of Table 3.2. In 'long' format we can write each subject's data as two data records, each represented as $(I, D, Y, X_{\mathrm{Test}})$, where the test-type identifier, X_{Test}, is equal to 1 in one record indicating that it relates to test type A, while X_{Test} is equal to 0 in the other record indicating that the record relates to test type B. Thus, when $X_{\mathrm{Test}} = 1$ the test result variable, Y, is the result of test A, $Y = Y_A$, and when $X_{\mathrm{Test}} = 0$ we have $Y = Y_B$. An illustration is provided in Table 3.4.

Table 3.4 *Wide and long data representation of some paired test data*

	Wide format				Long format		
Subject	Disease status	Result test A	Result test B	Subject	Disease status	Test result	Test type
I	D	Y_A	Y_B	I	D	Y	X_{Test}
1	1	1	1	1	1	1	1
2	1	1	0	1	1	1	0
3	0	0	0	2	1	1	1
4	0	0	1	2	1	0	0
				3	0	0	1
				3	0	0	0
				4	0	0	1
				4	0	1	0

One advantage of the 'long' data format, where subjects have records for each test type, is that it can accommodate settings where the number of tests performed varies across individuals. More importantly, it provides a general framework for statistical inference about the multiple marginal probability distributions that are of interest to us. That is, we re-emphasize that we are not interested in the performance of a combination of multiple tests. That would involve *joint* distributions of test results, $P[Y_A, Y_B, D]$. Rather, we are interested only in the performance of each test on its own, that is, in the *marginal* probabilities, $P[Y_A, D]$ and $P[Y_B, D]$, and functions of them.

With data arranged in long format, the procedures that produced the tabulations of Table 3.1 with unpaired data can be used to produce the same tabulation for paired data. The empirical estimates of comparative measures can, therefore, be calculated in the same way for both paired and unpaired data. The arrangement emphasizes that we seek to estimate the same population parameters with both paired and unpaired study designs.

3.3.4 *Large sample inference*

Distribution theory for empirical measures of relative performance must account for the within-subject correlation among tests. We assume that data from different subjects are independent. In the following result, due to Cheng and Macaluso (1997), we use TPPF to denote $P[Y_A = Y_B = 1|D = 1]$ and FPPF for $P[Y_A = Y_B = 1|D = 0]$.

Result 3.4

In large samples, $\log r\hat{\text{TPF}}(A, B)$ and $\log r\hat{\text{FPF}}(A, B)$ are independent and approximately normally distributed with

$$\text{var}(\log r\hat{\text{TPF}}(A, B)) = (n_D)^{-1}(\text{TPF}_A + \text{TPF}_B - 2\text{TPPF})/\text{TPF}_A\text{TPF}_B,$$
$$\text{var}(\log r\hat{\text{FPF}}(A, B)) = (n_{\bar{D}})^{-1}(\text{FPF}_A + \text{FPF}_B - 2\text{FPPF})/\text{FPF}_A\text{FPF}_B.$$

Using the notation of Table 3.2, these can be estimated consistently with

$$\hat{\text{var}}(\log r\hat{\text{TPF}}(A, B)) = (b + c)/(b + d)(c + d),$$
$$\hat{\text{var}}(\log r\hat{\text{FPF}}(A, B)) = (f + g)/(f + h)(g + h).$$

We note that the traditional McNemar's statistic can be used with paired data to test the null hypothesis of equality of true positives fractions $H_0: r\text{TPF}(A, B)$ = 1 and similarly to test $H_0: r\text{FPF}(A, B) = 1$ (Schatzkin *et al.*, 1987). In the notation of Table 3.2, the true positive fractions, say, are the marginal probabilities and $H_0: r\text{TPF}(A, B) = 1$ asserts that these are equal. McNemar's statistic is the standard test statistic for testing such a null hypothesis and is written as $M = (b - c)/(b + c)^{1/2}$, which is compared to a standard normal distribution. Interestingly, this test procedure is asymptotically equivalent to that based on confidence intervals for $r\text{TPF}(A, B)$ (see Exercise 5). Lachenbruch and Lynch

(1998) discuss a two degrees of freedom extension of McNemar's statistic to test the joint null hypothesis $H_0 : \mathrm{rTPF}(A, B) = 1$ and $\mathrm{rFPF}(A, B) = 1$. We reiterate, however, that we prefer procedures based on confidence intervals for $\mathrm{rTPF}(A, B)$ and $\mathrm{rFPF}(A, B)$. They are much more flexible in relation to the hypotheses that can be evaluated, as is discussed in detail in Chapter 8.

Consistency and asymptotic normality of the empirical estimators of the relative predictive value and diagnostic likelihood ratio measures also follow from the asymptotic normal approximation to the multinomial distribution of the frequencies in Table 3.2. They are, after all, simply functions of those frequencies. However, simple explicit expressions for the asymptotic variance structures have not yet been derived. In Sections 3.6.2 and 3.7.3 we discuss a straightforward method for estimating the asymptotic variances and covariances by embedding the estimation of these comparative statistics in the more general marginal regression modeling framework.

3.3.5 *Efficiency of paired versus unpaired designs*

Let us compare the efficiencies of the two designs, focusing on estimation of the $\mathrm{rTPF}(A, B)$ parameter, since similar considerations apply to $\mathrm{rFPF}(A, B)$. Consider the expression for $\mathrm{var}(\log \mathrm{r\hat{T}PF}(A, B))$ under the unpaired design with $n_D(A) = n_D(B) = n_D$. The expression given in Result 3.1 can be written as

$$\mathrm{var}(\log \mathrm{r\hat{T}PF}) = (n_D)^{-1}(\mathrm{TPF}_A + \mathrm{TPF}_B - 2\mathrm{TPF}_A\mathrm{TPF}_B)/\mathrm{TPF}_A\mathrm{TPF}_B .$$

The next result is easily derived using this expression and the corresponding one for the paired design in Result 3.4. Note that the paired and unpaired designs considered involve the same numbers of tests performed, although the numbers of subjects will be doubled when an unpaired design is employed.

Result 3.5

Suppose $n_D(A) = n_D(B) = n_D$ and let $V^{\mathrm{rTPF}}(\text{unpaired})$ and $V^{\mathrm{rTPF}}(\text{paired})$ denote $\mathrm{var}(\log \mathrm{r\hat{T}PF}(A, B))$ with unpaired and paired designs, respectively. Then

$$V^{\mathrm{rTPF}}(\text{unpaired}) - V^{\mathrm{rTPF}}(\text{paired}) = 2(n_D)^{-1}\left\{\frac{\mathrm{TPPF}}{\mathrm{TPF}_A\mathrm{TPF}_B} - 1\right\}. \qquad \blacksquare$$

Observe that when tests are conditionally independent, in the sense that $P[Y_A = 1, Y_B = 1|D] = P[Y_A = 1|D]P[Y_B = 1|D]$, then $\mathrm{TPPF} = \mathrm{TPF}_A\mathrm{TPF}_B$. In this setting the paired and unpaired designs are equally efficient.

The parameter

$$A_D(A, B) = \frac{\mathrm{TPPF}}{\mathrm{TPF}_A\mathrm{TPF}_B}$$

$\left\{\begin{array}{l} >1 \quad \textit{unpaired test is bet} \\ <1 \quad \textit{highly unlikely} \end{array}\right.$

can be interpreted as a measure of agreement or association between tests in diseased subjects. Indeed, since

$$A_D(A, B) = \frac{P[Y_A = 1, Y_B = 1|D = 1]}{P[Y_A = 1|D = 1]\, P[Y_B = 1|D = 1]}$$

$$= \frac{P[Y_B = 1 | Y_A = 1, D = 1]}{P[Y_B = 1 | D = 1]}$$

$$= \frac{P[Y_A = 1 | Y_B = 1, D = 1]}{P[Y_A = 1 | D = 1]},$$

it can be interpreted as the relative risk of a positive result with one test that is conferred by knowledge of a positive result from the other test.

We define a positive association between tests as one for which $A_D(A, B) > 1$. Positive associations are most common in practice. Clearly the paired design is more efficient for estimating $rTPF(A, B)$ than the unpaired design when $A_D(A, B) > 1$. With an obvious change of notation, paired designs are also more efficient for estimating $rFPF(A, B)$ when $A_{\bar{D}}(A, B) > 1$, where we define

$$A_{\bar{D}}(A, B) = \frac{FPPF}{FPF_A FPF_B}$$

$$= \frac{P[Y_A = 1, Y_B = 1 | D = 0]}{P[Y_A = 1 | D = 0] P[Y_B = 1 | D = 0]}$$

$$= \frac{P[Y_B = 1 | Y_A = 1, D = 0]}{P[Y_B = 1 | D = 0]}$$

$$= \frac{P[Y_A = 1 | Y_B = 1, D = 0]}{P[Y_A = 1 | D = 0]}.$$

3.3.6 Small sample properties

Tables 3.5 and 3.6 below show the results of some simulation studies to assess if inference based on large sample distribution theory is valid in small samples. See Cheng *et al.* (2000) for related results. We only show results for inference about classification probabilities because inference from paired data is not as well developed for predictive values and DLRs. Confidence interval coverage appears to be reasonably close to the nominal level for the configurations shown. The only point of concern is that confidence intervals cannot be calculated when the numerator or denominator of the estimate is 0 or 1. Thus, in Table 3.6, confidence intervals could not be calculated in up to 12% of the simulations when $n_{\bar{D}} = 50$ and $FPF_B = 0.05$. Obuchowski and Zhou (2002) suggest the rule of thumb that expected frequencies should be at least 5 in order to rely on large sample inference procedures. Our simulations suggest that for inference about rFPF or rTPF this rule of thumb is appropriate. When the expected numbers of false positives and false negatives are at least 5 for each test, large sample inference procedures are applicable in small samples.

3.3.7 The CASS study

We illustrate the methodology for paired data with a comparison of the exercise stress test (EST) and the chest pain history test (CPH) for diagnosing coronary artery disease (CAD), as measured in the CASS study. Refer back to Section 1.3.2 for a brief description of this study.

Table 3.5 *Coverage of 90% confidence intervals for* $\mathrm{rTPF}(A,B)$. *Results are based on 1000 simulations for each configuration. Shown are results for unpaired data* $(\mathcal{A}_D = 1)$ *as well as for paired data with maximum positive* $(\mathcal{A}_D > 1)$ *and negative* $(\mathcal{A}_D < 1)$ *correlation that is consistent with the marginal probabilities*

			Coverage (%) Number diseased (n_D)		
TPF(B)	rTPF(A,B)	$\mathcal{A}_D(A,B)$	25	50	100
0.5	1.2	1.00	90.1	89.7	91.2
0.5	1.2	0.33	91.3	89.6	90.7
0.5	1.2	1.67	88.2	88.9	89.8
0.5	1.5	1.00	91.0	91.0	90.0
0.5	1.5	0.67	90.5	89.4	89.1
0.5	1.5	1.33	89.4	89.6	89.8
0.5	1.9	1.00	86.3	89.7	89.0
0.5	1.9	0.95	91.0	89.6	89.1
0.5	1.9	1.05	88.5	90.4	90.8
0.7	1.2	1.00	90.5	90.0	89.8
0.7	1.2	1.00	89.6	90.1	89.9
0.7	1.2	0.92	88.3	89.8	89.3
0.7	1.4	1.00	86.8	89.4	90.4
0.7	1.4	1.14	92.5	88.6	89.5
0.7	1.4	1.00	87.8	89.5	89.8

Table 3.6 *Coverage of 90% confidence intervals for* $\mathrm{rFPF}(A,B)$. *Results are based on 1000 simulations for each configuration. Shown are results for unpaired data* $(\mathcal{A}_{\bar{D}} = 1)$ *as well as for paired data with maximum positive* $(\mathcal{A}_{\bar{D}} > 1)$ *and negative* $(\mathcal{A}_{\bar{D}} < 1)$ *correlation. In parentheses are the proportions of simulations that yielded 0 in the denominator of* $\mathrm{rFPF}(A,B)$

			Coverage (%) Number of subjects ($n_{\bar{D}}$)		
FPF(B)	rFPF(A,B)	$\mathcal{A}_{\bar{D}}(A,B)$	50	100	200
0.05	1.2	1.00	86.4 (8%)	91.2	90.7
0.05	1.2	0.00	86.5 (12%)	92.3	89.8
0.05	1.2	8.00	82.1 (10%)	89.5	90.6
0.05	1.9	1.00	87.4 (7%)	92.3	91.7
0.05	1.9	0.00	90.1 (7%)	91.8	91.7
0.05	1.9	8.00	81.6 (8%)	88.8	89.8
0.10	1.2	1.00	92.7	91.7	90.9
0.10	1.2	0.00	91.9	91.7	90.9
0.10	1.2	4.00	91.5	92.8	91.1
0.10	1.9	1.00	91.3	89.4	90.3
0.10	1.9	0.00	91.8	91.1	91.6
0.10	1.9	4.00	86.9	89.8	89.6

Example 3.2

Table 3.7(a) displays the data in the paired data format of Table 3.2, while Table 3.7(b) displays the same data in the format of Table 3.1 which ignores the pairing. The accuracy measures are calculated using the margins of Table 3.7(a) or directly, as for unpaired data, from the rows of Table 3.7(b).

We calculate $r\hat{T}PF(CPH, EST) = 1.19$ with 95% confidence interval (1.15, 1.23). Thus CPH appears to detect almost 20% more diseased subjects than EST. With 95% confidence the relative true positive fraction, $rTPF(CPH, EST)$, is at least 115%. On the other hand, the $r\hat{F}PF(CPH, EST) = 2.13$ with 95% confidence interval (1.79, 2.54). At least 1.8 times as many non-diseased subjects test positive with CPH as do so with EST, and the number could be as high as 2.5. As a joint statement we can say that with 90% confidence the $rFPF(CPH, EST)$ lies in $(1.79, 2.54)$ and the $rTPF(CPH, EST)$ lies in $(1.15, 1.23)$. The CPH test is clearly superior in the TPF dimension but clearly inferior in the FPF dimension. Equivalence in either dimension appears to be ruled out. It may be that the criteria for classifying a positive CPH test are too relaxed. One possibility might be to make the criteria more stringent, in order to reduce the false positive fraction and make it more in line with that of the EST test. More stringent criteria, however, will also be likely to reduce the true positive fraction relative to the EST test.

The paired design yields confidence intervals that are sufficiently narrow so as to make strong conclusions about the relative accuracies of the CPH versus EST tests in both the TPF and FPF dimensions. Let us anticipate the widths of the confidence intervals had an unpaired design been used, with the same total number of tests and therefore twice the number of subjects. The confidence intervals calculated using the formulae for unpaired data are $(1.15, 1.23)$ for the $rTPF(CPH, EST)$ and $(1.78, 2.55)$ for the $rFPF(CPH, EST)$. The confidence intervals are in fact changed very little, being only slightly wider with the unpaired design and thus suggesting that there is no gain in statistical efficiency by using a paired versus unpaired study design. Interestingly, the association

Table 3.7 *Data from the CASS study in the (a) paired data and (b) unpaired data formats*

(a)

	Diseased			Non-diseased		
	CPH = 0	CPH = 1		CPH = 0	CPH = 1	
EST = 0	25	183	208	151	176	327
EST = 1	29	786	815	46	69	115
	54	969	1023	197	245	442

(b)

	Diseased			Non-diseased		
	Y = 0	Y = 1		Y = 0	Y = 1	
CPH	54	969	1023	197	245	442
EST	208	815	1023	327	115	442

parameters $\mathcal{A}_D(\text{CPH}, \text{EST}) = 1.02$ and $\mathcal{A}_{\bar{D}}(\text{CPH}, \text{EST}) = 1.08$ are both close to 1, indicating that these tests are nearly conditionally independent. Note that the paired design has the advantage of including half the number of subjects that the unpaired design employs.

The CASS study was a cohort study, so that estimation of predictive values and their comparative statistics is possible. We calculate $r\hat{\text{PPV}}(\text{CPH}, \text{EST}) = 0.91$ and $r\hat{\text{NPV}}(\text{CPH}, \text{EST}) = 1.28$, suggesting that the CPH test has a lower positive predictive value but a higher negative predictive value than the EST test. Methods for calculating confidence intervals have not yet been described, but will be later in this chapter. We refer to Section 3.6.2. The 95% confidence intervals are $(0.89, 0.94)$ for $r\text{PPV}(\text{CPH}, \text{EST})$ and $(1.19, 1.39)$ for $r\text{NPV}(\text{CPH}, \text{EST})$. Again, the CPH test appears to perform better than the EST on one dimension but worse than the EST on the other. Given the results pertaining to the classification probabilities, this is to be expected for the predictive value measures (Result 2.9). ■

3.4   The regression modeling framework

We now turn to regression analysis methods for evaluating medical tests. As with other areas of biostatistics, regression modeling allows one to address a broad range of research questions. Moreover, it provides a richer, more sophisticated approach to the comparative analysis of tests. In this section we provide some general background on the importance of regression analysis in this setting.

3.4.1   *Factors potentially affecting test performance*

Regression analysis can be used to identify factors that influence the performance of a test. It is important to understand such factors in order to determine optimal and suboptimal conditions or populations for test performance. Insights can lead to modifications of a test to improve its performance. Alternatively, if we find that a factor does not influence test performance, we may be able to relax the conditions under which the test is performed.

Much of the applied literature on medical testing assumes that test performance is a constant entity. Begg (1987) and Kraemer (1992), amongst others, have lamented this state of affairs. It should be recognized that many factors can affect test performance. Table 3.8 lists some broad categories and examples.

Let us consider some specific examples of factors relating to the tested subject that can affect the test result. Firstly, the ability of mammography to detect breast cancer depends on the woman's age. Younger women have denser breast tissue which renders the mammogram more difficult to interpret. Secondly, in evaluating the exercise stress test, sex should be considered as a potential covariate because women and men differ in their abilities to perform physical exercise. Finally, the baby's health or neurologic condition could influence its ability to respond to an audiology test. The characteristics of study subjects must therefore be carefully considered when interpreting the performance of a test. A test that performs well in one population may not perform well in another.

Table 3.8 *Some factors that can affect test performance*

Factor	Examples
Subject or test unit	Age, gender
Tester	Experience, expertise
Test	Protocol, operating conditions
Environment	Location, health care resources
Disease manifestations	Severity, histology
Non-disease state	Normal or other abnormal condition

Most tests require an operator or tester to perform the test. Characteristics of the tester can affect test performance. For example, the expertise of persons performing the test can affect test results. A well-trained audiologist, experienced in the use of test equipment, will perform a more accurate and successful test than a poorly-trained inexperienced tester. The expertise of the radiologist in interpreting images has a great bearing on the success of an imaging test. Similar considerations pertain to pathologists reading histologic slides.

Variations on how the test is performed are also important covariates to be considered. The stimulus levels used for an audiology test can affect the test result. The method used for collecting, processing or storing a biological specimen can affect the result of a biomarker assay. The physical environment in which a test is performed should be considered in audiology, where ambient room noise plays a role, and in bacterial culture testing, where contamination in the clinic or laboratory is a concern. Non-physical environmental factors can also affect the test result. These include the availability of health care resources and disease prevalence, both of which can influence criteria for classifying a test result as positive. Positivity criteria may be more stringent in environments with less resources and/or higher disease prevalences.

Characteristics of disease will often affect the performance of the test. Typically, the more advanced or severe the disease, the easier it is to detect. It is surprising that this 'covariate' is so frequently ignored in practice. Other features of the disease can also influence ease of detection. These could include histology and grade in cancer detection and bacterial subtype in infectious disease testing. Non-diseased subjects can also be heterogeneous. Subjects who are hospitalized or attending the same medical clinic as the cases may have conditions that lead to false positive results. In prostate cancer research, for example, subjects with benign prostate tissue growth tend to have high PSA levels and hence will have a higher probability of false positive results than controls with normal prostate gland tissue. The influence of these characteristics should be investigated when evaluating the false positive fractions associated with a test.

3.4.2 *Questions addressed by regression modeling*

We have alluded to the need for evaluating factors that affect the performance of a diagnostic test. The simultaneous evaluation of multiple factors and interactions between factors can be accomplished through regression modeling.

We can also compare medical tests within the regression modeling framework. An advantage of using regression models for comparing tests is that the analysis can control for concomitant factors. In observational studies, this reduces the potential for confounding. Even in experimental studies, regression modeling can increase the precision with which relative accuracy is estimated. More complex questions can be addressed, such as whether or not relative accuracy varies with covariates. One test may perform better than another but only in certain settings, for example.

Finally, it may be of interest to determine the incremental value of a test over other information already available. For example, in the presence of information about clinical symptoms, is a bacterial culture test informative? When multiple tests are performed, does one test detect disease that is not already detected by another? These questions are also addressed within the general regression framework.

3.4.3 *Notation and general set-up*

We use Z to denote the covariate or set of covariates of interest. In addition, we let $X(Z)$ denote the specific numerical variables included in the regression model, i.e. $X(Z)$ is the coding chosen for quantifying the effect of the Z. We call $X(Z)$ the covariables that code for the covariate Z. For example, if Z denotes the covariate sex, then the statistical model might include a covariable $X(Z)$ coded as 0 for males and 1 for females. If Z denotes study site, of which there are 3, say, we could define $X(Z) = (X_1(Z), X_2(Z))$, where the dummy variable $X_i(Z) = 1$ for site i. If the covariate Z is age, $X(Z)$ might be an ordinal variable, where $X(Z) = k$ if the subject's age is in the kth interval, or $X(Z)$ might be age measured in years. We find it useful to distinguish between the entity Z and the manner in which we choose to code it in the regression model, $X(Z)$. To reduce notation we write X instead of $X(Z)$, with the understanding that by definition the covariables, X, are numerical functions of Z.

We assume that the data are arranged in 'long' form. That is, an observation consists of (I, D, Y, Z), where I is a subject identifier. There may be multiple observations for a subject, one observation for each test result. If only one test is under consideration, multiple observations can arise if a subject is tested at multiple sites (e.g. each of two ears) or at multiple times (e.g. annual screening for cervical cancer). If multiple tests are under consideration, there will be one observation for each test type and the covariables will include a component that indicates to which test type Y corresponds (see Section 3.3.3).

3.5   Regression for true and false positive fractions

First we consider regression models for classification probabilities. Key references are Coughlin *et al.* (1992), Diamond (1992), Smith and Hadgu (1992), Leisenring *et al.* (1997) and Sternberg and Hadgu (2001). We begin with a description of the general methodology and then provide illustrations on data that demonstrate how the methodology can address a variety of research questions.

3.5.1   *Binary marginal GLM models*

To model the true and false positive fractions, $\text{TPF}(Z) = \text{P}[Y = 1|D = 1, Z]$ and $\text{FPF}(Z) = \text{P}[Y = 1|D = 0, Z]$, a generalized linear model for binary outcomes can be used. Separate models for TPF and FPF can be employed:

$$g_D(\text{TPF}(Z_D)) = \beta_D X_D\,,$$
$$g_{\bar{D}}(\text{FPF}(Z_{\bar{D}})) = \beta_{\bar{D}} X_{\bar{D}}\,,$$

where the subscripts D and $\bar{D}$ denote components specific to the models for observations associated with diseased and non-diseased subjects, respectively. We write separate models since the populations to which they relate are different. Note that the modeled covariates Z_D and $Z_{\bar{D}}$ and link functions g_D and $g_{\bar{D}}$ may be different in the two models. Nevertheless, if the link functions are the same, and we drop the subscripts, a single model form can be written by including interactions with disease status:

$$g\left(\text{P}[Y = 1|D, Z_D \text{ or } Z_{\bar{D}}]\right) = \beta_{\bar{D}} X_{\bar{D}} I[D = 0] + \beta_D X_D I[D = 1]\,,$$

where $I[\cdot]$ denotes the indicator function.

Related models for ordinal-valued tests have been developed by Tosteson and Begg (1988) and Toledano and Gatsonis (1995). If covariate effects are equal for some common elements of $X_{\bar{D}}$ and X_D, a simpler, more parsimonious model may result.

Popular choices for link functions are the logit link, $g(t) = \log(t/(1 - t))$ and the probit link, $g(t) = \Phi^{-1}(t)$, where Φ denotes the standard normal cumulative distribution function. Another choice is the log link, $g(t) = \log t$. This link function has the disadvantage that fitted probabilities may exceed 1.0 (although our experience is that this rarely happens within the range of the observed data). The advantage of the log link is that the interpretation of model parameters is in terms of relative true and false positive fractions. For example, if $X_D = (1, X)$ and $\beta_D = (\beta_{0D}, \beta_{1D})$, the TPF model is $\log \text{TPF} = \beta_{0D} + \beta_{1D}X$. We see that $\exp \beta_{1D}$ is interpreted as the ratio of the TPF at covariable level X to the TPF at level $X - 1$. With the logit link, the interpretation is in terms of odds ratios, which are less appealing. With the probit link, the interpretation is even more obscure.

3.5.2   *Fitting marginal models to data*

The above models for the classification probabilities, TPF and FPF, are marginal generalized linear models (Liang and Zeger, 1986). Observe that the modeled probabilities, $P[Y = 1|D, Z]$, are marginal probabilities in the sense that they relate to single observations (Y, D, Z) from the population of observations. Even if subjects contribute multiple observations to the analysis, we have noted that their joint probabilities are not of interest here. Implicitly, we assume that sampling of data is such that observations are randomly sampled from the populations of diseased and non-diseased observations, conditional on covariates.

This allows us to make inferences about $P[Y = 1|D, Z]$ from the data collected. However, observations do not need to be statistically independent. Indeed, they will usually not be independent when subjects contribute multiple observations to the analysis. Recall that the paired data setting of Section 3.3 is one setting where this arises and we discussed sources and implications of correlations. Now note that those discussions are also relevant for the broader context of clustered data, where subjects provide observations at multiple sites, at multiple time points or under multiple conditions.

Assuming that, conditional on disease status and covariates, observations are sampled at random from the population, generalized estimating equations can be used to fit the models. This is a standard technique and we refer to Liang and Zeger (1986) for details. In all of our applications we use independence working covariance matrices in the estimating equations, although other forms may provide greater statistical efficiency. See Pepe and Anderson (1994) for some cautionary advice about choosing non-independence working covariance matrices.

If the TPF and FPF models are distinct, they can be fitted separately to the sets of observations from diseased and non-diseased subjects, assuming statistical independence between them. Fitting the models together requires a little more attention to the details of defining covariables, particularly when there are covariates that are not common to the TPF and FPF components. Consider the following simple illustration.

Example 3.3

It is thought that age might affect the chances of a positive test result in diseased and non-diseased subjects. In addition, more severe disease is easier to detect with the test. The covariate age enters into the models for both the FPF and TPF, while disease severity is relevant only to the TPF. The models to be fitted are

$$\log \mathrm{TPF(age, severity)} = \beta_{0D} + \beta_{1D}X_{\mathrm{age}} + \beta_{2D}X_{\mathrm{sev}}$$

and

$$\log \mathrm{FPF(age)} = \beta_{0\bar{D}} + \beta_{1\bar{D}}X_{\mathrm{age}},$$

where X_{age} = age in years and X_{sev} = a numerical measure of disease severity (that is meaningless when $D = 0$). Define $X_1 = X_{\mathrm{age}} \times (1 - D)$, $X_2 = X_{\mathrm{age}} \times D$ and $X_3 = X_{\mathrm{sev}} \times D$. Fitting the following composite model simultaneously gives estimates of the parameters in both the TPF and FPF models:

$$\log P[Y = 1|D, \mathrm{age, severity}] = \beta_{0\bar{D}} + \alpha D + \beta_{1\bar{D}}X_1 + \beta_{1D}X_2 + \beta_{2D}X_3,$$

where $\alpha = \beta_{0D} - \beta_{0\bar{D}}$.   ∎

An advantage of fitting a composite model to the combined data, rather than separately fitting the TPF model to diseased observations and the FPF model to non-diseased observations, is that one can test if covariates that are common to both models have the same effects in the TPF and FPF models. If so, a reduced model that requires estimation of fewer parameters can result. With fewer parameters to be estimated, they are likely to be estimated with greater precision. In the example above, one could determine if $\alpha = 0$. If so, the number of parameters to be estimated in the reduced composite model is one less than the number to be estimated when the TPF and FPF models are fitted separately.

3.5.3   Illustration: factors affecting test accuracy

Example 3.4

Consider test A in the neonatal audiology study described in Section 1.3.7. Its performance might be affected by the gestational age of the child and by the location in which the test is performed. For hearing-impaired individuals, their degree of hearing impairment might affect the chances of a response to the hearing test. Consider the covariables

$$X_{\text{age}} = \text{age (weeks)} - 35\,,$$
$$X_{\text{loc}} = I[\text{the test is performed in a sound booth}]\,,$$
$$X_{\text{sev}} = (\text{hearing threshold (dB)} - 30)/10$$

and the models

$$\log \text{TPF}(\text{age}, \text{location}, \text{severity}) = \beta_1 + \beta_2 X_{\text{age}} + \beta_3 X_{\text{loc}} + \beta_4 X_{\text{sev}}\,,$$
$$\log \text{FPF}(\text{age}, \text{location}) = \alpha_1 + \alpha_2 X_{\text{age}} + \alpha_3 X_{\text{loc}}\,.$$

Observe that interpretations for model parameters are in terms of relative positive fractions (rFPF, rTPF), because the log link function is used. The estimated parameter values are displayed in Table 3.9. Both test location and degree of hearing impairment affect the capacity of the test to detect hearing-impaired ears. The TPF in a sound booth is 1.19 times that of the test conducted in a standard room, with a 95% confidence interval for the rTPF of $(1.04, 1.37)$. In addition, the TPF increases by a multiplicative factor of 1.07 for each 10 dB increase in the severity of hearing impairment.

The gestational age of the child does not appear to affect the likelihood of a positive response to the test, either for hearing-impaired ears $(p = 0.77)$ or for normally-hearing ears $(p = 0.50)$. Although location does not have a statistically significant impact on the FPF, there is a suggestion that the FPF is increased in a sound booth.

We fitted a reduced model that excludes age and calculated the fitted true and false positive fractions displayed in Table 3.10. This table of setting specific (FPF, TPF) values might be the final data summary of most interest to audiology researchers.   ∎

Table 3.9 *Regression analysis of TPF and FPF for audiology test A*

Factor	Parameter	Estimate	p value	Relative fraction	95% CI
Constant	β_1	−0.548	–	–	–
Age (weeks)	β_2	−0.002	0.77	1.00	$(0.98, 1.01)$
Location (booth vs room)	β_3	0.176	0.01	1.19	$(1.04, 1.37)$
Severity (per 10 dB)	β_4	0.070	0.01	1.07	$(1.02, 1.13)$
Constant	α_1	−1.01	–	–	–
Age (weeks)	α_2	0.007	0.50	1.01	$(0.99, 1.03)$
Location (booth vs room)	α_3	0.170	0.12	1.18	$(0.96, 1.46)$

Table 3.10 *Fitted TPF and FPF values, with 90% confidence intervals in parentheses*

Location	Severity	TPF	FPF
Room	30 dB	0.58 $(0.52, 0.64)$	0.37 $(0.32, 0.42)$
Room	40 dB	0.62 $(0.57, 0.68)$	0.37 $(0.32, 0.42)$
Room	50 dB	0.67 $(0.60, 0.74)$	0.37 $(0.32, 0.42)$
Booth	30 dB	0.69 $(0.63, 0.75)$	0.43 $(0.38, 0.49)$
Booth	40 dB	0.74 $(0.69, 0.79)$	0.43 $(0.38, 0.49)$
Booth	50 dB	0.79 $(0.73, 0.85)$	0.43 $(0.38, 0.49)$

This dataset illustrates a few points about model formulation and fitting. First, the test unit in this example is not a study subject, but rather an ear. That is, each observation (I, D, Y, Z) pertains to the test performed on an ear. The models, therefore, also pertain to test performance on hearing-impaired ears (TPF) and normally-hearing ears (FPF) rather than on study subjects. Performance on a per ear basis is sought in audiology research. However, in other research areas, where subjects are tested at multiple sites, measures of overall test performance in terms of the individual rather than the specific test unit are sought. Such is the case in breast cancer research, for example. In such settings the overall test result would need to be defined as an appropriate composite of results at multiple sites. In breast cancer, a positive mammogram in either breast would be regarded as a screen positive result for the individual. Second, subjects contribute observations for each ear tested. Some subjects contribute observations to both the TPF and the FPF analyses. Therefore the models should be fitted simultaneously in order that the standard errors, calculated with the 'robust' sandwich variance–covariance matrix, properly account for all the clustering of observations in the data.

3.5.4 *Comparing tests with regression analysis*

Suppose that there are two types of tests, labeled A and B, that are applied to individuals. Associated with each test result Y we define the covariate 'Test', which is the test type to which Y corresponds (see Section 3.3.3). Define the covariable

$$X_{\text{Test}} = \begin{cases} 1 & \text{for test A}; \\ 0 & \text{for test B}, \end{cases}$$

and consider the regression models

$$\log \text{TPF(Test)} = \beta_0 + \beta_1 X_{\text{Test}},$$
$$\log \text{FPF(Test)} = \alpha_0 + \alpha_1 X_{\text{Test}}.$$

Observe that

$$\text{TPF}_B = e^{\beta_0}, \quad \text{TPF}_A = e^{\beta_0 + \beta_1}, \quad \text{rTPF}(A, B) = e^{\beta_1},$$
$$\text{FPF}_B = e^{\alpha_0}, \quad \text{FPF}_A = e^{\alpha_0 + \alpha_1}, \quad \text{rFPF}(A, B) = e^{\alpha_1}.$$

In particular, we can use the regression modeling framework to estimate $\text{rTPF}(A, B)$ and $\text{rFPF}(A, B)$. The estimators from this approach are exactly the same empirical estimators described in Sections 3.2 and 3.3. The confidence intervals are not precisely the same in small samples but are asymptotically equivalent.

Example 3.5

Fitting the above models to the CASS data yielded the following estimates and univariate 95% confidence intervals:

$$\text{r}\widehat{\text{TPF}}(\text{CPH}, \text{EST}) = 1.19 \quad (1.15, 1.23),$$
$$\text{r}\widehat{\text{FPF}}(\text{CPH}, \text{EST}) = 2.13 \quad (1.79, 2.54).$$

These are precisely the same as those calculated using the paired data methodology of Section 3.3.7.   ∎

One attractive feature of using the regression methodology is that there is a great deal of flexibility in the types of data structures that can be accommodated. Data can be unpaired, paired or subjects can even have variable numbers of tests performed. As in the neonatal audiology study, subjects can simultaneously contribute to both the rTPF and rFPF calculations, and correlations between their observations will be properly accounted for.

With paired data, we noted previously that McNemar's test can be used to test for equality of true positive fractions (or of false positive fractions). Leisenring *et al.* (1997) shows that the generalized score test for $H_0 : \beta_1 = 0$ from fitting the rTPF(Test) model with a single binary covariate to paired data is, in fact, equal to McNemar's test. Therefore, one can think of this score test as a generalization of McNemar's test that accommodates variable numbers of tests among study subjects.

Example 3.6

Consider a comparison of tests A and B from the neonatal audiology study. The raw data are shown in Table 3.11. Note that, due to incomplete testing, the simple cross-classification of the two tests is restricted only to the subsets of ears for which both tests were performed.

Test A detects more hearing-impaired ears than test B, the rTPF from Table 3.11 being 1.11 with 95% confidence interval $(1.03, 1.21)$ using the regression model framework with the log link function and the binary covariate X_{Test}. Although not statistically significant $(p = 0.15)$, the tests also appear to differ in their FPFs, with test A having the higher value, $rFPF(A, B) = 1.09$ (95% confidence interval $(0.97, 1.22)$). There is no clear conclusion about which test is better based on this simple analysis.

We saw earlier that the location in which the test is performed and the degree of hearing impairment both influence the classification probabilities for test A. We next performed a more in depth analysis by fitting regression models that incorporated these covariates into the comparison of the tests. Results are shown in Table 3.12.

Consider Table 3.12(a). The test × location parameter quantifies the ratio

$$\frac{rTPF(A, B) \text{ in a booth}}{rTPF(A, B) \text{ in a room}}, \qquad (3.10)$$

which is estimated at 1.20 (95% CI $(1.01, 1.42)$). This indicates that the relative performance of test A to test B for detecting disease is substantially higher in a sound booth than in a room. When conducted in a hospital room the tests detect similar numbers of ears with hearing impairment. The $rTPF(A, B)$ in a room $= 1.03$ (95% CI $(0.89, 1.18)$), while in a booth the $rTPF(A, B)$ is increased to $1.20 \times 1.03 = 1.24$.

The degree of hearing impairment has an impact on the ability of both tests to detect impairment. The impact is similar on both tests, as indicated by the

Table 3.11 *Results of tests A and B from the neonatal audiology study. (a) Data using the unpaired marginal data representation. (b) The cross-classification of test results which is restricted to ears for which both test results are available*

		Hearing-impaired ears		Normally-hearing ears	
(a)		Negative	Positive	Negative	Positive
	Test B	159	251	407	236
	Test A	129	277	380	253

		Test B		Test B	
(b)		Negative	Positive	Negative	Positive
Test A	Negative	72	33	228	55
	Positive	48	166	87	111

Table 3.12 *Regression model fit to neonatal audiology data for tests A and B using (a) the model for TPF and (b) the model for FPF*

(a)

Covariate	Estimate	Relative positive fraction	95% CI
Constant	−0.575	–	–
Test (A vs B)	0.028	1.03	$(0.89, 1.18)$
Location (booth vs room)	−0.009	0.99	$(0.85, 1.16)$
Severity (per 10 dB)	0.094	1.10	$(1.03, 1.17)$
Test × location	0.182	1.20	$(1.01, 1.42)$
Test × severity	−0.025	0.97	$(0.91, 1.05)$

(b)

Covariate	Estimate	Relative positive fraction	95% CI
Constant	−0.981	–	–
Test (A vs B)	−0.018	0.98	$(0.82, 1.17)$
Location (booth vs room)	−0.044	0.96	$(0.77, 1.19)$
Test × location	0.204	1.22	$(0.97, 1.55)$

test × severity parameter. The TPF of test B increases by a multiplicative factor of 1.10 for each 10 dB increase in hearing loss, while the TPF of test A increases by 0.97 of that amount, i.e. by 1.07.

Table 3.12(b) suggests that location influences the rFPFs of the tests. The interaction between test type and location indicates that

$$\frac{\text{rFPF}(A, B) \text{ in a booth}}{\text{rFPF}(A, B) \text{ in a room}} = 1.22, \tag{3.11}$$

although the confidence interval does contain the null value of 1.0. The disparity between the tests is greater in a sound booth. Closer examination of Table 3.12 indicates that location only appears to influence the FPF of test A and not that of test B. We see that $\text{FPF}_B(\text{booth})/\text{FPF}_B(\text{room}) = 0.96$, while $\text{FPF}_A(\text{booth})/\text{FPF}_A(\text{room}) = 1.22 \times 0.96 \times 0.98/0.98 = 1.17$. Indeed, when comparing the tests performed in a hospital room, their false positive fractions are essentially equal, $\text{rFPF}(A, B)$ in a room $= 0.98$. In a sound booth the $\text{rFPF}(A, B)$ is estimated to be $1.22 \times 0.98 = 1.20$.

The overall conclusion then is that the two tests have essentially equal performance when conducted in a hospital room. Either test might be chosen for use in facilities that do not have sound booths. For facilities that do have sound booths, test A will detect a greater number of hearing-impaired ears, but at the expense of falsely classifying a larger number of normal-hearing ears than will test B.   ■

The important methodological point to glean from this illustration is that one should explore how covariates affect test performance and if the relative performance of several tests differs with covariates. Our initial analysis that ignored test location found that overall test A has higher true and false positive fractions. The regression analysis clarified that the disparity only occurs when tests are performed in sound booths and that the relative performance is similar across all levels of hearing impairment.

3.6   Regression modeling of predictive values

3.6.1   *Model formulation and fitting*

Covariate effects on predictive values can also be modeled with marginal probability generalized linear models. Consider the model

$$g(\mathrm{P}[D=1|Y,Z]) = \alpha_0 + \alpha_1 Y + \alpha_2 X + \alpha_3 YX, \qquad (3.12)$$

where $X = X(Z)$ are the covariables coding the covariates Z.

Covariates that affect either disease prevalence or test performance can affect predictive values. Interpretations of covariate effects are therefore a little more complex here than they are for classification probability models. Moreover, covariates specific to diseased or non-diseased states cannot be included in models for predictive values.

As is well known in epidemiologic risk assessment, the link function, g, must be of logistic form if a case-control study design is used. This ensures that the parameters quantifying covariate effects will be valid, although the fitted predictive values will not be. With cohort designs there is more flexibility in the link functions that can be employed. A log link function yields interpretations in terms of relative predictive values.

Generalized estimating equations can be used to fit models with data in 'long' form. We note, however, that there are some important differences with standard GEE methods for correlated data, as originally described by Liang and Zeger (1986). First, in the original formulation of GEE, the outcome variable varies across observations from an individual and the modeled probabilities are conditional on the entire set of predictors from an individual. In contrast, we see that the outcome variable in the predictive value models, D, is typically constant across observations from an individual (or at least across those from a test unit). It is the predictors, including Y, that vary from observation to observation from a subject. Pepe *et al.* (1999) call these models *marginal with respect to covariates*.

Second, an independence working covariance matrix is generally required. This is because the Pepe–Anderson condition that is required for consistent parameter estimation when non-diagonal matrices are used (Pepe and Anderson, 1994; Pan and Louis, 2000) is likely to fail. In particular, let (I, D, Y, Z) and (I, D, Y^*, Z^*) denote two observations for individual I. The Pepe–Anderson condition in our setting is that

$$\mathrm{P}[D=1|Y,Z,Y^*,Z^*] = \mathrm{P}[D=1|Y,Z]. \qquad (3.13)$$

This will rarely hold. For example, if Y and Y^* are results of two different tests, Y^* is likely to be informative about D even in the presence of knowledge about Y.

3.6.2 Comparing tests

Similar to Section 3.5.4, by defining a covariate 'Test' that indicates test type, A or B, we can use the regression framework to compare the PPV of two tests and to compare their NPVs. To set the analysis of PPVs and NPVs in the same model we need to define a model for agreement between D and Y rather than simply a model for the probability of disease (3.12). The agreement model is

$$\log P[D = Y|Y, \text{Test}] = \alpha_0 + \alpha_1 Y + \alpha_2 X_{\text{Test}} + \alpha_3 Y X_{\text{Test}}, \qquad (3.14)$$

where X_{Test} is the binary covariable indicating test type. Observe that $\text{rPPV}(A, B) = e^{\alpha_2 + \alpha_3}$ and $\text{rNPV}(A, B) = e^{\alpha_2}$.

Fitting this model to data with GEE yields the empirical values as estimates of the relative predictive values. These are the same as the estimates of Sections 3.2 and 3.3. An advantage of the regression framework is that it provides standard errors for estimates of α_2 and $\alpha_2 + \alpha_3$. Hence it yields confidence intervals for $\text{rPPV}(A, B)$ and $\text{rNPV}(A, B)$. We noted earlier that simple explicit expressions for asymptotic variances of $\log \text{r}\hat{\text{P}}\text{PV}(A, B)$ and $\log \text{r}\hat{\text{N}}\text{PV}(A, B)$ have not yet been derived. Thus the regression framework offers an elegant solution to confidence interval calculation. The analysis of the CASS data (Section 3.3.7) provided confidence intervals for $\text{rPPV}(\text{CPH}, \text{EST})$ and $\text{rNPV}(\text{CPH}, \text{EST})$ that were calculated using this regression modeling framework.

Leisenring et al. (2000) developed a test statistic for testing the null hypothesis $H_0 : \text{PPV}_A = \text{PPV}_B$. It is the generalized score test for $\alpha_1 = 0$ in the regression model

$$g(\text{P}[D = 1|Y = 1, \text{Test}]) = \alpha_0 + \alpha_1 X_{\text{Test}}, \qquad (3.15)$$

fitted with GEE under an independence working correlation matrix. Observe that this model is fitted using all observations for which the test result is positive. With a paired design each subject contributes either 1, 2 or 0 observations to the analysis. The resultant generalized score test statistic does not depend on the link function chosen, and indeed it is proportional to $\hat{\text{P}}\text{PV}_A - \hat{\text{P}}\text{PV}_B$. This test statistic was compared with the Wald test for $H_0 : \alpha_1 = 0$, which is equivalent to a test based on the confidence interval for $\text{rPPV}(A, B)$ containing the null value of 1.0. Although the Wald and generalized score tests are asymptotically equivalent, small sample properties of the generalized score statistic were found to be better (Leisenring et al., 2000).

3.6.3 The incremental value of a test for prediction

Regression models provide a convenient framework for evaluating the incremental predictive value of a test beyond information contained in other sources. For example, suppose that the result of a simple test, denoted by Y_A, is available and that another test Y_B can be performed in addition. One can quantify the additional information provided by the second test as $\text{P}[D = 1|Y_A = 1, Y_B]$ compared with $\text{P}[D = 1|Y_A = 1]$. One can also compare $\text{P}[D = 1|Y_A = 0, Y_B]$

with $P[D = 1|Y_A = 0]$. For example, by comparing $P[D = 1|Y_A = 1, Y_B]$ with $P[D = 1|Y_A = 1]$, we determine, amongst subjects testing positive with Y_A, if Y_B provides additional predictive information.

To do this we consider a composite model that simultaneously models $P[D = 1|Y_A = 1]$ and $P[D = 1|Y_A = 1, Y_B]$. Two data records are constructed for each observation (D, Y_A, Y_B) from subjects that test positive with test A. We use a labeling covariate L that indicates if the test result Y_B is to be included in the model for that record, and code $X_L = 0$ (for no) in one record and $X_L = 1$ (for yes) in the other. Now consider the model

$$g\left(P[D = 1|Y_A = 1, Y_B, L]\right) = \alpha_0 + \beta_1 X_L(1 - Y_B) + \beta_2 X_L Y_B . \qquad (3.16)$$

When $X_L = 0$, Y_B is not included as a covariate. If g is the log link function, we see that

$$e^{\alpha_0} = P[D = 1|Y_A = 1]$$

is simply the positive predictive value based on Y_A alone. When $X_L = 1$, Y_B is included and we have

$$e^{\beta_1} = \frac{P[D = 1|Y_A = 1, Y_B = 0]}{P[D = 1|Y_A = 1]} ,$$

$$e^{\beta_2} = \frac{P[D = 1|Y_A = 1, Y_B = 1]}{P[D = 1|Y_A = 1]} .$$

Thus β_2 quantifies the increase in the PPV of test A associated with the addition of the information that Y_B is positive, and β_1 quantifies the decrease due to the information that Y_B is negative. This model can again be fitted with GEE.

Example 3.7

Consider the EST and CPH tests from the CASS study. Suppose that a subject is known to have a positive history of chest pain, $Y_{CPH} = 1$. We fit model (3.16) using observations for those with $Y_{CPH} = 1$. The estimates and 90% confidence intervals are

$$e^{\hat{\alpha}_0} = 0.80 ,$$

$$e^{\hat{\beta}_1} = 0.64 \quad (0.59, 0.69) ,$$

$$e^{\hat{\beta}_2} = 1.15 \quad (1.13, 1.17) .$$

Thus, the positive predictive value of CPH alone is 0.80. If subjects that test positive with CPH are also tested with the EST test, a positive result increases their risk by a factor of 1.13 to 1.17 ($p < 0.001$). A negative EST test decreases the risk by a multiplicative factor of 59% to 69% ($p < 0.001$). Thus the EST test provides statistically significant incremental predictive information to the CPH test.   ∎

3.7 Regression models for DLRs

3.7.1 *The model form*

Covariate effects on test accuracy can also be quantified in terms of their associations with DLR parameters. Similar to Sections 3.5 and 3.6, we model a function of the accuracy parameter as a linear form:

$$g^+(\text{DLR}^+(Z)) = \beta_0 + \beta_1 X, \qquad (3.17)$$

$$g^-(\text{DLR}^-(Z)) = \alpha_0 + \alpha_1 X, \qquad (3.18)$$

where g^+ and g^- are specified link functions.

Since DLRs are not probabilities, link functions with domains in $(0,1)$ such as logit or probit forms are not appropriate. Leisenring and Pepe (1998) suggest using the log link function because DLRs are restricted to the positive real line $(0,\infty)$. Recall that the DLR by definition relates to both diseased and non-diseased populations, $\text{DLR}^+ = \text{P}[Y = 1|D = 1]/\text{P}[Y = 1|D = 0]$ and $\text{DLR}^- = \text{P}[Y = 0|D = 1]/\text{P}[Y = 0|D = 0]$. Therefore, when defined conditionally on a covariate Z, $\text{DLR}(Z)$ relates to the diseased and non-diseased populations at the same covariate level Z. In a sense, they quantify the separation between test results in diseased and non-diseased populations, at covariate level Z. The regression analysis seeks to determine how this separation changes with Z.

3.7.2 *Fitting the DLR model*

Observe that because DLR^+ and DLR^- are not expectations of random variables, models (3.17) and (3.18) are not generalized linear models in the classical sense. This contrasts with classification probabilities and predictive values which are expectations of binary random variables and so can be fitted with standard GLM methods. The DLR models require alternative strategies for model fitting.

The strategy proposed by Leisenring and Pepe (1998) is based on the observation that the models (3.17) and (3.18) induce expressions for the classification probabilities as follows:

$$\text{P}[Y = 1|D = 1, Z] = \frac{\text{DLR}^+(Z)\{1 - \text{DLR}^-(Z)\}}{\text{DLR}^+(Z) - \text{DLR}^-(Z)},$$

$$\text{P}[Y = 1|D = 0, Z] = \frac{1 - \text{DLR}^-(Z)}{\text{DLR}^+(Z) - \text{DLR}^-(Z)}.$$

The parameters $\theta = (\alpha, \beta)$ can then be estimated from the derivative of the log-likelihood, which is easily expressed in terms of the classification probabilities. We refer to Leisenring and Pepe (1998) for further details.

3.7.3 *Comparing DLRs of two tests*

The regression framework can be used to compare two tests with regard to their DLR parameters by defining a covariable that indicates test type. We have already used this approach for comparing classification probabilities and for comparing predictive values. Consider the models

$$\log \mathrm{DLR}^+(\text{Test}) = \beta_0 + \beta_1 X_{\text{Test}}, \qquad (3.19)$$

$$\log \mathrm{DLR}^-(\text{Test}) = \alpha_0 + \alpha_1 X_{\text{Test}}. \qquad (3.20)$$

The rDLRs are parameterized as $\mathrm{rDLR}^+(A,B) = e^{\beta_1}$ and $\mathrm{rDLR}^-(a,B) = e^{\alpha_1}$. In Section 3.2 we derived the asymptotic distribution theory for empirical estimates of $\mathrm{rDLR}^+(A,B)$ and $\mathrm{rDLR}^-(A,B)$ only when data were unpaired and independent. The regression framework here allows us to make inferences, at least in large samples, for paired data, or for more general clustered data.

Example 3.8

Let us compare the DLR^+s of the CPH and EST tests using the CASS data. The empirical values are

$$\hat{\mathrm{DLR}}^+(\mathrm{CPH}) = 1.71,$$

$$\hat{\mathrm{DLR}}^+(\mathrm{EST}) = 3.06.$$

With the regression model (3.19) the $\mathrm{rDLR}^+(\mathrm{CPH},\mathrm{EST})$ is estimated to be $e^{\beta_1} = 0.56$ with 90% confidence interval equal to $(0.48, 0.65)$. Clearly the EST test has a superior DLR^+ $(p < 0.001)$. ∎

Further applications of the DLR regression methodology to real data can be found in Leisenring and Pepe (1998).

3.7.4 *Relationships with other regression models*

The DLRs have explicit relationships with classification probabilities and with predictive values that were delineated in Chapter 2. Similarly, there are relationships between covariate effects on DLRs and covariate effects on (FPF, TPF) and on (PPV, NPV) that are noteworthy.

First, suppose that classification probability models with the log link function are used to quantify covariate effects as follows:

$$\log \mathrm{TPF}(Z) = \beta_{0D} + \beta_{1D}X,$$

$$\log \mathrm{FPF}(Z) = \beta_{0\bar{D}} + \beta_{1\bar{D}}X.$$

That is, $\exp \beta_{1D}$ and $\exp \beta_{1\bar{D}}$ are the relative TPF and FPF covariate parameters, respectively. Because $\mathrm{DLR}^+ = \mathrm{TPF}/\mathrm{FPF}$, the induced model for $\mathrm{DLR}^+(Z)$ is

$$\log \mathrm{DLR}^+(Z) = \beta_{0D} - \beta_{0\bar{D}} + (\beta_{1D} - \beta_{1\bar{D}})X.$$

If $\beta_{1D} = \beta_{1\bar{D}}$, then the covariate has no effect on the DLR^+ parameter. That is, if a covariate has the same effect on the TPF and FPF on a multiplicative scale, then it does not influence the positive DLR. It will, however, influence the negative DLR, and in a nonlinear complex fashion, since

$$\log \mathrm{DLR}^-(Z) = \log\{1 - \exp(\beta_{0D} + \beta_{1D}X)\} - \log\{1 - \exp(\beta_{0\bar{D}} + \beta_{1\bar{D}}X)\}.$$

Turning now to predictive values, recall that covariates can affect predictive values if they affect disease prevalence or if they affect classification probabilities.

Indeed, the relationship between DLRs and predictive values summarized in Result 2.2 indicates that

$$\text{logit P}[D = 1|Y = 1, Z] = \log \text{DLR}^+(Z) + \text{logit P}[D = 1|Z],$$
$$\text{logit P}[D = 1|Y = 0, Z] = \log \text{DLR}^-(Z) + \text{logit P}[D = 1|Z].$$

Thus covariate effects on predictive value odds can be explicitly decomposed into two additive components. The second component relates to covariate effects on prevalence, whereas the first component relates to covariate effects on accuracy, as parameterized by the DLR models. Then, in assessing predictive value models, it might be of interest to evaluate covariate effects separately on the prevalence and on the DLRs in order to gain insights into the sources of effects.

3.8 Concluding remarks

This chapter completes the discussion of basic statistical techniques for making inferences about the diagnostic accuracy of binary tests. Methods for comparing tests were first introduced and then generalized to regression modeling methodology. Not only does the regression framework incorporate the comparison of tests as a special case, but it similarly allows one to compare the performance of a single test in different populations or under different conditions. In addition, it provides tools for making such comparisons while controlling for concomitant or confounding variables, for evaluating covariate effects on comparisons (with interactions) and for determining the incremental value of a test in the presence of other diagnostic information. The statistical techniques are fairly standard and are applied routinely in other areas of medical research. I hope that their application in diagnostic testing studies will become more commonplace, so that biomarkers and diagnostic tests receive thorough evaluation before being applied in medical practice. Such is not the case at present (see Feinstein, 2002 and related editorials and commentaries).

Statistical inference is described for population level measures of test performance. The classification probabilities and predictive values are defined as 'marginal probabilities' (see Sections 3.3.2, 3.3.3 and 3.5.2). In Exercise 3 below we introduce the concept of individual level models for classification probabilities. Parameters in these models do not relate to the relative performance of tests in the population, but rather they relate to comparisons between test results in an individual. I feel strongly that the population level performance of tests is ultimately most relevant to public health. Hence, marginal models are emphasized almost exclusively in this book. Individual level comparisons between tests however may be of interest in secondary analyses and random effect models can be employed for that purpose.

Data from diagnostic testing studies is typically clustered, with multiple test results available per subject. Indeed, locating a dataset from an unpaired research study proved impossible and ultimately hypothetical data were generated for the illustration in Example 3.1. The key assumption needed with clustered data is that observations are randomly sampled from the relevant population. Technical details about fitting marginal models to clustered data are not described in great depth in this chapter. The recent edition of the text by Diggle *et al.* (2002) is a good source for technical discussion, as are the papers cited in this chapter.

3.9 Exercises

1. Using the delta method or otherwise, provide formal proofs of Results 3.1 and 3.4 that give expressions for the variances of $\log r\hat{\text{TPF}}(A, B)$ and $\log r\hat{\text{FPF}}(A, B)$ in large samples based on unpaired and paired data, respectively.

2. Calculate a 90% confidence interval for the absolute difference in true positive fractions for the EST and CPH tests, namely $\Delta\text{TPF}(\text{EST}, \text{CPH})$ in the notation of Table 2.5, with the CASS data. Describe the result for a clinical audience. Calculate a 90% confidence interval for the $r\text{TPF}(\text{EST}, \text{CPH})$ using the same data and contrast its description with that for the $\Delta\text{TPF}(\text{EST}, \text{CPH})$ interval.

3. When multiple tests are performed on a test unit we have defined the classification probabilities in a marginal probability sense. Let D_i denote a test subject's disease status and (Y_{iA}, Y_{iB}) denote results of two different tests. Suppose that instead of the marginal population level model, a subject specific model is postulated. With α_i and γ_i denoting subject specific random variables, let $\text{TPF}_i(\text{Test}) = P[Y_i = 1 | D_i = 1, \alpha_i, \text{Test}]$ and $\text{FPF}_i(\text{Test}) = P[Y_i = 1 | D_i = 0, \gamma_i, \text{Test}]$, and consider the models

$$g(\text{TPF}_i(\text{Test})) = \alpha_i + \beta_D X_{\text{Test}},$$
$$g(\text{FPF}_i(\text{Test})) = \gamma_i + \beta_{\bar{D}} X_{\text{Test}}.$$

   (a) Let g be the log link function. Provide interpretations for $\exp\beta_D$ and $\exp\beta_{\bar{D}}$ and contrast them with those for the $r\text{TPF}$ and $r\text{FPF}$ measures defined in the sense of marginal population level probabilities.

   (b) Let g be the logit link function. Use the conditional likelihood methods, as described in Breslow and Day (1980), to estimate β_D and $\beta_{\bar{D}}$ with the CASS data. Observe that only observations for which $Y_{\text{CPH}} \neq Y_{\text{EST}}$ enter into the analysis.

4. Consider $C(\text{testing})$, the per subject expected cost of the disease to the population in the presence of screening, as an overall measure of test performance (Section 2.3.4). Given a disease with prevalence ρ and two screening tests that cost C_A and C_B, describe a statistical procedure to compare their expected costs using data from a case-control study. You can use data from the CASS study and postulate cost components and prevalence to illustrate your approach.

5. Consider testing the hypothesis $H_0 : \text{rTPF}(A, B) = 1$ using a confidence interval for $\text{rTPF}(A, B)$. Show that, with paired data, McNemar's test is asymptotically equivalent to this procedure. You can use the marginal GLM framework and note that Leisenring *et al.* (1997) showed that McNemar's test statistic is the generalized score statistic for the marginal model.

6. In eqn (3.16) suppose that the link function is the logit function. Show that $\text{DLR}^- = \exp \beta_1$ and that $\text{DLR}^+ = \exp \beta_2$, where these DLRs are defined conditional on $Y_A = 1$. That is, within the population testing positive on test A, these are the DLRs associated with test B.

4

THE RECEIVER OPERATING CHARACTERISTIC CURVE

In this chapter we consider medical tests with results that are not simply positive or negative, but that are measured on continuous or ordinal scales. The receiver operating characteristic (ROC) curve is currently the best-developed statistical tool for describing the performance of such tests. ROC curves have been in use for a long time, having arisen in the context of signal detection theory which was developed in the 1950s and 1960s (Green and Swets, 1966; Egan, 1975). Their potential for medical diagnostic testing was recognized as early as 1960 (Lusted, 1960), although it was in the early 1980s, after publication of the text by Swets and Pickett (1982), that they became popular, especially in radiology. Today they enjoy broader applications in medicine (Hanley, 1989; Shapiro, 1999).

4.1 The context

4.1.1 *Examples of non-binary tests*

Most tests have some quantitative aspect. Biomarkers for cancer, such as PSA and CA-125, are measured as serum concentrations. Other standard biochemical measures, such as bilirubin for liver disease and creatinine for kidney malfunction, are also measured as concentrations in serum. Cell counts, antibody levels, serum glucose, serum cholesterol, temperature and blood pressure are all familiar quantitative clinical measures that are used for diagnostic purposes. Even the results of neonatal audiology tests are quantitative, the 'signal-to-noise ratio' being the output parameter most frequently considered.

Tests that involve an element of subjective assessment are often ordinal in nature. The radiologist's reading of an image results in a classification of his or her suspicion that disease is present. The classification might be 'definitely', 'probably', 'possibly' or 'definitely not'. Clinical symptoms are used as diagnostic tools and are often classified as 'severe', 'moderate', 'mild' or 'not present'. Behaviors are also used as diagnostic measures. In psychology, for example, they are often classified according to their frequency using an ordinal scale such as 'always', 'often', 'sometimes', 'rarely' and 'never'.

4.1.2 *Dichotomizing the test result*

By convention we assume that larger values of the test result, Y, are more indicative of disease. Even if the result on its original scale does not satisfy this requirement, a transformation of it usually does. For example, in neonatal audiology, a lower signal-to-noise ratio (SNR) indicates poorer response to an auditory stimulus, so we define $Y = -\text{SNR}$ in order to satisfy our convention.

The notion of using Y to define a dichotomous decision rule is fundamental to the evaluation of medical tests. This stems from the fact that diagnostic tests are used ultimately to make medical decisions. Should the patient be treated or not? Should a biopsy be taken or not? The decision rule is based on whether or not the test result (or some transformation of it) exceeds a threshold value. Some conventional thresholds are 4.0 ng/ml for serum PSA, 126 mg/dL for fasting blood glucose, 1.3 mg/dL for serum creatinine and 200 mg/dL for cholesterol.

The choice of a suitable threshold will vary with circumstances. It will depend on options for working-up or treating subjects and on the availability of health care resources. If health care resources are abundant, a lower (more lenient) threshold may be feasible because the system can afford work-up for many individuals. If work-up or treatment is invasive, a higher, more restrictive threshold will be used. The perceived gravity of the condition will also play a role in setting the threshold. A more conservative approach, that is a lower threshold, would be set for more serious disease.

Implicitly, the choice of threshold depends on the trade-off that is acceptable between failing to detect disease and falsely identifying disease with the test. The acceptable trade-off varies with the circumstances under which the test is done. The ROC curve is a device that simply describes the range of trade-offs that can be achieved by the test.

4.2 The ROC curve for continuous tests

In this section we focus mostly on continuous ROC curves. However, when it is possible to accommodate both continuous and discrete tests in the same discussion, we do so. Our notation will indicate definitions and results that accommodate discrete tests.

4.2.1 *Definition of the ROC*

Using a threshold c, define a binary test from the continuous test result Y as

$$\begin{cases} \text{positive if } Y \geq c, \\ \text{negative if } Y < c. \end{cases}$$

Let the corresponding true and false positive fractions at the threshold c be $\text{TPF}(c)$ and $\text{FPF}(c)$, respectively, where

$$\text{TPF}(c) = P[Y \geq c | D = 1] \tag{4.1}$$

$$\text{FPF}(c) = P[Y \geq c | D = 0]. \tag{4.2}$$

The ROC curve is the entire set of possible true and false positive fractions attainable by dichotomizing Y with different thresholds. That is, the ROC curve is

$$\text{ROC}(\cdot) = \{(\text{FPF}(c), \text{TPF}(c)), \ c \in (-\infty, \infty)\}. \tag{4.3}$$

Observe that, as the threshold c increases, both $\text{FPF}(c)$ and $\text{TPF}(c)$ decrease. At one extreme, $c = \infty$, we have $\lim_{c \to \infty} \text{TPF}(c) = 0$ and $\lim_{c \to \infty} \text{FPF}(c) = 0$.

At the other, $c = -\infty$, we have $\lim_{c \to -\infty} \mathrm{TPF}(c) = 1$ and $\lim_{c \to -\infty} \mathrm{FPF}(c) = 1$. Thus, the ROC curve is a monotone increasing function in the positive quadrant. This is illustrated in Fig. 4.1. We also write the ROC curve as

$$\mathrm{ROC}(\cdot) \;=\; \{(t, \mathrm{ROC}(t)),\; t \in (0,1)\}, \tag{4.4}$$

where the ROC function maps t to $\mathrm{TPF}(c)$, and c is the threshold corresponding to $\mathrm{FPF}(c) = t$.

4.2.2 *Mathematical properties of the ROC curve*

The ROC curve is a monotone increasing function mapping $(0,1)$ onto $(0,1)$. An uninformative test is one such that Y is unrelated to disease status. That is, the probability distributions for Y are the same in the diseased and non-diseased populations, and therefore for any threshold c we have $\mathrm{TPF}(c) = \mathrm{FPF}(c)$. The ROC curve for a useless test is therefore $\mathrm{ROC}(t) = t$, which is a line with unit slope.

A perfect test on the other hand completely separates diseased and non-diseased subjects. That is, for some threshold c we have $\mathrm{TPF}(c) = 1$ and $\mathrm{FPF}(c) = 0$. Its ROC curve is along the left and upper borders of the positive unit quadrant.

Most tests have ROC curves that lie between those of the perfect and useless tests. Better tests have ROC curves closer to the upper left corner. See Fig. 4.2, where test A, the better of the two tests, is such that at any false positive fraction its corresponding true positive fraction is higher than that of test B. Similarly, if we choose thresholds c_A and c_B for which $\mathrm{TPF}_A(c_A) = \mathrm{TPF}_B(c_B)$,

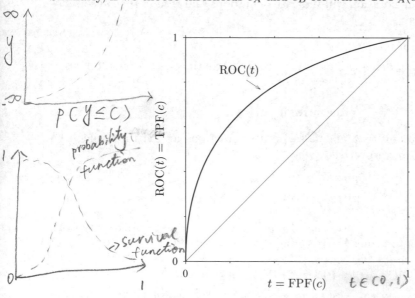

FIG. 4.1. An example of an ROC curve

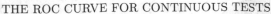

$FPF_{AC}(c_A) \stackrel{?}{=} FPF_B(c_B)$

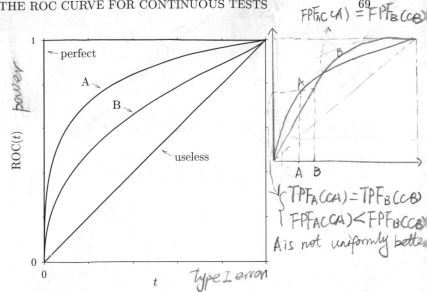

power

ROC(t)

perfect

A

B

useless

0

0

t *Type I error*

$TPF_A(c_A) = TPF_B(c_B)$
$FPF_A(c_A) < FPF_B(c_B)$
A is not uniformly better

A B

Fig. 4.2. ROC curves for two tests, A and B, where test A is unequivocally better. Also shown are ROC curves for the useless and perfect tests for comparison $TPF_A > TPF_B$

the corresponding false positive fractions are ordered in favor of test A, so that $\mathrm{FPF}_A(c_A) < \mathrm{FPF}_B(c_B)$.

Some formal properties of the ROC curve are stated in the next set of results. They are somewhat technical and some readers may choose to proceed directly to Section 4.2.3 at this point.

Result 4.1

The ROC curve is invariant to strictly increasing transformations of Y.

Proof Let $(\mathrm{FPF}(c), \mathrm{TPF}(c))$ be a point on the ROC curve for Y. Let h be a strictly increasing transformation and let $W = h(Y)$ and $d = h(c)$. Then $P[W \geqslant d|D = 0] = P[Y \geqslant c|D = 0]$ and $P[W \geqslant d|D = 1] = P[Y \geqslant c|D = 1]$. Thus the same point exists on the ROC curve for W. A similar argument shows that each point on the ROC curve for W is also on that for Y. ∎

Result 4.2

Let S_D and $S_{\bar{D}}$ denote the survivor functions for Y in the diseased and non-diseased populations: $S_D(y) = P[Y \geqslant y|D = 1]$ and $S_{\bar{D}}(y) = P[Y \geqslant y|D = 0]$. The ROC curve has the following representation:

$$\mathrm{ROC}(t) = S_D(S_{\bar{D}}^{-1}(t)), \quad t \in (0,1). \tag{4.5}$$

Proof This follows simply from the definition of the ROC curve. Let $c = S_{\bar{D}}^{-1}(t)$. That is, c is the threshold corresponding to the false positive fraction

t, so that $P[Y \geqslant c|D = 0] = t$. The corresponding true positive fraction is $P[Y \geqslant c|D = 1] = S_D(c)$. So the TPF that corresponds to the FPF $= t$ is

$$\mathrm{ROC}(t) = S_D(c) = S_D(S_{\bar{D}}^{-1}(t)).$$ ∎

Another representation is given in the next result which follows as a simple corollary to Result 4.2. This result applies only to continuous tests.

Result 4.3

The ROC curve is the function on $(0, 1)$ with $\mathrm{ROC}(0) = 0$, $\mathrm{ROC}(1) = 1$ and which has slope

$$\frac{\partial \mathrm{ROC}(t)}{\partial t} = \frac{f_D(S_{\bar{D}}^{-1}(t))}{f_{\bar{D}}(S_{\bar{D}}^{-1}(t))}, \tag{4.6}$$

where f denotes the probability density of Y.

Proof We have

$$\frac{\partial S_D(S_{\bar{D}}^{-1}(t))}{\partial t} = \frac{\partial S_D(S_{\bar{D}}^{-1}(t))}{\partial S_{\bar{D}}^{-1}(t)} \cdot \frac{\partial S_{\bar{D}}^{-1}(t)}{\partial t}$$

$$= -f_D(S_{\bar{D}}^{-1}(t)) \cdot \frac{\partial S_{\bar{D}}^{-1}(t)}{\partial t},$$

and the result follows because

$$\frac{\partial S_{\bar{D}}^{-1}(t)}{\partial t} = 1 \bigg/ \frac{\partial}{\partial w}(S_{\bar{D}}(w)) = \frac{1}{-f_{\bar{D}}(w)},$$

which is evaluated at $w = S_{\bar{D}}^{-1}(t)$. ∎

Observe that the slope can be interpreted as the likelihood ratio $\mathcal{L}R(c) = P[Y = c|D = 1]/P[Y = c|D = 0]$ at the threshold c corresponding to the point $(t, \mathrm{ROC}(t))$, i.e. at $c = S_{\bar{D}}^{-1}(t)$. In many settings one will expect that the likelihood ratio $\mathcal{L}R(c) = f_D(c)/f_{\bar{D}}(c)$ will increase with c, since by convention higher values of the test result are more indicative of disease.

The likelihood ratio function has an important place in the evaluation of medical tests. Later, in Chapter 9, we use some results about the $\mathcal{L}R$ function to develop optimal combinations of tests. Here we simply give a key mathematical result from signal detection theory about the function $\mathcal{L}R(Y)$ that is essentially the Neyman–Pearson lemma (Neyman and Pearson, 1933; McIntosh and Pepe, 2002). A full account is provided by Green and Swets (1966) and Egan (1975) who provide other optimality properties of $\mathcal{L}R(Y)$.

Result 4.4

The optimal criterion based on Y for classifying subjects as positive for disease is

$$\mathcal{LR}(Y) > c \qquad (4.7)$$

in the sense that it achieves the highest true positive fraction among all possible criteria based on Y with false positive fractions $t = \mathrm{P}[\mathcal{LR}(Y) > c | D = 0]$. ∎

Moreover, we note the following implications:

(i) If the test result Y is such that $\mathcal{LR}(\cdot)$ is monotone increasing, then decision rules based on Y exceeding a threshold are optimal because they are equivalent to rules based on $\mathcal{LR}(Y)$ exceeding a threshold.

(ii) The ROC curve for $W = \mathcal{LR}(Y)$ is uniformly above all other ROC curves based on Y. It is therefore the optimal ROC curve.

(iii) The optimal ROC curve is concave. This is because, if we define $L = \mathcal{LR}(Y)$, its ROC curve has slope $\mathrm{P}[L = x | D = 1]/\mathrm{P}[L = x | D = 0] = x$ at the threshold value x (Exercise 1), which, by definition, is monotone increasing in x. Therefore, as a function of $t = \mathrm{P}[L > x | D = 0]$, the slope of the ROC curve is monotone decreasing.

If the $\mathcal{LR}$ function were known, one could transform Y to its optimal scale, i.e. $\mathcal{LR}(Y)$. In practice we do not know $\mathcal{LR}$. It could be estimated from data in order to approximate the optimal transformation. We will pursue this approach in Chapter 9 when we consider tests with multiple results and how they can be combined into a single optimal score.

For the most part, however, when Y has only one dimension, we consider Y without transformation. In many practical settings, the biological or biophysical theory behind the test implies that $\mathcal{LR}(Y)$ is monotone increasing in Y. Consider such examples as cancer biomarkers or audiometric responses ($-$SNR) to hearing stimuli. Indeed, our convention that larger values of Y are more indicative of disease is essentially a statement that $\mathcal{LR}(Y)$ is monotone increasing. In such cases, the above results state that transformations are unnecessary and that decisions based on Y exceeding a threshold are optimal.

4.2.3 *Attributes of and uses for the ROC curve*

As a descriptive device, the ROC curve depicts the entire set of operating characteristics (FPF, TPF) possible with the test. Reporting of the (FPF, TPF) attained at only a single threshold is clearly very limited. Unfortunately this occurs all too often in practice. Moreover, such reporting makes it difficult to compare different studies of the same test, particularly when different thresholds are employed. By reporting the entire ROC curve, information about a test can be compared and possibly combined across studies.

The choice of threshold value can be suggested in part by displaying the ROC curve. Informally, acceptable (FPF, TPF) values on the ROC curve can be selected and the corresponding thresholds determined. Formally, if one defines a cost or utility function that combines the (FPF, TPF) values, then the values of (FPF, TPF) that optimize the utility can be determined. See also Metz (1978).

Result 4.5

Using the notation of Section 2.3.4, consider the cost of a screening program based on Y when operating the test at an FPF $= t$:

$$\text{Cost}(t) = C + C_D^+ \text{ROC}(t)\rho + C_D^-(1 - \text{ROC}(t))\rho + C_{\bar{D}}^+ t(1 - \rho).\qquad(4.8)$$

The threshold that minimizes the cost function is the threshold that corresponds to

$$\frac{\partial \text{ROC}(t)}{\partial t} = \left(\frac{1 - \rho}{\rho}\right)\frac{C_{\bar{D}}^+}{C_D^- - C_D^+}.\qquad(4.9)$$

■

Compelling motivation for ROC curves arises particularly in the context of comparing medical tests. When test results are measured in different units or on different scales, it is meaningless to compare the raw data measurements themselves. The ROC curve transforms tests to a common scale. Moreover, the scale to which they are transformed is one that is relevant to their performances as diagnostic tests. Meaningful comparisons between tests are possible on the ROC scale.

Example 4.1

Data shown in Figs 4.3 and 4.4 are from an audiology study comparing the DPOAE and ABR tests (Norton *et al.*, 2000). In fact, these data came from the

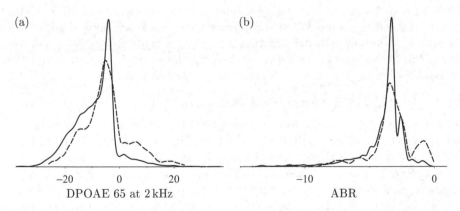

FIG. 4.3. Probability distributions of test results for the (a) DPOAE and (b) ABR tests among hearing-impaired ears (dashed lines) and normally-hearing ears (solid lines)

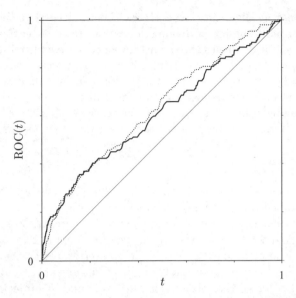

FIG. 4.4. ROC curves for the DPOAE (dotted line) and ABR (solid line) tests

realized screening study for which the previously analyzed hypothetical binary data of Leisenring *et al.* (1997) were generated at the planning phases. The output from the DPOAE test is a signal-to-noise ratio measured on a scale from about −40 to 40 in this study. The ABR test result is an F-statistic. For both tests we multiply the results by −1 so that the result is larger for hearing-impaired subjects, in accordance with our convention. The ABR test result is therefore negative, ranging from −14 to −0.18 in these data.

It is difficult to discern from the raw distributions if one test better distinguishes between hearing-impaired and normally-hearing ears than does the other. The ROC curves in Fig. 4.4 clearly show that the tests are quite similar in this regard. In Chapter 5 we will discuss methods for comparing curves statistically.
■

Table 4.1 summarizes the four points made above about the use of ROC

Table 4.1 *Some attributes of ROC curves for evaluating diagnostic tests*

(1) Provides a complete description of potential performance
(2) Facilitates comparing and combining information across studies of the same test
(3) Guides the choice of threshold in applications
(4) Provides a mechanism for relevant comparisons between different non-binary tests

curves for evaluating diagnostic tests. It has been noted that they can also be useful in applications outside of diagnostic testing. In essence, the ROC curve is a statistical tool that describes the separation between two distributions, S_D and $S_{\bar{D}}$, and so it can be useful in any setting where separations between distributions are of interest. For example, such a description can be valuable for evaluating treatment effects on an outcome in a clinical trial or for evaluating risk factors for disease. Although our focus is on ROC curves for evaluating medical tests, we provide one illustration of their potential application in evaluating a therapeutic agent.

Example 4.2

A parallel-arm clinical trial randomized subjects with cystic fibrosis to receive intermittent inhaled tobramycin or placebo for a period of 20 weeks (Ramsey *et al.*, 1999). The primary outcome measure was the percentage change in FEV_1 from baseline to 4 weeks after treatment was initiated. FEV_1 is a measure of lung function, a key clinical parameter that deteriorates as the cystic fibrosis disease progresses. Figure 4.5 displays the distributions of the outcome measure in subjects that received the tobramycin antibiotic and in subjects that received placebo.

Let D denote the treatment group, where $D = 1$ for tobramycin and $D = 0$ for placebo, and let Y be the percentage change in FEV_1. The corresponding ROC curve provides another visual display of the separation between the treated and untreated groups. It shows that the distribution of Y in the treated group is shifted towards larger improvements than for the placebo group. Consider, for example, the median change in the placebo group, which is indexed at 0.5 on the horizontal axis of the ROC plot. The corresponding point on the ROC curve is

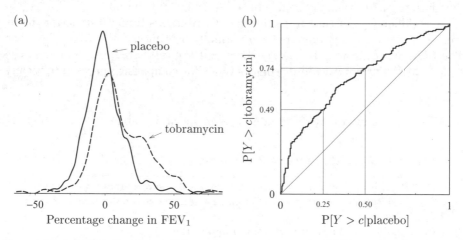

FIG. 4.5. (a) Distributions of the percentage change in FEV_1 in the placebo and treatment arms of the TOBI clinical trial. Shown in (b) is the corresponding ROC curve

75%. Therefore 75% of the treatment group had improvements above the median for the placebo group. Similarly, the ROC point $(0.25, 0.50)$ indicates that 50% of the tobramycin group were above the 75th percentile of the placebo group. The ROC curve provides a visual comparison between the two study arms and interestingly this comparison is independent of the scale on which the outcome is measured.   ∎

4.2.4   Restrictions and alternatives to the ROC curve

In some settings only part of the ROC curve is of interest (McClish, 1989; Thompson and Zucchini, 1989). For example, if the test is for use as a population screening test, it can only be applied in practice using thresholds corresponding to false positive fractions in the lowest part of the $(0, 1)$ domain. The ROC curve with domain restricted to $(0, t_0)$, where t_0 is the maximal acceptable false positive fraction for screening, would provide an appropriate description of the potential performance of a screening test.

Similarly, there are settings where maintaining a high TPF is the priority (Jiang et al., 1996). For example, among those that screen positive on a PSA test for prostate cancer, a large proportion do not have cancer. A non-invasive medical test is currently sought to be applied in men that are PSA positive which will select the subset of them that are truly diseased. It is important that the new test does not erroneously eliminate any of the true cancers but that it only eliminates non-cancers from further work-up. That is, the new test must have a very high TPF in the population to which it is to be applied. Restricting attention to the ROC curve for the test where its TPF range is acceptably high therefore seems appropriate.

Although the ROC curve as we have described it here is most popular, a few alternative measures of test performance have been proposed for continuous tests. Kraemer (1992) suggests the quality ROC curve, the so-called QROC curve. This is a plot of standardized sensitivity, denoted by qTPF, versus standardized specificity (or true negative fraction TNF $= 1 - $ FPF), denoted by qTNF, where for a binary test these are defined as

$$qTPF = (TPF - P[Y = 1])/(1 - P[Y = 1]),$$
$$qTNF = (TNF - P[Y = 0])/P[Y = 1].$$

Rationale for the standardization of TPF is as follows. In the numerator the subtraction of $P[Y = 1]$ serves to distinguish the probability of a positive result in diseased subjects from the background probability in the population as a whole. That is, the numerator is a measure of the excess chance of a positive result due to the presence of disease. The denominator is the maximal value that the numerator can attain. Thus qTPF is interpreted as the positivity probability of the test in diseased subjects beyond chance relative to that of the perfect test. It is the chance-corrected TPF, and it takes values on the scale $(0, 1)$. Similar considerations apply to the standardization of the specificity,

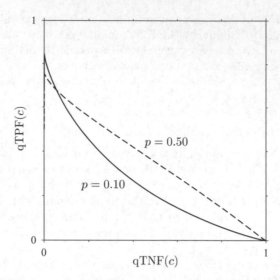

FIG. 4.6. The QROC curves that correspond to the ROC curve of Fig. 4.1 with prevalences of $p = 0.10$ and $p = 0.50$

TNF = 1 − FPF, which can be interpreted as a chance-corrected TNF. Kraemer (1992) draws analogies between components of the Kappa statistic for agreement in a two-by-two table and the chance-corrected (qTNF, qTPF) values. One appealing feature of qTNF and qTPF is that interchanging the roles of D and Y yields the same pair of values. That is, if qTNF* and qTPF* are the chance-corrected true negative and true positive values, respectively, when the roles of D and Y are interchanged, one can show that qTNF* = qTPF and qTPF* = qTNF.

A plot of the points (qTNF(c), qTPF(c)) for dichotomized tests corresponding to different threshold values c is Kraemer's QROC curve. Note that the QROC is not necessarily a smooth monotone curve. In general it is a scatterplot of points in the positive unit quadrant. Figure 4.6 plots the QROC corresponding to the ROC curve of Fig. 4.1. The QROC curve has not (yet) become a popular tool for evaluating diagnostic tests, perhaps because its interpretation is not as straightforward as that of the ROC curve. Additionally, it is functionally dependent on disease prevalence and is not easy to estimate from case-control studies. We mention it here for completeness and refer the interested reader to Kraemer (1992) for an extensive discussion with illustrations.

4.3   Summary indices

Numerical indices for ROC curves are often used to summarize the curves. When it is not feasible to plot the ROC curve itself, such summary measures convey important information about the curve. This is similar to the use of summary measures such as the mean and variance to describe a probability distribution.

Summary indices are particularly useful when many tests are under consideration. Moreover, they can be used as the basis of inferential statistics for comparing ROC curves.

4.3.1   The area under the ROC curve (AUC)

The most widely used summary measure is the area under the ROC curve defined
as

$$\text{AUC} = \int_0^1 \text{ROC}(t)\,dt. \tag{4.10}$$

A perfect test, one with the perfect ROC curve, has the value AUC $= 1.0$.
Conversely, an uninformative test, with $\text{ROC}(t) = t$, has AUC $= 0.5$. Most
tests have values falling in between. Clearly, if two tests are ordered with test A
uniformly better than test B in the sense that

$$\text{ROC}_A(t) \geqslant \text{ROC}_B(t) \quad \forall t \in (0,1) \tag{4.11}$$

(see Fig. 4.2), then their AUC statistics are also ordered:

$$\text{AUC}_A \geqslant \text{AUC}_B.$$

However, the converse is not necessarily true.

The AUC has an interesting interpretation. It is equal to the probability that
test results from a randomly selected pair of diseased and non-diseased subjects
are correctly ordered, namely $P[Y_D > Y_{\bar{D}}]$ (Bamber, 1975; Hanley and McNeil,
1982). An informal proof is displayed in Fig. 4.7 for a continuous test.

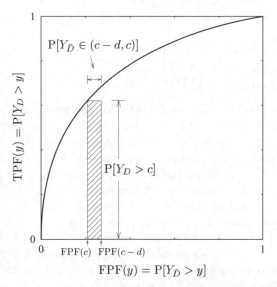

FIG. 4.7. A visual proof that AUC $= P[Y_D > Y_{\bar{D}}]$

This proof relies on approximating the AUC by a sum of the areas of the rectangles below it, each of width $P[Y_{\bar{D}} \in (c-d,c)]$ and height $P[Y_D > c]$. Each rectangle has area $P[Y_D > c]P[Y_{\bar{D}} \in (c-d,c)] = P[Y_D > c, Y_{\bar{D}} \in (c-d,c)]$ by the statistical independence of Y_D and $Y_{\bar{D}}$. Therefore the summation across all rectangles yields $P[Y_D > Y_{\bar{D}}]$. We now provide a more formal proof for continuous tests.

Result 4.6

The following result holds:

$$\text{AUC} = P[Y_D > Y_{\bar{D}}], \qquad (4.12)$$

where Y_D and $Y_{\bar{D}}$ correspond to independent and randomly chosen test results from the diseased and non-diseased populations, respectively.

Proof We have

$$\text{AUC} = \int_0^1 \text{ROC}(t)\,dt = \int_0^1 S_D(S_{\bar{D}}^{-1}(t))\,dt$$

$$= \int_\infty^{-\infty} S_D(y)\,dS_{\bar{D}}(y)$$

$$= \int_{-\infty}^\infty P[Y_D > y]\,f_{\bar{D}}(y)\,dy\,,$$

using the change of variable from t to $y = S_{\bar{D}}^{-1}(t)$ in the second line and where $f_{\bar{D}}$ denotes the probability density function for $Y_{\bar{D}}$ in the third line. Thus, by statistical independence of Y_D and $Y_{\bar{D}}$, we can write

$$\text{AUC} = \int_{-\infty}^\infty P[Y_D > y, Y_{\bar{D}} = y]\,dy$$

$$= P[Y_D > Y_{\bar{D}}]\,. \qquad \blacksquare$$

Although the interpretation of the AUC as the probability of 'correctly ordering diseased and non-diseased subjects' is interesting, it does not necessarily provide the best interpretation of this summary measure. The clinical relevance of the correct ordering is not particularly compelling for the applications that we consider. Rather, it is a more natural quantity to consider in the so-called forced-choice experiment that is sometimes conducted in radiology. In the forced-choice experiment a radiologist is provided with pairs of images, one from each of a diseased and a non-diseased subject, and chooses that which he/she assumes to be most likely from the diseased subject. In such experiments the proportion of correct choices is $P[Y_D > Y_{\bar{D}}]$, where Y is his/her suspicion about the presence of disease. Again this quantity does not seem particularly relevant for clinical practice, although it does provide a natural summary of discrimination in the experiment.

We prefer to interpret the AUC as an average TPF, averaged uniformly over the whole range of false positive fractions in $(0, 1)$. Dodd (2001) suggests calculating a weighted average, weighting certain parts of the false positive fraction domain more than others. This idea could be developed further.

4.3.2 The $\mathrm{ROC}(t_0)$ and partial AUC

If there is particular interest in a specific false positive fraction, t_0 say, then the corresponding TPF value, $\mathrm{ROC}(t_0)$, provides a relevant summary index. For instance, available resources may be able to accommodate a false positive fraction of t_0. Comparing tests when their thresholds are such that each yields this acceptable $\mathrm{FPF} = t_0$ is accomplished by comparing their $\mathrm{ROC}(t_0)$ values. The $\mathrm{ROC}(t_0)$ has an interpretation that is easily grasped by non-statisticians, namely the proportion of diseased subjects with test results above the $1 - t_0$ quantile for non-diseased observations. If t_0 is small, e.g. $t_0 = 5\%$ or 1%, the quantile is often interpreted as the upper limit of the 'normal' range for Y. Therefore $\mathrm{ROC}(t_0)$ is interpreted as the proportion of diseased subjects with test values above the normal range. Such summaries of test performance are intuitively appealing and are already well established for many clinical laboratory tests.

A problem with $\mathrm{ROC}(t_0)$, however, is that it ignores much of the information in the ROC curve. Values of $\mathrm{ROC}(t)$ for $t < t_0$ may be of interest, even if values for $t > t_0$ are not. Moreover, for two tests that have $\mathrm{ROC}_A(t_0) = \mathrm{ROC}_B(t_0)$, if $\mathrm{ROC}_A(t) \geqslant \mathrm{ROC}_B(t)$ over the range $t \in (0, t_0)$ then it will often be reasonable to rank test A higher than test B with regards to overall performance. The partial area under the curve, $\mathrm{pAUC}(t_0)$, is a summary index that restricts attention to FPFs at and below t_0, and which uses all points on the ROC curve in that range of FPFs. It can be considered as striking a compromise between the full AUC and $\mathrm{ROC}(t_0)$ (McClish, 1989; Thompson and Zucchini, 1989). It is defined as

$$\mathrm{pAUC}(t_0) = \int_0^{t_0} \mathrm{ROC}(t)\, \mathrm{d}t\,. \tag{4.13}$$

Its values range from $t_0^2/2$ for a completely uninformative test, $\mathrm{ROC}(t) = t$, to t_0 for a perfect test. The normalized value, $\mathrm{pAUC}(t_0)/t_0$, which ranges from $t_0/2$ to 1, has the following interpretation:

$$\mathrm{pAUC}(t_0)/t_0 = \mathrm{P}[Y_D > Y_{\bar{D}} | Y_{\bar{D}} > S_{\bar{D}}^{-1}(t_0)]\,, \tag{4.14}$$

which can be proven using arguments similar to Result 4.6 (Dodd, 2001). In words, $\mathrm{pAUC}(t_0)/t_0$ is the probability of correctly ordering a disease and a non-disease observation chosen at random given that the non-disease observation is in the range above the $1 - t_0$ quantile of the non-disease distribution. The clinical relevance of this interpretation is not very strong and in practical terms the interpretation as the average TPF in the relevant range of FPF is sufficient.

4.3   Summary indices

A 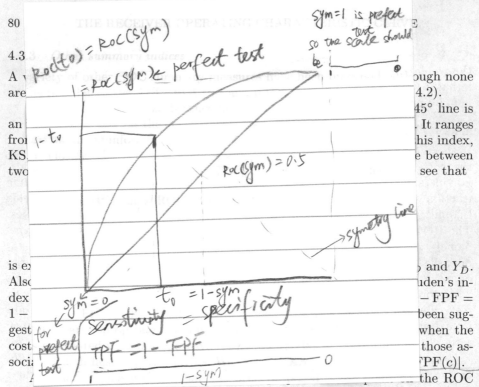 ough none
are 4.2).
an 45° line is
fro It ranges
KS his index,
two e between
see that

is e and $Y_{\bar{D}}$.
Also den's in-
dex $- \text{FPF} =$
$1 -$ been sug-
gest when the
cost those as-
soci PF$(c)|$.

the ROC
curve where sensitivity is equal to specificity, TPF $= 1 -$ FPF. Visually this is
the intersection of the negative 45° line with the ROC curve. Although Moses *et
al.* (1993) use Q^* for its notation, we call it the symmetry point and denote this
measure by 'Sym'. Mathematically, Sym is defined by

$$\text{ROC}(\text{Sym}) = 1 - \text{Sym}.$$

Table 4.2 *Summary indices for ROC Curves*

Index name	Notation	Definition	Interpretations*
Area under the curve	AUC	$\int_0^1 \text{ROC}(t)\,dt$	(i) $P[Y_D > Y_{\bar{D}}]$ (ii) Average TPF across all possible FPF
Specific ROC point	ROC(t_0)	ROC(t_0)	$P[Y_D > q]$
Partial area under the curve	pAUC(t_0)	$\int_0^{t_0} \text{ROC}(t)\,dt$	(i) $t_0 P[Y_D > Y_{\bar{D}} \mid Y_{\bar{D}} > q]$ (ii) Average TPF across FPF $\in (0, t_0)$
Symmetry point	Sym	ROC$(\text{Sym}) = $ Sym	Sensitivity $=$ specificity
Kolmogorov–Smirnov	KS	$\sup |\text{ROC}(t) - t|$	$\max |S_D(c) - S_{\bar{D}}(c)|$

*$q = 1 - t_0$ quantile for $Y_{\bar{D}}$

Note that if $b = 1$, then the binormal ROC curve is concave everywhere. To see this, observe that the slope of the ROC curve at t is the likelihood ratio at the corresponding threshold c, which can be written as

$$\frac{f_D(c)}{f_{\bar{D}}(c)} = \left(\frac{\sigma_{\bar{D}}}{\sigma_D}\right) \exp\left\{\frac{-(c - \mu_D)^2}{2\sigma_D^2} + \frac{(c - \mu_{\bar{D}})^2}{2\sigma_{\bar{D}}^2}\right\}.$$

When $b = 1$, we have $\sigma_D = \sigma_{\bar{D}}$ and the common value is denoted by σ. The likelihood ratio then reduces to $\exp\left\{c(\mu_D - \mu_{\bar{D}})/\sigma^2 - (\mu_D^2 - \mu_{\bar{D}}^2)/2\sigma^2\right\}$. As c decreases (t increases), we see that the slope decreases because $\mu_D > \mu_{\bar{D}}$. Thus, when $b = 1$ the slope of the ROC curve is monotone decreasing in t.

On the other hand, if $b \neq 1$ the monotonicity criterion fails. For $b > 1$, the likelihood ratio decreases and then increases. Conversely, for $b < 1$ the likelihood ratio increases and then decreases as t ranges from 0 to 1. This produces anomalies in the ROC curve where it falls below the uninformative test ROC curve, $\mathrm{ROC}(t) = t$. For some $\varepsilon > 0$, this occurs at the lowest part of the range $t \in (0, \varepsilon)$ when $b > 1$, and at the highest part of the range $t \in (1 - \varepsilon, 1)$ when $b < 1$.

Such anomalies in the ROC curve are very unlikely for most real diagnostic tests. Indeed, a monotone likelihood ratio function is intuitively reasonable for most tests and the fact that the binormal curve does not have a monotone likelihood ratio raises some concern about using it to approximate real data. However, Swets (1986) and Hanley (1988, 1996) conclude that the binormal ROC curve provides a good approximation to a wide range of ROC curves that occur in practice. This may be because the undesirable behavior of the approximating binormal ROC usually occurs over a very small part of the ROC curve. Moreover, non-diseased subjects often tend to have more homogenous test results than do diseased subjects, so that $b < 1$. This implies that the anomalies in the ROC approximation occur at the higher end of the $(0, 1)$ false positive range, which as we have pointed out is often of little interest for practical purposes.

4.4.2 The binormal AUC

The AUC summary measure has a simple analytic form when the ROC curve is binormal.

Result 4.8

The AUC for the binormal ROC curve is

$$\mathrm{AUC} = \Phi\left(\frac{a}{\sqrt{1 + b^2}}\right).$$

$b\uparrow$ the control is more spread

$a\uparrow$ mean difference is bigger

Proof Recall that $\mathrm{AUC} = P[Y_D > Y_{\bar{D}}] = P[Y_D - Y_{\bar{D}} > 0]$. Let $W = Y_D - Y_{\bar{D}}$. Then

$$W \sim N\left(\mu_D - \mu_{\bar{D}}, \sigma_D^2 + \sigma_{\bar{D}}^2\right)$$

and

$$P[W > 0] = 1 - \Phi\left(\frac{-\mu_D + \mu_{\bar{D}}}{\sqrt{\sigma_D^2 + \sigma_{\bar{D}}^2}}\right)$$

$$= \Phi\left(\frac{\mu_D - \mu_{\bar{D}}}{\sqrt{\sigma_D^2 + \sigma_{\bar{D}}^2}}\right)$$

$$= \Phi\left(\frac{\mu_D - \mu_{\bar{D}}}{\sigma_D} \middle/ \sqrt{1 + \frac{\sigma_{\bar{D}}^2}{\sigma_D^2}}\right)$$

$$= \Phi\left(\frac{a}{\sqrt{1 + b^2}}\right).$$

We see that the AUC is an increasing function of a and a decreasing function of b. Unfortunately, a simple analytic expression does not exist for the pAUC summary measure. It must be calculated using numerical integration or a rational polynomial approximation. Nor is there a simple expression for the Kolmogorov–Smirnov summary measure. Interestingly, the symmetry point on the ROC curve can be written as a simple analytic expression (Exercise 5), which is similar in form to the AUC.

4.4.3 The binormal assumption

We have seen that the ROC curve is invariant to monotone increasing data transformations. Therefore if Y_D and $Y_{\bar{D}}$ have normal probability distributions and we transform them to

$$W_D = h(Y_D), \quad W_{\bar{D}} = h(Y_{\bar{D}}),$$

where h is a monotone strictly increasing function, then the ROC curve for W_D and $W_{\bar{D}}$ is also the binormal ROC curve

$$\mathrm{ROC}(t) = \Phi\left(a + b\Phi^{-1}(t)\right).$$

Conversely, to say that the ROC curve for Y_D and $Y_{\bar{D}}$ is binormal is simply to say that, for some strictly increasing transformation h, $h(Y_D)$ and $h(Y_{\bar{D}})$ have normal distributions. We can go further and define the function h that transforms the data to normality.

Result 4.9

If the ROC curve for Y_D and $Y_{\bar{D}}$ is of the binormal form (4.15), namely

$$\mathrm{ROC}(t) = \Phi\left(a + b\Phi^{-1}(t)\right),$$

and we define

$$h(y) = -\Phi^{-1}\left(S_{\bar{D}}(y)\right),$$

probability of FP

where $S_{\bar{D}}$ is the survivor function for $Y_{\bar{D}}$, then ~~binormal ROC~~

$$h(Y_{\bar{D}}) \sim \mathrm{N}(0,1)\,, \quad h(Y_D) \sim \mathrm{N}\left(\frac{a}{b}, \frac{1}{b^2}\right).$$

$$\hookrightarrow \frac{\mu_D - \mu_{\bar{D}}}{\delta D} \cdot \frac{\delta D}{\delta \bar{D}} = \frac{\mu_D - \mu_{\bar{D}}}{\delta \bar{D}}$$

Proof We have

$$\mathrm{P}[h(Y_{\bar{D}}) < y] = \mathrm{P}[S_{\bar{D}}(Y_{\bar{D}}) > \Phi(-y)] = \mathrm{P}[F_{\bar{D}}(Y_{\bar{D}}) < \Phi(y)] = \Phi(y)\,,$$

since $F_{\bar{D}}(Y_{\bar{D}}) \equiv 1 - S_{\bar{D}}(Y_{\bar{D}})$ has a uniform distribution. Then

$$\begin{aligned}
\mathrm{P}[h(Y_D) > y] &= \mathrm{P}[Y_D > S_{\bar{D}}^{-1}(\Phi(-y))] \\
&= S_D S_{\bar{D}}^{-1}\left(\Phi(-y)\right) \\
&= \mathrm{ROC}\left(\Phi(-y)\right) \\
&= \Phi(a - by) = 1 - \Phi\left(\frac{y - a/b}{1/b}\right).
\end{aligned}$$

Thus $h(Y_{\bar{D}})$ has a standard normal distribution and $h(Y_D)$ has a normal distribution with mean a/b and variance $1/b^2$. ∎

The binormal assumption, therefore, states that some monotone transformation of the data exists to make Y_D and $Y_{\bar{D}}$ normally distributed. This is considered to be a fairly weak assumption. The raw data can look decidedly non-Gaussian while the binormal model still holds (Swets and Pickett, 1982; Hanley, 1996). It re-emphasizes the fact that ROC curves have nothing to do with the particular distributions of the test results but rather that they quantify the *relationships* between distributions.

4.5 The ROC for ordinal tests

4.5.1 *Tests with ordered discrete results*

So far we have mostly considered tests where the result Y is measured on a continuous scale. Some tests yield results on a discrete scale. Laboratory tests often report the dilution, among a discrete set tested, at which the desired response is observed. For example, the minimal inhibitory concentration of an antibiotic is a standard measure of bacterial resistance. Questionnaires that ask for the numeric frequency at which an event occurs also yield discrete numeric results.

Many tests are not numeric at all. We mentioned earlier in this chapter subjective assessments that yield qualitative results on an ordinal scale. Examples include the severity or qualitative frequency with which symptoms occur. A very important example is the assessment of an image by a radiologist, where his/her suspicion that disease is present is classified on an ordinal scale. The BIRADS (American College of Radiology, 1995) classification for mammograms is shown in Table 4.3.

A key difference between qualitative assessments that are measured on ordinal scales and quantitative assessments made on numeric (often continuous)

Table 4.3 *The BIRADS classification of mammograms (American College of Radiology, 1995)*

Category*	Description
1	Cancer not present
2	Benign lesion, no follow-up required
3	Unclear, six month follow-up recommended
4	Possibly malignant, biopsy recommended
5	Highly suspicious for cancer, biopsy recommended

*A category 0 is sometimes used to denote that additional assessments are needed before a final classification can be made

scales is the recognition that different assessors can use the ordinal scale differently. An image considered 'highly suspicious for cancer' (BIRADS = 5) by one radiologist may be considered 'possibly malignant' (BIRADS = 4) by another, even though they both have the same perception of the image. ROC analysis has been extremely popular for use with rating data. Indeed, historically most of the statistical development of ROC analysis has been in this context (Hanley, 1989; Gatsonis *et al.*, 1995). One reason for its popularity is that it purports to disentangle the inherent discriminatory capacity of the test or imaging device from the particular use of the scale by an assessor or rater. We will elaborate on this in the next section.

4.5.2 The latent decision variable model

A popular conceptual framework for the subjective assessment of an image in radiology is as follows. Assume that there is an unobserved latent continuous variable L corresponding to the assessor's perception of the image. The reader has some cut-points or threshold values that correspond to his classification or rating of the image. That is, with Y denoting the reported classification, the idea is that

$$Y = y \quad \Longleftrightarrow \quad c_{y-1} < L < c_y, \qquad y = 1, \ldots, P, \qquad (4.16)$$

where $c_0 = -\infty$ and $c_P = \infty$. The reader classifies the image in the yth category if L falls within the interval corresponding to his implicit definition for the yth category (c_{y-1}, c_y).

Different raters might perceive an image in the same way but classify it differently because their implicit decision thresholds are different. For example, one radiologist might be more conservative than another, in which case his/her decision thresholds for higher categories would be lower (Fig. 4.8).

4.5.3 Identification of the latent variable ROC

Of interest is the ROC curve for L, the latent decision variable. The discriminatory value of an imaging modality is often quantified by how well the distribution of L in diseased subjects is separated from that in the non-diseased population. Although L itself is not observed, it turns out that we can identify $P + 1$ points

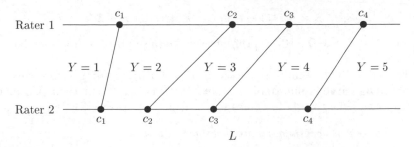

FIG. 4.8. Implicit decision thresholds for two raters with rater 2 more conservative than rater 1

on its ROC curve on the basis of Y. By interpolation we therefore can identity the ROC curve for L.

In particular, since

$$Y \geqslant y \iff L > c_{y-1}$$

and we can identify $P[Y \geqslant y | D = 1]$ and $P[Y \geqslant y | D = 0]$ from the data, we have the true and false positive fractions corresponding to the threshold c_{y-1} for L, which are written as $\text{TPF}(c_{y-1})$ and $\text{FPF}(c_{y-1})$, respectively. The set of $P + 1$ points from the ROC curve for L are therefore identifiable from the distributions of the observed ordinal-valued Y in diseased and non-diseased subjects:

$$\{(\text{FPF}(c_{y-1}), \text{TPF}(c_{y-1})), \ y = 1, \dots, P+1\}. \tag{4.17}$$

If the ROC curve follows a parametric form, then that can dictate how interpolation is performed between observable points. For example, if the binormal model holds then only two non-degenerate points are required, namely $(t_1, \text{ROC}(t_1))$ and $(t_2, \text{ROC}(t_2))$. Since $\text{ROC}(t_k) = \Phi(a + b\Phi^{-1}(t_k))$, the parameters a and b are given by

$$a = \Phi^{-1}(\text{ROC}(t_1)) - b\Phi^{-1}(t_1)$$

and

$$b = \frac{\Phi^{-1}(\text{ROC}(t_2)) - \Phi^{-1}(\text{ROC}(t_1))}{\Phi^{-1}(t_2) - \Phi^{-1}(t_1)}.$$

We note that *some* assumptions are required, though not necessarily parametric ones, in order to recreate the entire ROC curve for L from the observable points, (4.17), derived from Y.

By convention we can assume that L has a standard normal distribution in the non-diseased population. We have seen in Result 4.9 that test results can always be transformed to achieve this. Moreover, because L is only a conceptual construct, this assumption does not impose any real restrictions. It simply provides a convenient scale for the cut-points $(c_1, \dots, c_{P-1})$ and a conceptual scale for L. We therefore can define the cut-points for L as

$$c_k = \Phi^{-1}(1 - t_{k+1}), \quad k = 1, \ldots, P - 1,$$

where $t_k = P[Y \geqslant k | D = 0]$ are the observable false positive fractions based on the discrete Y.

Observable ROC points are shown in Fig. 4.9(b). Assuming that the latent variable ROC curve is binormal, we can construct the latent variable model in Fig. 4.9(a) and the threshold values follow from the observed FPFs.

4.5.4   *Changes in accuracy versus thresholds*

Consider an educational intervention that purports to improve a radiologist's reading of mammograms. We use a subscript A for pre-intervention classification probabilities and B for post-intervention values. Let $\text{FPF}_A(y) = P[Y_A \geqslant y | D = 0]$ and $\text{TPF}_A(y) = P[Y_A \geqslant y | D = 1]$, for $y = 2, \ldots, P$, denote the false and true positive fractions, respectively, before intervention and similarly define $\{(\text{FPF}_B(y), \text{TPF}_B(y)), \ y = 2, \ldots, P\}$ for the post-intervention values. Figure 4.10 displays two possible effects of intervention on the classification probabilities.

In Fig. 4.10(a) the ROC curve passing through the pre-intervention points is the same as that for the post-intervention points. Thus the separation between diseased and non-diseased distributions for L is unchanged by intervention. The inherent accuracy of the test, characterized by the ROC curve for L, remains the same. However, the observed operating points appear to have shifted along the ROC curve. That is, the reader's cut-points that define the observed test result Y appear to have been changed.

In Fig. 4.10(b) the thresholds have also been changed by intervention since the set of FPFs post-intervention are different from those before intervention. In addition, the inherent accuracy of the reader for discriminating between diseased

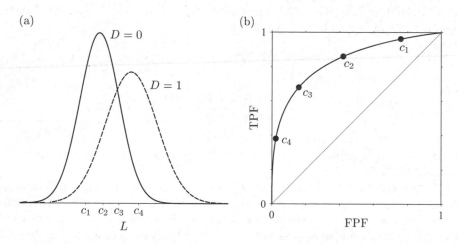

FIG. 4.9. The (a) latent variable model and (b) identifiable points on its ROC curve

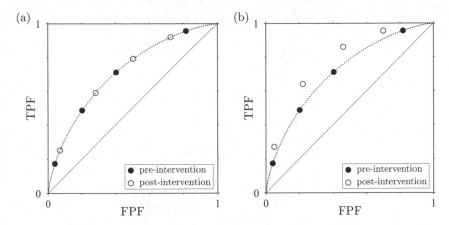

FIG. 4.10. (a) Intervention affects thresholds only and (b) intervention affects accuracy. Shown are (FPF, TPF) points before and after intervention

and non-diseased images is improved by the intervention. The post-intervention ROC curve shows better discrimination than the pre-intervention curve. This may be due to improved perception or judgement about the mammograms. In a sense, in Fig. 4.10(b) the change in the TPF values is not completely accounted for by changes in the thresholds that define the categories for Y, whereas changes in thresholds alone do explain the changes in TPF values in Fig. 4.10(a).

This attribute of the ROC curve for disentangling changes in threshold from changes in inherent accuracy is one reason why ROC curves have been so popular in radiology. The value goes beyond the evaluation of intervention effects. It allows one to compare different imaging modalities, for example, again disentangling differences in inherent accuracy from differences in how the reader interprets the particular classification categories for the imaging modalities.

If ROC curves are similar across multiple readers, though their thresholds and hence their FPFs differ, the ROC framework provides a way of pooling their data appropriately. Simply pooling raw data for Y across readers can lead to false impressions about accuracy (Fig. 4.11). We will return to this later in Chapter 6 (see Result 6.1). For now we simply reiterate that the ROC framework allows one to separate the discriminatory capacity of a test from the way in which the test is used to classify a positive result, and this is particularly useful when raters use the same scale differently. This has long been recognized as an important issue for subjective ordinal tests.

4.5.5   The discrete ROC curve

The latent variable framework with decision thresholds that give rise to observed test results, Y, is an appealing conceptual model that is well established in some settings. However, there are drawbacks to this framework. First and foremost, the latent variable, L, is not a well-defined entity. It does not have an explicit

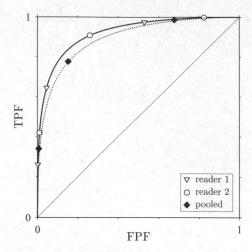

FIG. 4.11. Reader-specific ROC (solid line) and that based on pooled classifications (dotted line)

clinical meaning. Thus interpretations of the ROC curve for L are somewhat dubious. Second, the ROC curve for the latent variable is not fully identifiable. All that is available is the set of discrete observable points on the ROC curve. Points between those observed are based purely on a speculated model. In Fig. 4.12 we show two different ROC curves that have the same observable ROC points. One cannot choose between the two in a scientifically objective fashion.

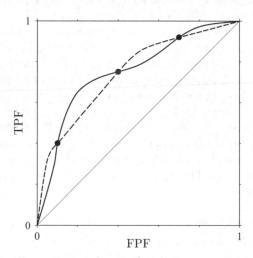

FIG. 4.12. Two different ROC curves for L with the same observable points

Another approach to ROC analysis for ordinal data is to simply define the ROC curve as a discrete function, namely the following set of observed points:

$$\text{ROC} = \{(t_y, \text{ROC}(t_y)),\ y = 1, \ldots, P + 1\}, \tag{4.18}$$

where $t_y = \text{P}[Y \geqslant y | D = 0]$ and $\text{ROC}(t_y) = \text{P}[Y \geqslant y | D = 1]$. (Note that the two points at $y = 1$ and $y = P + 1$ are by definition the corner points $(0, 0)$ and $(1, 1)$.) This definition corresponds exactly to that given in Section 4.2.1 for continuous tests. The difference here is that the domain, the set of possible false positive fractions, is finite.

The mathematical properties of ROC curves noted in Section 4.2.2 also apply, for the most part, to the discrete ROC function. The one exception to this is Result 4.3 which pertains to the slope of the ROC curve, and this is clearly only relevant for continuous ROC curves. A result that we use extensively in Chapter 6 is the identity

$$\text{ROC}(t_y) = S_D\left(S_{\bar{D}}^{-1}(t_y)\right),$$

and we note here that this mathematical result applies equally well to the discrete ROC function as it does to continuous ROC curves (see Result 4.2).

A parametric model can be used for the discrete ROC function. For example,

$$\text{ROC}(t_y) = \Phi\left(a + b\Phi^{-1}(t_y)\right), \quad y = 1, \ldots, P + 1$$

is of the binormal form, with discrete domain $T = \{t_y, y = 1, \ldots, P + 1\}$. For visual display one might even plot the continuous curve, $\{(t, \Phi(a + b\Phi^{-1}(t))), t \in (0, 1)\}$, upon which the ROC points lie. However, this curve is not interpreted as an ROC curve for a continuous decision variable. It serves more as a visual aid to viewing the discrete ROC function associated with the discrete observed decision variable Y. In addition to the parameters $\{a, b\}$ the domain $T = \{t_y, y = 2, \ldots, P\}$ is required to completely characterize the discrete ROC function.

Strictly speaking, two discrete ROC functions differ if their domains differ, even if their points lie on the same smooth curve. Consider again an intervention to improve radiologists' reading and now use the discrete ROC functions before and after the intervention. One might consider a shifting of points along a single curve as 'no effect' if one considers that the changes in FPFs compensate fully for the corresponding changes in TPFs. However, this is a qualitative subjective judgement. In general, such shifts in operating points are of consequence and the intervention cannot be considered as having 'no effect'. Indeed, there are settings where one would consider such intervention effects to be important. For example, in Fig. 4.13 the intervention appears to decrease the false positive fractions with little loss in the true positive fractions, indicating a net benefit. The discrete ROC framework requires one to consider the FPFs that are attainable with the test (i.e. the domain for the discrete ROC function) in addition to the trade-offs between the true and false positive fractions. For a discrete test both should be considered, whereas for a continuous test all FPF values in the range $(0, 1)$ are attainable so only the trade-off is of concern.

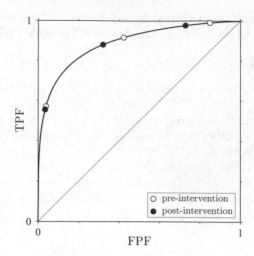

FIG. 4.13. Shifting points along a single ROC curve may constitute an important effect on accuracy for a discrete test

4.5.6   Summary measures for the discrete ROC curve

The ROC summary indices defined in Section 4.3 apply to continuous curves and hence can be applied to the ROC curves that arise from the latent decision variable framework. In contrast, for discrete ROC functions the summary measures do not apply directly. A summary of the ROC points can be calculated by first joining the points either with a curved parametric function or linearly, and then calculating the ROC summary measure relative to the resulting curve. These are not summary measures for ROC curves and are somewhat hard to interpret in general. Interestingly, when a linear interpolation between points is employed, the area under that curve has the interpretation as the probability of correctly ordering diseased and non-diseased observations. We conclude this section on discrete ROC functions with the following result, the proof of which is left as an exercise.

Result 4.10

When the test result is discrete, the area under the ROC function based on linear interpolation between points (AUC) is

$$\mathrm{AUC} = \mathrm{P}[Y_D > Y_{\bar{D}}] + \frac{1}{2}\mathrm{P}[Y_D = Y_{\bar{D}}].\qquad\blacksquare$$

4.6   Concluding remarks

In this chapter the ROC curve has been defined and both its conceptual attributes and mathematical properties were described. A variety of ROC summary indices were defined (Table 4.2), which can be viewed essentially as measures of distance between two distributions. Next, the form of the ROC curve for normally distributed test results, Y_D and $Y_{\bar{D}}$, was investigated. This binormal curve applies much more generally, in fact, to any setting where a monotone transformation h exists that renders $h(Y_D)$ and $h(Y_{\bar{D}})$ normally distributed. For ordinal-valued tests the binormal curve is often assumed to hold for an underlying latent decision variable. The classic latent decision variable framework was presented. Finally, an alternative perspective for dealing with ordinal-valued tests was presented. That is, to consider a discrete ROC function for observed test results. This definition corresponds directly with that for the ROC curve for continuous tests. The next two chapters will proceed to describe how statistical inference about the ROC curve and its summary indices can be accomplished.

The ROC curve is the most popular approach for describing the accuracy of a continuous or ordinal-valued test. It naturally generalizes notions of false and true positive fractions to non-binary tests. In Chapters 2 and 3 predictive values (PPV, NPV) and diagnostic likelihood ratios (DLR$^+$, DLR$^-$) were discussed as alternatives to the classification probabilities (FPF, TPF) for describing test accuracy. To date these entities have not been generalized for use with continuous or ordinal-valued tests. Obvious analogies of the ROC curve are plots of PPV versus NPV and DLR$^+$ versus DLR$^-$ for tests dichotomized at various thresholds. We have not found them to be particularly insightful in the few applications that we have explored. Nevertheless, they may be useful in some settings and may be worthy of further development. At this point statistical methods for making inferences about such curves are not available. We consider only ROC curves in this book, for which inference is reasonably well developed.

The ROC curve has been popular for a long time in radiology and psychometric research, where test results are quantified on ordinal scales. Their application to continuous-valued tests is emphasized here, in part perhaps because of my experience with applications to biomarkers and other quantitative tests. A recent text by Zhou et al. (2002) on the other hand emphasizes ordinal-valued tests and complements the discussion here. Interestingly, a recent trend in radiology reading studies is to solicit a continuous-valued probabilistic assessment of the image from the reader, rather than an ordinal classification. This may provide more sensitive tools for research. Moreover, problems with unstable numerical procedures for statistical inference about ordinal ratings that arise because of low-frequency categories may be alleviated by replacing ordinal classifications with quantitative assessments.

The ROC curve provides a description of separation between distributions, and we have alluded to the fact that they might also be useful in clinical trials research. The area under the ROC curve is already used in a variety of non-diagnostic testing settings, albeit with different nomenclature. See Hauck et al. (2000) for application in clinical trials, Fine and Bosch (2000) for application in toxicology, Foulkes and DeGruttola (2002) for application in evaluating drug resistance in HIV research, and literature in material science where it is known as the reliability index (Simonoff et al., 1986). The use of the ROC curve itself may be worth exploring too in these settings.

Although the scale for the AUC of a test is $(0.5, 1.0)$, surprisingly small differences in the AUC can correspond to substantial differences in ROC curves. Suppose, for example, that two ROC curves are equal over most of $(0, 1)$ but differ by 0.3 over the interval $(0.0, 0.2)$. This very substantial difference in test accuracy corresponds to a difference of only 0.06 in the AUCs. The magnitudes of AUC that constitute adequate diagnostic accuracy and the magnitudes of change in AUC that constitute substantial change in performance will need careful consideration in practice. Swets (1988) presents representative values of the AUC from a variety of application areas within and outside of diagnostic testing, including materials testing, weather forecasting and polygraph testing.

The binormal ROC curve described in Section 4.4 is the classic parametric model. Other parametric forms for the ROC curve are easy to motivate too (see Exercise 6, for example). One weakness of the binormal model, $\text{ROC}(t) = \Phi(a + b\Phi^{-1}(t))$, mentioned in Section 4.4.1, is that it is not concave over the whole domain $t \in (0, 1)$. The requirement that ROC curves be concave or 'proper' (Egan, 1975) is reasonable in most practical settings. In particular, if the likelihood ratio function is monotone in Y, then the ROC curve for Y is the same as that for $\mathcal{LR}(Y)$, which is concave (see the implications following from Result 4.4). Parametric models for the ROC curve that constrain it to be 'proper' have been proposed. The interested reader is referred to Dorfman et al. (1997) and Metz and Pan (1999).

4.7   Exercises

1. Show that the likelihood ratio of the likelihood ratio is the likelihood ratio, $\mathcal{LR}(\mathcal{LR}(Y)) = \mathcal{LR}(Y)$. See Green and Swets (1966, p. 26).

2. Prove rigorously Result 4.5, which gives the operating point for a test in order to minimize the cost associated with disease in the population. Can you provide intuitive reasoning for why the result makes sense?

3. Interpret the AUC for the ROC curve in Example 4.2 that displays the difference in outcome measures for patients in the two arms of the tobramycin clinical trial.

4. Show that Kraemer's standardized sensitivity and specificity values are invariant to the labeling of D and Y for a dichotomous test. Suppose that the test is dichotomous but that disease is measured on a continuum. What do you think of plotting the QROC curve that dichotomizes D according to varying thresholds?

5. Show that for the binormal ROC curve, $\text{ROC}(t) = \Phi(a + b\Phi^{-1}(t))$, the symmetry point summary index is $\text{Sym} = \Phi(a/(1 + b))$. Contrast this expression with that for the binormal AUC summary index.

6. Show that if the distributions of Y_D and $Y_{\bar{D}}$ follow a location-scale model $Y_D = \mu_D + \sigma_D \varepsilon$ and $Y_{\bar{D}} = \mu_{\bar{D}} + \sigma_{\bar{D}} \varepsilon$, where ε has survivor function, S_0,

with mean 0 and variance 1, then the ROC curve has the form $\text{ROC}(t) = S_0(a + bS_0^{-1}(t))$. Indicate how this generalizes the binormal ROC form derived in Result 4.7.

7. Consider a test which has a discrete unordered outcome with P categories. Each possible subset of categories can be used to define a positive result and hence defines an (FPF, TPF) point in ROC space. This yields a cloud of points rather than a curve.

    (i) Use the likelihood ratio principle to define an ordered categorical test result.

    (ii) In what sense is it optimal?

    (iii) Generate data and illustrate your answers.

8. Provide a proof of Result 4.10 using either a formal mathematical or informal pictorial approach.

9. An ordinal test has the following distributions for diseased and non-diseased observations:

Category	Non-diseased	Diseased
1	25%	2%
2	30%	3%
3	20%	5%
4	10%	10%
5	15%	80%

    (i) Calculate the observed (FPF, TPF) points.

    (ii) Plot them on a normal probability scale. Does the binormal model appear to hold?

    (iii) Estimate the binormal intercept and slope using a simple linear fit to the points.

Exercise 1:

$g_{(i)}$ denots polf of L

$Y = LR^{-1}(\ell)$

$g(\ell) = f(LR^{-1}(\ell)) \left| \frac{dLR^{-1}(\ell)}{d\ell} \right|$

$LR(\ell) = \frac{g_D(\ell)}{g_{\bar{D}}(\ell)} = \frac{f_D(LR^{-1}(\ell)) \left| \frac{dLR^{-1}(\ell)}{d\ell} \right|}{f_{\bar{D}}(LR^{-1}(\ell)) \left| \frac{dLR^{-1}(\ell)}{d\ell} \right|}$

$= f_D / f_{\bar{D}}$

5

ESTIMATING THE ROC CURVE

5.1 Introduction

5.1.1 *Approaches*

Having defined the ROC curve and explored some of its properties in the previous chapter, we turn now in this chapter to statistical methodology for making inferences about the ROC curve from data. We consider three approaches for estimating the ROC curve and its summary indices. The first is to apply non-parametric empirical methods to the data to obtain the empirical ROC curve, from which empirical summary measures can be calculated. Empirical methods have been the popular choice for settings involving continuous test results. The second approach uses statistical models for the distributions of Y_D and $Y_{\bar{D}}$. Parameters in these distributions are estimated and the induced ROC curve together with summary measures are calculated. Although it is a natural approach, this 'modeling distributions' approach is not popular, in part because it requires strong assumptions about the forms of the distributions of test results. This is an unnecessary nuisance because the ROC curve is concerned only with the relationship between the distributions of Y_D and $Y_{\bar{D}}$, and not with the distributions themselves. The third approach rectifies this nuisance by modeling the ROC curve, rather than the probability distributions, as a smooth parametric function. The parameters are estimated from the rankings of the test results for diseased and non-diseased subjects. We call it the 'parametric distribution-free' approach, since the ROC curve is parameterized but only the ranks and not the test results themselves enter into the estimation. This general approach has been most popular for use with tests that have ordinal results. We will also present the recent development of such methods for continuous data.

Although the focus in this chapter is on estimating ROC curves, many of the concepts will be relevant for material discussed in the next chapter on fitting regression models to ROC curves. In particular, the distinction between the conceptual frameworks for the 'parametric distributions' and 'parametric distribution-free' approaches will arise again in Chapter 6. We lay the groundwork for that discussion here.

5.1.2 *Notation and assumptions*

We assume that the data can be represented as test results for n_D cases and $n_{\bar{D}}$ controls:

$$\{Y_{Di}, \; i = 1, \ldots, n_D\} \quad \text{and} \quad \{Y_{\bar{D}j}, \; j = 1, \ldots, n_{\bar{D}}\}.$$

Either cohort or case-control sampling can be used to obtain the data. We assume that the $\{Y_{Di}, i = 1, \ldots, n_D\}$ are identically distributed with the population survivor function $S_D(y) = P[Y_{Di} \geqslant y]$, and similarly $\{Y_{\bar{D}j}, j = 1, \ldots, n_{\bar{D}}\}$ are such that $S_{\bar{D}}(y) = P[Y_{\bar{D}j} \geqslant y]$. In words, we assume that Y_{Di} and $Y_{\bar{D}j}$ are selected randomly from the populations of test results associated with diseased and non-diseased states, respectively.

In some specific instances, notably when deriving asymptotic distribution theory, we will assume that observations are independent. However, for the most part, observations may be dependent, as is the case for example when an individual subject gives rise to several test results. It is important to remember that the distributions and ROC curves we consider are interpreted as marginal entities, in the sense that they pertain to S_D and $S_{\bar{D}}$ defined above for randomly selected Y_{Di} and $Y_{\bar{D}j}$, respectively. There may be statistical clustering in the population due to correlation between multiple observations from an individual, say. Such clustering does not interfere with estimation of the (marginal) ROC curve itself, $\text{ROC}(t) = S_D(S_{\bar{D}}^{-1}(t))$, but must be accommodated when assessing sampling variability of the estimates. These same considerations arose in Chapters 2 and 3 with regards to statistical inference about binary tests. In summary, there are three key points to keep in mind:

(i) probabilities and hence accuracy parameters are defined in a marginal probability sense;

(ii) estimation of parameters ignores correlation between data records; and

(iii) sampling variability in parameter estimates explicitly acknowledges clustering.

5.2 Empirical estimation

5.2.1 The empirical estimator

The empirical estimator of the ROC curve simply applies the definition of the ROC curve to the observed data. Thus, for each possible cut-point c, the empirical true and false positive fractions are calculated as follows:

$$\hat{\text{TPF}}(c) = \sum_{i=1}^{n_D} I[Y_{Di} \geqslant c] / n_D,$$

$$\hat{\text{FPF}}(c) = \sum_{j=1}^{n_{\bar{D}}} I[Y_{\bar{D}j} \geqslant c] / n_{\bar{D}}.$$

The empirical ROC curve is a plot of $\hat{\text{TPF}}(c)$ versus $\hat{\text{FPF}}(c)$ for all $c \in (-\infty, \infty)$. Equivalently, we can write the empirical ROC, $\hat{\text{ROC}}_e$, as

$$\hat{\text{ROC}}_e(t) = \hat{S}_D(\hat{S}_{\bar{D}}^{-1}(t)), \tag{5.1}$$

where $\hat{S}_D$ and $\hat{S}_{\bar{D}}$ are the empirical survivor functions for Y_D and $Y_{\bar{D}}$, respectively (see Result 4.2).

Observe that, technically, $\hat{\text{ROC}}_e$ is a discrete function because $\hat{\text{FPF}}(c)$ can only take values in $\{0, 1/n_{\bar{D}}, 2/n_{\bar{D}}, \ldots, 1\}$. In practice, points are joined linearly. If there are no ties in the data, this yields an increasing step function with vertical jumps of size $1/n_D$ corresponding to test results for observations from diseased test units and horizontal jumps of size $1/n_{\bar{D}}$ corresponding to observations for non-diseased units. Ties between test results for diseased observations and ties between non-diseased observations yield larger jumps. Ties between results for diseased and non-diseased observations produce diagonal line segments corresponding to simultaneous vertical and horizontal jumps.

Example 5.1

For illustration consider the following data from the ovarian cancer gene expression array study described in Section 1.3.6. The relative gene expression intensities of a particular gene are displayed below for 23 non-diseased ovarian tissues and 30 ovarian tumor tissues.

Normal tissues:	0.442, 0.500, 0.510, 0.568, 0.571, 0.574, 0.588, 0.595, 0.595, 0.595, 0.598, 0.606, 0.617, 0.628, 0.641, 0.641, 0.680, 0.699, 0.746, 0.793, 0.884, 1.149, 1.785
Cancer tissues:	0.543, 0.571, 0.602, 0.609, 0.628, 0.641, 0.666, 0.694, 0.769, 0.800, 0.800, 0.847, 0.877, 0.892, 0.925, 0.943, 1.041, 1.075, 1.086, 1.123, 1.136, 1.190, 1.234, 1.315, 1.428, 1.562, 1.612, 1.666, 1.666, 2.127

If the expression of this gene is different in the two tissue types, this could possibly lead to insights about the biology of ovarian cancer. To see the separation in the distributions of the expression levels between the two tissues, the empirical ROC curve is shown in Fig. 5.1. The separation is substantial but not complete. From a technical point of view, we see that the curve depends only on the ranks of the data. Also, observe the larger jumps at tied data points or where points with adjacent ranks are derived from the same tissue type. Diagonal components occur where there are ties between tumor and non-tumor data. ∎

The empirical ROC curve is a function only of the ranks of the data. That is, it only depends on the relative orderings of the test results and their status as being from diseased or non-diseased individuals. It is, therefore, invariant to strictly increasing transformations of the data. This is a basic property of the ROC function (Result 4.1), but, as we will see, it is not shared by all estimators of the ROC curve.

We next consider sampling variability for the empirical ROC curve. Sampling variability can be assessed from several points of view. One can consider the threshold c as fixed and assess variability in the corresponding point on the ROC curve $(\text{FPF}(c), \text{TPF}(c))$. Alternatively, one can consider the false positive fraction, t, as fixed and consider sampling variability in $\hat{\text{ROC}}_e(t)$, which occurs in a vertical direction only. Yet another point of view is to consider the true

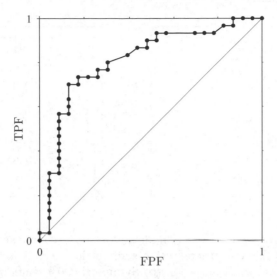

FIG. 5.1. The empirical ROC curve for the ovarian gene expression data

positive fraction as fixed and consider sampling variability of the ROC curve in the horizontal direction. Finally, one can consider the entire curve and quantify variability with confidence bands, say. We will consider these various points of view in the next two sections.

5.2.2 *Sampling variability at a threshold*

In this section we consider the threshold c as fixed. Writing the binary test result, $Y(c) = I[Y \geqslant c]$, as that which dichotomizes the test at threshold c, we see that the corresponding point on $\hat{\mathrm{ROC}}_e$ is $(\hat{\mathrm{FPF}}(c), \hat{\mathrm{TPF}}(c))$, the estimated false and true positive fractions for the binary test $Y(c)$. A joint confidence region for $(\mathrm{FPF}(c), \mathrm{TPF}(c))$ can be constructed using methods described in Section 2.2.2 for binary tests, when observations are independent. A rectangle or a series of rectangles corresponding to different thresholds shows variability in Fig. 5.2(a) (Hilgers, 1991; Campbell, 1994). When observations are dependent, confidence intervals and corresponding rectangles can be found using bootstrap resampling (Efron and Tibshirani, 1993).

5.2.3 *Sampling variability of* $\hat{\mathrm{ROC}}_e(t)$

In this section we assume that the test result is measured on a continuous scale. Suppose that, instead of fixing the threshold, we fix the false positive fraction t. The value of $\hat{\mathrm{ROC}}_e(t)$ can be thought of as being calculated in two steps. First, we determine the estimated threshold corresponding to t. Second, we determine the proportion of diseased observations with test values above that threshold. The first step uses only data for the $n_{\bar{D}}$ non-diseased observations to calculate the threshold, while the second uses only data for the n_D diseased observations

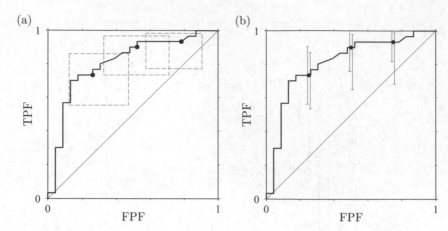

FIG. 5.2. Ovarian gene expression data. (a) 90% confidence rectangles for
$(\mathrm{FPF}(c), \mathrm{TPF}(c))$ constructed using symmetric intervals for the logit transform at $c = 0.57,\ 0.61$ and 0.70. (b) Symmetric 90% confidence intervals for
$\mathrm{ROC}(t)$ at $t = 0.25,\ 0.50$ and 0.75 based on normality for $\hat{\mathrm{ROC}}_e(t)$, and
asymmetric intervals based on normality for $\mathrm{logit}\,\hat{\mathrm{ROC}}_e(t)$

and the estimated threshold.

We see therefore that sampling variability in both non-diseased and diseased
observations enters into variability in $\hat{\mathrm{ROC}}_e(t)$. Schematically we write

$$
t \;\xrightarrow{\;n_{\bar{D}}\;}\; \left(\begin{array}{c} \text{estimated threshold} \\ = \hat{S}_{\bar{D}}^{-1}(t) \end{array} \right) \;\xrightarrow{\;n_D\;}\; \left(\begin{array}{c} \hat{\mathrm{ROC}}_e(t) \\ = \hat{S}_D\big(\hat{S}_{\bar{D}}^{-1}(t)\big) \end{array} \right).
$$

A formal derivation of the asymptotic variability in $\hat{\mathrm{ROC}}_e(t)$ was provided
as early as 1950 by Greenhouse and Mantel (1950). A more recent derivation
that includes uniform consistency and weak convergence of the whole process
$\{\hat{\mathrm{ROC}}_e(t),\ t \in (0,1)\}$ can be found in Hsieh and Turnbull (1996). We provide
the result and a heuristic proof for a single point $(t, \mathrm{ROC}(t))$. The following result
only concerns the case of independent continuous test results, with f_D and $f_{\bar{D}}$
denoting the probability densities for Y_D and $Y_{\bar{D}}$, respectively, and $\mathcal{LR} = f_D/f_{\bar{D}}$
is assumed to be finite. The proof is given at the end of this chapter in Section
5.8.

Result 5.1

For large values of n_D and $n_{\bar{D}}$, we can approximate the distribution of $\hat{\mathrm{ROC}}_e(t)$
by a normal distribution with mean $\mathrm{ROC}(t)$ and variance given by

$$
\mathrm{var}\left(\hat{\mathrm{ROC}}_e(t)\right) = \frac{\mathrm{ROC}(t)\,(1 - \mathrm{ROC}(t))}{n_D} + \left(\frac{f_D(c^*)}{f_{\bar{D}}(c^*)}\right)^2 \frac{t(1-t)}{n_{\bar{D}}}, \qquad (5.2)
$$

where $c^* = S_{\bar{D}}^{-1}(t)$. ∎

The result is interesting in that it breaks down the variance of $\hat{\text{ROC}}_e(t)$ into the sum of two components. The second component derives from estimating the threshold $S_{\bar{D}}^{-1}(t)$, while the first derives from the binomial variability of the estimated true positive fraction when the threshold is fixed. We noted the contribution of both sources of variability earlier in this section. Now we see that they contribute in an additive fashion.

For t close to 0 or 1 the variance is small—a consequence of the ROC function being close to 0 or 1 at those points. We recognize that the likelihood ratio $\mathcal{L}\text{R}(c^*) = f_D(c^*)/f_{\bar{D}}(c^*)$ enters into the variance. Recall that this represents the slope of the ROC curve at t (Result 4.3). Thus the larger the slope, the higher the variability in $\hat{\text{ROC}}_e(t)$. This makes sense on an intuitive level. If a small change in t has a large effect on $\text{ROC}(t)$, then the component of variability due to estimating the threshold should be emphasized.

The next point of view from which to investigate sampling variability in $\hat{\text{ROC}}_e$ is to consider horizontal variability at a fixed point on the vertical scale. Suppose that we fix the true positive fraction at v and consider the estimate of the corresponding false positive fraction $\hat{\text{ROC}}_e^{-1}(v)$. We see that $\hat{\text{ROC}}_e^{-1}(v) = \hat{S}_{\bar{D}}(\hat{S}_D^{-1}(v))$. Therefore, by analogy with Result 5.1 and by exchanging the labels for D and $\bar{D}$, we can approximate its variance with

$$\text{var}\left(\hat{\text{ROC}}_e^{-1}(v)\right) = \frac{\text{ROC}^{-1}(v)(1 - \text{ROC}^{-1}(v))}{n_{\bar{D}}} + \left(\frac{f_{\bar{D}}(c^*)}{f_D(c^*)}\right)^2 \frac{v(1-v)}{n_D}. \quad (5.3)$$

This yields horizontal variability in the empirical ROC curve.

Observe that, if (t, v) is a point on the ROC with $v = \text{ROC}(t)$ and $t = \text{ROC}^{-1}(v)$ and we write $\hat{v}(t) = \hat{\text{ROC}}_e(t)$ and $\hat{t}(v) = \hat{\text{ROC}}_e^{-1}(v)$, then the above result and Result 5.1 indicate that

$$\text{var}\left(\hat{v}(t)\right) = \left(\frac{f_D(c^*)}{f_{\bar{D}}(c^*)}\right)^2 \text{var}\left(\hat{t}(v)\right). \quad (5.4)$$

An intuitive explanation is that a small perturbation in $\hat{t}$ induces a perturbation in $\hat{v}$ which is magnified by approximately $\partial\text{ROC}(t)/\partial t$ for large n. This same reasoning suggests that the above relationship between $\text{var}(\hat{v}(t))$ and $\text{var}(\hat{t}(v))$ will hold when other estimators of the ROC curve are used. Henceforth, we just consider variability of estimators of $v = \text{ROC}(t)$ in the vertical direction and use (5.4) for variability in the horizontal direction.

Example 5.1 (continued)

Figure 5.2(b) displays confidence intervals based on the asymptotic normal approximation to the distribution of $\hat{\text{ROC}}_e(t)$. Symmetric confidence intervals centered at $\hat{\text{ROC}}_e(t)$ are of the form

$$\hat{\text{ROC}}_e(t) \pm \Phi^{-1}\left(1 - \frac{\alpha}{2}\right)\sqrt{\hat{\text{var}}\left(\hat{\text{ROC}}_e(t)\right)}.$$

The variance was estimated by substituting estimates for $\text{ROC}(t)$ and the likelihood ratio at c^*. We used kernel density estimates for f_D and $f_{\bar{D}}$.

As with any binomial proportion, symmetric intervals work poorly when t or ROC(t) are close to 0 or 1. We have found that asymmetric confidence intervals based on the logistic transform have better properties, and these are also displayed in Fig. 5.2. These confidence intervals, derived from symmetric intervals for logit ROC(t) that are of the form

$$\text{logit}\,\hat{\text{ROC}}_e(t) \pm \Phi^{-1}\left(1 - \frac{\alpha}{2}\right) \frac{\sqrt{\hat{\text{var}}(\hat{\text{ROC}}_e(t))}}{\hat{\text{ROC}}_e(t)\left(1 - \hat{\text{ROC}}_e(t)\right)},$$

are then back-transformed to yield the corresponding intervals for ROC(t). ∎

Up to this point, we have considered confidence intervals for ROC(t) (or $\hat{\text{ROC}}^{-1}(v)$) at a fixed point t (or v). The final point of view for assessing sampling variability is to consider the entire curve. A confidence band for the ROC curve can be based on the results of Hsieh and Turnbull (1996) concerning the asymptotic distribution of the process $\hat{\text{ROC}}_e(\cdot)$. For completeness we state the result.

Result 5.2

Let B_1 and B_2 be two independent Brownian bridges. That is, mean 0 Gaussian processes with variance–covariance function, $\text{cov}(B_k(t), B_k(s)) = s(1 - t)$ for $s \leqslant t$. Then, if the empirical ROC curve is based on independent observations, the following approximation holds:

$$\sqrt{\frac{n_D n_{\bar{D}}}{n_D + n_{\bar{D}}}}\left(\hat{\text{ROC}}_e(t) - \text{ROC}(t)\right)$$
$$\doteq \lambda^{1/2} B_1(\text{ROC}(t)) + (1 - \lambda)^{1/2} \frac{f_D(S_{\bar{D}}^{-1}(t))}{f_{\bar{D}}(S_{\bar{D}}^{-1}(t))} B_2(t),$$

where $\lambda = n_{\bar{D}}/(n_D + n_{\bar{D}})$. ∎

Unfortunately, confidence bands based on the nonparametric ROC curve are not used widely in practice yet. Standard procedures for calculating bands using the asymptotic theory are not in place. One approach is to base the calculation on the distribution of $\sup |\hat{\text{ROC}}_e(t) - \text{ROC}(t)|$, which can be calculated using Result 5.2. Observe that estimates of the likelihood ratio function, $\mathcal{LR} = f_D/f_{\bar{D}}$, over the support of $Y_{\bar{D}}$ are required for this. One can assume that $\mathcal{LR}$ is a smooth function and use kernel density estimates for f_D and $f_{\bar{D}}$. Alternatively, one could model the risk function $\text{P}[D = 1|Y]$ with standard logistic regression methods, and use the relationship between $\mathcal{LR}$ and the risk function (see also Result 9.4) to derive the estimated $\mathcal{LR}$ function:

$$\log \mathcal{LR} = \log\left(\frac{f_D(y)}{f_{\bar{D}}(y)}\right) = \log\left(\frac{\text{P}[D = 1|Y = y]}{\text{P}[D = 0|Y = y]}\right) - \log\left(\frac{\text{P}[D = 1]}{\text{P}[D = 0]}\right)$$
$$= \text{logit}\,\text{P}[D = 1|Y = y] - \text{logit}\,\text{P}[D = 1].$$

Further work is needed to develop and evaluate procedures for constructing nonparametric confidence bands for the ROC curve.

We have mentioned four points of view from which variability in the non-parametric ROC curve can be assessed. Which should be reported in practice? In circumstances where a particular threshold is specified in advance, a joint confidence region for the associated (FPF, TPF) is appropriate. For example, since 4.0 ng/ml and 10.0 ng/ml are standard thresholds for defining a positive PSA test for prostate cancer, the rectangular confidence region discussed in Section 5.2.2 should be reported. However, when a specific threshold is not specified in advance, confidence intervals or confidence bands for the ROC curve seem more relevant. If one can specify a particular FPF that would be acceptable for the test, then a vertical confidence interval for the associated TPF would be of interest. In Chapter 8 we discuss the design of studies that seek to estimate $\text{ROC}(\text{FPF}_0)$, where FPF_0 is some minimally acceptable value, and use the pointwise confidence intervals based on $\hat{\text{ROC}}_e(\text{FPF}_0)$. Similarly, if a minimally acceptable TPF value, TPF_0, can be specified, the confidence interval for $\text{ROC}^{-1}(\text{TPF}_0)$ would be of interest. However, if the purpose of the analysis is simply to describe the ROC curve, a confidence band seems most appropriate.

5.2.4 *The empirical AUC and other indices*

Estimates of the ROC summary measures described in Chapter 4 can be calculated by applying their definitions to the empirical curve, $\hat{\text{ROC}}_e$. Thus

$$\hat{\text{AUC}}_e = \int_0^1 \hat{\text{ROC}}_e(t)\,\mathrm{d}t\,,$$

$$\text{p}\hat{\text{AUC}}_e(t_0) = \int_0^{t_0} \hat{\text{ROC}}_e(t)\,\mathrm{d}t\,,$$

$$\vdots$$

and so forth. There is an interesting relationship between some of these estimators and two-sample rank test statistics. The best known result is the following.

Result 5.3

The area under the empirical ROC curve is the Mann–Whitney U-statistic

$$\hat{\text{AUC}}_e = \sum_{j=1}^{n_{\bar{D}}} \sum_{i=1}^{n_D} \left\{ I\left[Y_{Di} > Y_{\bar{D}j}\right] + \frac{1}{2} I\left[Y_{Di} = Y_{\bar{D}j}\right] \right\} \Big/ n_D n_{\bar{D}}. \tag{5.5}$$

Proof The proof is evident from the plot shown in Fig. 5.3. Suppose first that there are no ties between diseased and non-diseased observations. Then the horizontal step in $\hat{\text{ROC}}_e$ corresponding to the point $Y_{\bar{D}j}$ adds a rectangular area of size $(1/n_{\bar{D}}) \times \hat{\text{TPF}}(Y_{\bar{D}j}) = (1/n_{\bar{D}}) \times \sum_i I[Y_{Di} > Y_{\bar{D}j}]/n_D$. The result then follows because $\hat{\text{AUC}}_e$ is the sum (over j) of these $n_{\bar{D}}$ rectangular areas. When there are ties, between $Y_{\bar{D}j}$ and Y_{Di} say, this adds a triangular area with horizontal side of length $1/n_{\bar{D}}$ and vertical side of length $1/n_D$, i.e. an area of $1/2(1/n_D \times 1/n_{\bar{D}})I[Y_{Di} = Y_{\bar{D}j}]$.   ∎

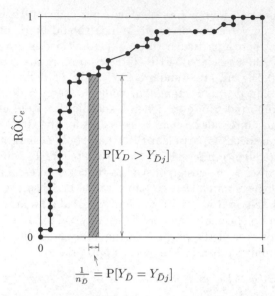

$$\frac{1}{n_{\bar{D}}} = P[Y_{\bar{D}} = Y_{\bar{D}j}]$$

FIG. 5.3. Proof of Result 5.3

The Kolmogorov–Smirnov two-sample rank statistic for comparing the distributions of Y_D and $Y_{\bar{D}}$ is also a summary of $\hat{ROC}_e$ (Gail and Green, 1976). In particular, it is written as $\max |\hat{S}_D(c) - \hat{S}_{\bar{D}}(c)|$, or by transforming to $t = \hat{S}_{\bar{D}}(c)$ an equivalent representation is

$$\hat{KS} = \max |\hat{ROC}_e(t) - t|.$$

This is the Kolmogorov–Smirnov ROC measure described in Section 4.3.3 applied to the empirical ROC curve. That is, it is the maximum vertical or horizontal distance from $\hat{ROC}_e$ to the 45° line. Incidentally, Campbell (1994) uses this statistic as the basis for constructing a confidence band for the ROC curve.

Other two-sample rank statistics can also be written in terms of functionals of $\hat{ROC}_e$ (Exercise 1). Since such statistics summarize the distance between $\hat{S}_D$ and $\hat{S}_{\bar{D}}$ on the rank scale and $\hat{ROC}_e$ provides the same information, the existence of a relationship is not too surprising.

5.2.5 *Variability in the empirical AUC*

The variance of a summary measure of $\hat{ROC}_e$ is often complicated and in practice we frequently apply the bootstrap to calculate confidence intervals. This strategy is also a valid approach when data are clustered, as occurs when individuals contribute multiple data records to the analysis, in which case the resampling unit is at the cluster level.

Analytic expressions for asymptotic variance have been derived for the $\hat{AUC}_e$ measure when observations are independent. The following result can be found in Hanley and McNeil (1982). It is proven by calculating the expectations of the cross-products of the summations involved, in a first principles expansion of the variance. This and subsequent discussions assume that there are no ties between diseased and non-diseased observations, so that formula (5.5) simplifies to $\hat{\text{AUC}}_e = \sum_{j=1}^{n_{\bar{D}}} \sum_{i=1}^{n_D} I[Y_{Di} \geqslant Y_{\bar{D}j}]/n_D n_{\bar{D}}$.

Result 5.4

The following result holds:

$$\text{var}\left(\hat{\text{AUC}}_e\right) = (n_D n_{\bar{D}})^{-1} \left\{ \text{AUC}(1 - \text{AUC}) + (n_D - 1)(Q_1 - \text{AUC}^2) \right.$$
$$\left. + (n_{\bar{D}} - 1)(Q_2 - \text{AUC}^2) \right\}, \quad (5.6)$$

where

$$Q_1 = \text{P}[Y_{Di} \geqslant Y_{\bar{D}j}, Y_{Di'} \geqslant Y_{\bar{D}j}],$$
$$Q_2 = \text{P}[Y_{Di} \geqslant Y_{\bar{D}j}, Y_{Di} \geqslant Y_{\bar{D}j'}]$$

and $(Y_{Di}, Y_{Di'})$ and $(Y_{\bar{D}j}, Y_{\bar{D}j'})$ denote random pairs of observations from the diseased and non-diseased populations, respectively.   ∎

Observe that the first component in expression (5.6) is of order $1/(n_D n_{\bar{D}})$, whereas the second and third components are of order $1/n_{\bar{D}}$ and $1/n_D$, respectively, so that in large samples the contribution of the first component is minimal. Empirical estimates of each component are easily calculated to yield a variance estimator.

An alternative representation of the asymptotic variance was derived by De-Long et al. (1988) and some interesting insights into it are given by Hanley and Hajian-Tilaki (1997). See Bamber (1975) for yet another approximation to the variance. We develop the DeLong et al. (1988) derivation here, in part because it allows us to introduce the notion of a *placement value*, which we consider to be fundamental to ROC analysis. Placement values will be further discussed later in Section 5.5.2, and especially in relation to ROC regression methods in Chapter 6, but it is useful to define the concept here as it relates to the empirical AUC.

If we consider the distribution of $Y_{\bar{D}}$ as the reference distribution, then the placement value for a test result y in the non-diseased distribution is defined as

$$\text{non-disease placement value} = \text{P}[Y_{\bar{D}} \geqslant y] = S_{\bar{D}}(y), \quad (5.7)$$

the non-disease survivor function at y. The placement value concept is a familiar way of standardizing measurements relative to an appropriate reference distribution. For example, a child's weight is standardized for age and gender by reporting his/her placement value in a healthy population of children of the same age and gender (Hamill et al., 1977). We speak of his/her weight percentile being at say the 75th percentile for age and gender, which means that his/her placement value is 0.25. The placement value literally marks the placement of y in the reference distribution. The empirical placement value is $\hat{S}_{\bar{D}}(y)$.

One interpretation for the ROC curve is that it is the distribution function for diseased subjects of their non-disease placement values:

$$P[S_{\bar{D}}(Y_D) \leqslant t] = S_D(S_{\bar{D}}^{-1}(t)) = \text{ROC}(t).$$

Similarly, the empirical ROC can be written as the empirical distribution of the empirical non-disease placement value (Exercise 2). Interestingly, the AUC (and $\hat{\text{AUC}}_e$) can be written in terms of the expectations of placement values. Indeed, it is easy to see that $E(S_{\bar{D}}(Y_D)) = 1 - \text{AUC}$, and

$$\hat{\text{AUC}}_e = 1 - \sum_{i=1}^{n_D} \frac{\hat{S}_{\bar{D}}(Y_{Di})}{n_D}.$$

In an analogous fashion, using the distribution of Y_D as the reference distribution, the placement for y in the diseased population is defined as

$$\text{disease placement value} = P[Y_D \geqslant y] = S_D(y), \qquad (5.8)$$

and the empirical placement value is defined by $\hat{S}_D(y)$. It quantifies the proportion of diseased observations that exceed y. We can also write $\hat{\text{AUC}}_e$ as the sample average of empirical disease placement values for non-disease observations:

$$\hat{\text{AUC}}_e = \sum_{j=1}^{n_{\bar{D}}} \frac{\hat{S}_D(Y_{\bar{D}j})}{n_{\bar{D}}}. \qquad (5.9)$$

The DeLong *et al.* (1988) expression for $\text{var}(\hat{\text{AUC}}_e)$ is in terms of the variability of placement values. This is given in the next result, which is proven in Section 5.8. See Result 8.2 for further elaboration.

Result 5.5

In large samples

$$\text{var}(\hat{\text{AUC}}_e) \doteq \frac{\text{var}\,(S_{\bar{D}}(Y_D))}{n_D} + \frac{\text{var}\,(S_D(Y_{\bar{D}}))}{n_{\bar{D}}}, \qquad (5.10)$$

which is estimated with

$$\frac{\hat{\text{var}}(\hat{S}_{\bar{D}}(Y_{Di}))}{n_D} + \frac{\hat{\text{var}}(\hat{S}_D(Y_{\bar{D}j}))}{n_{\bar{D}}},$$

where $\hat{\text{var}}$ denotes the sample variances for the empirical placement values. ∎

This result, due to DeLong *et al.* (1988), provides a nice computational algorithm for estimating the variance of $\hat{\text{AUC}}_e$, and an interpretation for it. The variance is directly a function of the variability in the placement values of diseased observations within the non-diseased reference distribution and of the non-diseased within the reference distribution of diseased observations. A confidence interval for the AUC can be based on

$$A\hat{U}C_e \pm \Phi^{-1}\left(1 - \frac{\alpha}{2}\right)\sqrt{\text{v\^{a}r}(A\hat{U}C_e)}.$$

However, since the scale for the AUC is restricted to $(0, 1)$, an asymmetric confidence interval that guarantees an interval in $(0, 1)$ might be preferred. Using a logistic transform, a confidence interval for logit $AUC = \log(AUC/(1 - AUC))$ is

$$\log\left(\frac{A\hat{U}C_e}{1 - A\hat{U}C_e}\right) \pm \Phi^{-1}\left(1 - \frac{\alpha}{2}\right)\frac{\sqrt{\text{var}(A\hat{U}C_e)}}{A\hat{U}C_e(1 - A\hat{U}C_e)}.$$

In Section 5.2.7 we illustrate the calculation of these confidence intervals on data from the pancreatic cancer biomarker study. Table 5.1 displays the results of some simulation studies to evaluate the performance of 90% symmetric and asymmetric confidence intervals based on $A\hat{U}C_e$. It appears that coverage is quite good for both confidence intervals, even with 50 test results for diseased and non-diseased subjects. With smaller sample sizes the intervals based on logit $A\hat{U}C_e$ perform better than the symmetric intervals, at least for more accurate tests, i.e. those with values of AUC close to 1. Obuchowski and Lieber (2002) discuss *exact* confidence intervals when AUCs are close to 1. In practice we recommend that the *logit*-based transform be used for calculating confidence intervals.

5.2.6 *Comparing empirical ROC curves*

Summary indices are often used to compare ROC curves (Shapiro, 1999). The most commonly used statistic for comparing two ROC curves when test results are continuous is based on the difference in empirical AUC estimates. We denote

Table 5.1 *Coverage of 90% confidence intervals for the AUC using symmetric intervals based on asymptotic normality of $A\hat{U}C_e$ and asymmetric intervals based on asymptotic normality of logit $A\hat{U}C_e$. The DeLong et al. (1988) variance estimator was used. Data were generated from the binormal model* $\text{ROC}(t) = \Phi(a + b\Phi^{-1}(t))$, *with* $n_D = n_{\bar{D}}$

$n_D = n_{\bar{D}}$	AUC = 0.777 ($a = 1, b = 0.85$)		AUC = 0.927 ($a = 2, b = 0.95$)	
	Symmetric	Asymmetric	Symmetric	Asymmetric
20	0.88	0.92	0.83	0.90
50	0.89	0.90	0.88	0.91
100	0.91	0.91	0.89	0.90
200	0.90	0.90	0.89	0.90
500	0.90	0.91	0.90	0.90

the two curves by ROC_A and ROC_B, use the same indexing A and B for the AUCs, and write

$$\Delta A\hat{U}C_e = A\hat{U}C_{Ae} - A\hat{U}C_{Be}.$$

The null hypothesis $H_0 : \text{ROC}_A = \text{ROC}_B$ is tested by comparing the value of $\Delta A\hat{U}C_e / \sqrt{\{\text{var}(\Delta A\hat{U}C_e)\}}$ with a standard normal distribution.

If data for the two ROC curve estimates are derived from independent samples, then

$$\text{var}(\Delta A\hat{U}C_e) = \text{var}(A\hat{U}C_{Ae}) + \text{var}(A\hat{U}C_{Be})$$

and estimators of the two variance components have already been described. Frequently, data for the two curves will be derived from the same sample. For example, when they represent different tests and the study design is paired. In this case the variance of $\Delta A\hat{U}C_e$ is derived using the DeLong *et al.* (1988) method.

Result 5.6

For a paired study design, with test results $\{(Y_{Di,A}, Y_{Di,B}), i = 1, \ldots, n_D\}$ for n_D independent diseased observations and $\{(Y_{\bar{D}j,A}, Y_{\bar{D}j,B}), j = 1, \ldots, n_{\bar{D}}\}$ for $n_{\bar{D}}$ independent non-diseased observations, in large samples

$$\text{var}(\Delta A\hat{U}C_e) \doteq \frac{\text{var}\left(S_{\bar{D},A}(Y_{D,A}) - S_{D,B}(Y_{D,B})\right)}{n_D}$$
$$+ \frac{\text{var}\left(S_{D,A}(Y_{\bar{D},A}) - S_{D,B}(Y_{\bar{D},B})\right)}{n_{\bar{D}}},$$

which is estimated with

$$\frac{\hat{\text{var}}\left(\hat{S}_{\bar{D},A}(Y_{Di,A}) - \hat{S}_{\bar{D},B}(Y_{Di,B})\right)}{n_D} + \frac{\hat{\text{var}}\left(\hat{S}_{D,A}(Y_{\bar{D}j,A}) - \hat{S}_{D,B}(Y_{\bar{D}j,B})\right)}{n_{\bar{D}}}. \quad \blacksquare$$

This result is analogous to that of Result 5.5, with the difference in placement values taking the role of the placement values themselves. Given the representation of the $A\hat{U}C_e$ as an average of placement values, we can write the difference as an average of *differences* in placement values:

$$\Delta A\hat{U}C_e = A\hat{U}C_{Ae} - A\hat{U}C_{Be}$$
$$= \sum_{i=1}^{n_D} \frac{\hat{S}_{\bar{D},A}(Y_{Di,A}) - \hat{S}_{\bar{D},B}(Y_{Di,B})}{n_D}$$
$$= \sum_{j=1}^{n_{\bar{D}}} \frac{\hat{S}_{D,A}(Y_{\bar{D}j,A}) - \hat{S}_{D,B}(Y_{\bar{D}j,B})}{n_{\bar{D}}},$$

and so the result follows. Moreover, the interpretation of the $\Delta A\hat{U}C_e$ statistic afforded by this representation is interesting. For each diseased observation, the placement of the first test result in the non-diseased reference distribution for that test is compared with the analogous standardization of the second test result. Alternatively, we can think of the two test results for a non-diseased observation as being compared after being appropriately standardized by the reference distribution provided by the diseased observations.

Nonparametric statistics other than differences in $\mathrm{A\hat{U}C}_e$ can be used to compare ROC curves. Statistics based on differences in empirical estimates of partial AUCs have been advocated (Wieand et al., 1989) for settings where interest is focused on FPF or TPF values in subintervals of (0,1). Asymptotic variance expressions are more complex for partial AUC test statistics and we instead bootstrap the data for inference. Any of the other summary indices, estimated empirically, can likewise be used as the basis for a nonparametric comparison of ROC curves, with resampling methods employed for formal statistical inference.

5.2.7   *Illustration: pancreatic cancer biomarkers*

Example 5.2

Consider data from the pancreatic cancer biomarker study described in Section 1.3.3. The empirical ROC curves are shown in Fig. 5.4. They indicate that discrimination between patients with pancreatic cancer and the controls is better achieved with the CA-19-9 marker than it is with CA-125. The empirical AUC statistics are 0.86 and 0.71, respectively. Using the logit transform a 95% confidence interval for the AUC associated with CA-19-9 is $(0.79, 0.91)$, while that for

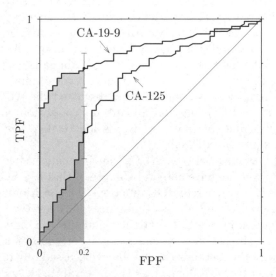

FIG. 5.4. Empirical ROC curves for two pancreatic cancer biomarkers. Data from Wieand *et al.* (1989). Shown also are 90% confidence intervals for ROC(*t*) at $t = 0.20$

CA-125 is $(0.61, 0.79)$. The difference, $\Delta A\hat{U}C_e$, which is based on paired data, is statistically significantly different from 0 ($p = 0.007$).

Wieand *et al.* (1989) focused their comparison on the range of FPFs below 0.20. This region is shaded in Fig. 5.4. Confidence intervals for the ROC at $t = 0.20$ are shown. A test for equality of the ROC curves based on $\hat{ROC}_{Ae}(0.2) - \hat{ROC}_{Be}(0.2)$ and percentiles of its bootstrap distribution rejects the null hypothesis of equality ($p = 0.04$). We also undertook a comparison that accumulated differences over the whole range $t \in (0, 0.2)$. The empirical partial AUC statistics are 0.14 for CA-19-9 and 0.05 for CA-125. The difference is highly significantly different from 0 based on the bootstrap distribution ($p < 0.001$). Accumulating the difference over the range of interest leads to a stronger conclusion than that based on the ROC value at $t = 0.2$ alone. ∎

5.2.8 *Discrete ordinal data ROC curves*

Empirical methods can also be used to estimate discrete ROC functions for tests with ordinal results. The $\hat{ROC}_e$ is defined as in Section 5.2.1, except that linear interpolation between estimated ROC points $\{(\hat{FPF}(y), \hat{TPF}(y)), y = 1, \ldots, P\}$ is not performed. That is, we recognize the discreteness of the ROC function and its finite discrete domain. Sampling variability of the ROC point associated with any fixed threshold can be assessed, as described in Section 5.2.2. Rectangular joint confidence intervals for $(FPF(y), TPF(y))$ can be displayed for each y.

However, the methods of Section 5.2.3 that describe sampling variability for points on the curve, $ROC(t)$, do not seem to be relevant when the test result is discrete. In finite samples one will not know what false positive fractions are attainable with a discrete test. Hence fixing t and making inferences about $ROC(t)$ is not feasible in the same way that it is for a continuous test.

The empirical AUC index is usually calculated using a linear interpolation between ROC points and the trapezoidal rule. Although, it is not interpreted as an area under the curve (because the ROC for an ordinal test is a discrete function, not a curve), we have nevertheless discussed the AUC as a summary index for the discrete ROC function and its interpretation as the probability $P[Y_D \geqslant Y_{\bar{D}}]$. The empirical value, $A\hat{U}C_e$, is identical to the Mann–Whitney U-statistic, as was proven in Result 5.3.

Similarly, comparisons between AUCs can be made using the methods of Section 5.2.6. However, we have noted in Chapter 4 that it is not always sensible to compare AUCs for two discrete ROC functions. The positioning of the attained FPFs dramatically affect the AUCs. Differences between two AUCs may exist that are simply caused by the fact that their domains are different.

In summary, empirical methods can be used for continuous or ordinal test result data. A few of the methods that we have discussed rely on the ROC curve being defined as a curve with domain on the interval $(0, 1)$, and therefore apply only to ROCs for continuous tests. This completes our discussion of empirical nonparametric methods for estimating and comparing ROC curves. In the next sections we consider methods that impose some structure on the ROC curve, first by modeling the distributions of Y_D and $Y_{\bar{D}}$ and then by modeling only the ROC curve.

5.3 Modeling the test result distributions

5.3.1 *Fully parametric modeling*

One approach for estimating the ROC curve, $\mathrm{ROC}(t) = S_D(S_{\bar{D}}^{-1}(t))$, is to estimate the constituent distribution functions parametrically and to calculate the induced ROC curve estimate. Suppose that we model each distribution as a parametric distribution with parameters α and γ for the non-diseased and diseased populations, respectively:

$$S_{\bar{D}}(y) = S_{\alpha,\bar{D}}(y) \quad \text{and} \quad S_D(y) = S_{\gamma,D}(y). \tag{5.11}$$

We estimate α from non-disease test result data and γ from the disease test result data. The resultant ROC estimate is

$$\hat{\mathrm{ROC}}_{\hat{\alpha},\hat{\gamma}}(t) = S_{\hat{\gamma},D}\left(S_{\hat{\alpha},\bar{D}}^{-1}(t)\right).$$

A standard error for $\hat{\mathrm{ROC}}(t)$ can be calculated using the variance of $(\hat{\alpha}, \hat{\gamma})$ and the delta method. Observe that, if the parameters are estimated with maximum likelihood methods, then the ROC estimate will be fully efficient, assuming that the models (5.11) are correctly specified. We illustrate this fully parametric approach with an example.

Example 5.3

Let us suppose that $Y_D \sim \mathrm{N}(\mu_D, \sigma_D^2)$ and $Y_{\bar{D}} \sim \mathrm{N}(\mu_{\bar{D}}, \sigma_{\bar{D}}^2)$. In the notation of (5.11), $\alpha = (\mu_{\bar{D}}, \sigma_{\bar{D}}^2)$ and $\gamma = (\mu_D, \sigma_D^2)$. Estimating the means and variances with their sample values, denoted by $\hat{\mu}_D$, $\hat{\mu}_{\bar{D}}$, $\hat{\sigma}_D^2$ and $\hat{\sigma}_{\bar{D}}^2$, yields estimates of the distribution functions for Y_D and $Y_{\bar{D}}$. We know then from Result 4.7 that the induced estimate of the ROC curve is

$$\hat{\mathrm{ROC}}(t) = \Phi\left(\frac{\hat{\mu}_D - \hat{\mu}_{\bar{D}}}{\hat{\sigma}_D} + \left(\frac{\hat{\sigma}_{\bar{D}}}{\hat{\sigma}_D}\right)\Phi^{-1}(t)\right).$$

Moreover, the AUC summary index is estimated with

$$\hat{\mathrm{AUC}} = \Phi\left(\frac{\hat{\mu}_D - \hat{\mu}_{\bar{D}}}{\sqrt{\hat{\sigma}_D^2 + \hat{\sigma}_{\bar{D}}^2}}\right).$$

Wieand *et al.* (1989) provides an explicit analytic expression for the variance of the $\hat{\mathrm{AUC}}$ that is derived using the delta method. ∎

To compare ROC curves in this framework one cannot simply compare parameters. The same ROC curve can result from different pairs of constituent test result distributions. Consider, for example, that if $Y_{\bar{D}}^* \sim \mathrm{N}(\mu_D + C, \sigma_D^2)$ and

$Y_{\bar{D}}^* \sim N(\mu_{\bar{D}} + C, \sigma_{\bar{D}}^2)$ for some constant C in the illustration of Example 5.3, then the ROC curve is unchanged although the parameters of the distributions are not the same. So comparing parameters of the distributions α_A versus α_B and γ_A versus γ_B for two curves indexed by A and B does not achieve a comparison of ROC curves. Rather, a summary ROC index can be estimated for each ROC curve, and compared. Wieand *et al.* (1989) evaluated the comparison of two ROC curves, with the difference in AUC indices estimated with the fully parametric normal models described above. They compared this approach with that based on the nonparametric $\Delta A\hat{U}C_e$. As expected, the parametric model-based comparison is more efficient but, interestingly, only slightly so.

The fully parametric method makes strong assumptions about the forms of the distributions, S_D and $S_{\bar{D}}$. More flexible parametric distributional forms than Gaussian might be considered (see Chapter 6). In the next section we describe a model that is flexible in that it is only partly parameterized.

5.3.2 *Semiparametric location-scale models*

Consider the semiparametric location-scale model for the test results:

$$Y_{Di} = \mu_D + \sigma_D \varepsilon_i ,$$
$$Y_{\bar{D}j} = \mu_{\bar{D}} + \sigma_{\bar{D}} \varepsilon_j , \tag{5.12}$$

where ε are independent, mean 0 and variance 1 random variables with survivor function S_0. When S_0 is standard normal this corresponds to the normal model described in Example 5.3. In this section we leave S_0 unspecified.

Under the location-scale model the ROC curve is written as

$$\text{ROC}(t) = S_0 \left((\mu_{\bar{D}} - \mu_D)/\sigma_D + (\sigma_{\bar{D}}/\sigma_D) S_0^{-1}(t) \right), \tag{5.13}$$

as was indicated in Chapter 4 (Exercise 6). Estimates of the location-scale parameters can be calculated using sample means and variances. A nonparametric estimate of S_0 can then be based on the residuals

$$\left\{ (Y_{Di} - \hat{\mu}_D)/\hat{\sigma}_D, \ i = 1, \ldots, n_D ; \quad (Y_{\bar{D}j} - \hat{\mu}_{\bar{D}})/\hat{\sigma}_{\bar{D}}, \ j = 1, \ldots, n_{\bar{D}} \right\}.$$

The empirical survivor function

$$\hat{S}_0(y) = \frac{1}{n_D + n_{\bar{D}}} \left\{ \sum_i I \left[\frac{Y_{Di} - \hat{\mu}_D}{\hat{\sigma}_D} \geqslant y \right] + \sum_j I \left[\frac{Y_{\bar{D}j} - \hat{\mu}_{\bar{D}}}{\hat{\sigma}_{\bar{D}}} \geqslant y \right] \right\}$$

is a consistent estimator of S_0. Thus

$$\hat{\text{ROC}}(t) = \hat{S}_0 \left((\hat{\mu}_{\bar{D}} - \hat{\mu}_D)/\hat{\sigma}_D + (\hat{\sigma}_{\bar{D}}/\hat{\sigma}_D) \hat{S}_0^{-1}(t) \right)$$

is an estimator of the ROC curve at t.

The ROC model (5.14) is semiparametric because the form of the function $S_0(\cdot)$ is not specified. We therefore call $\hat{\text{ROC}}(t)$ the semiparametric ROC estimator and refer to Pepe (1998) for further discussion.

Asymptotic distribution theory for the estimator does not appear to be available at this time, so inference is made with resampling techniques instead. Again, confidence intervals for ROC(t), for the entire curve, and for summary indices can be made with resampling methods. Comparisons between ROC curves can be based on summary indices calculated from the estimated curves.

Example 5.4

For the pancreatic cancer data we transformed the marker values CA-125 and CA-19-9 to a natural logarithmic scale and calculated means and standard deviations as $(\mu_D, \sigma_D, \mu_{\bar{D}}, \sigma_{\bar{D}}) = (3.26, 0.99, 2.67, 0.78)$ for CA-125 and $(5.42, 2.34, 2.47, 0.86)$ for CA-19-9. The semiparametric ROC curve estimates are shown in Fig. 5.5. These are more smooth than the empirical ROC curves.

At $t = 0.20$, 90% confidence intervals for ROC(t) based on the bootstrap distribution for $\hat{ROC}(t)$ are shown. Interestingly, these are slightly wider than the intervals shown in Fig. 5.4 for the empirical estimator. The explanation is that resampling methods generate wider confidence intervals than those based on asymptotic theory. Intervals produced from $\hat{ROC}_e(t)$, but using the bootstrap rather than asymptotic theory, gave rise to intervals close to or wider than the semiparametric ones in Fig. 5.5.

A formal comparison of the ROC curves at $t = 0.2$ can be based on the difference of the semiparametric ROC estimates. The p value from the bootstrap distribution using 5000 bootstrapped samples is 0.002. ∎

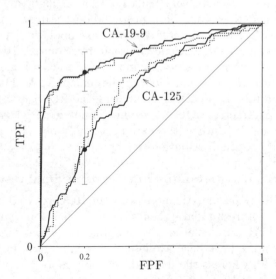

FIG. 5.5. ROC curves for the pancreatic cancer biomarkers estimated with semiparametric location-scale models for log transformed data (solid lines). Empirical ROC curves are included (dotted lines). Shown also are 90% confidence intervals for ROC(t) at $t = 0.20$

5.3.3 *Arguments against modeling test results*

In my opinion, the idea of modeling test results in order to estimate the ROC curve is somewhat unnatural. The basic rationale for the ROC curve is to quantify the relationship between S_D and $S_{\bar{D}}$ in a distribution-free manner. Thus, by definition, the ROC curve is invariant to monotone increasing transformations of the test result measurement. However, the parametric and semiparametric methods that model the test results in order to estimate the ROC are not invariant to such data transformations. They are not distribution free in the sense that the ROC curve relies on the distributional forms for both $S_{\bar{D}}$ and S_D, not just on their relationship or separation. There is a sort of philosophical rift between the ROC estimator produced by the 'modeling test result' approach and the basic framework of ROC analysis.

Modeling the test results can be restated as modeling the quantiles of S_D and $S_{\bar{D}}$. Estimation of the parameters is dictated by the bulk of the data. This implies that data towards the middle of the distributions are used to make inferences about quantiles at the extremes. One should be cautious about such model-based extrapolation in general.

The main advantages of the approach that models test results over the empirical methods described in Section 5.2 are that (i) the ROC curves are more smooth, and (ii) there is potential for increased statistical efficiency. On the latter point, the gain for estimating or comparing AUCs does not appear to be substantial (Wieand *et al.*, 1989; Dodd, 2001). We suspect that efficiency may be gained for estimates of ROC(t), particularly at low or high values of t. However, as mentioned earlier, there may be concerns about estimates derived from the modeling approach being heavily influenced by extrapolation. The usual statistical tension between bias and efficiency arises in this context. Regarding the first point, smooth ROC curves are certainly more aesthetically appealing. Moreover, smoothness is a reasonable assumption. In the remainder of this chapter we discuss the third and final approach to estimating the ROC curve. These methods produce smooth parametric ROC curves but do not require that test result distributions are modeled. Rather, they are based only on the ranks of the data. We call it the parametric distribution-free approach.

5.4 Parametric distribution-free methods: ordinal tests

We now consider fully parametric models for the ROC curve that do not require modeling of the test result data themselves. We begin our discussion of the parametric distribution-free methods with applications to ordinal test results in mind. Such techniques have been available for ordinal data for a long time and are well established, whereas the methods are only more recently developed for continuous tests. Recall from Chapter 4 that one can adopt the latent decision variable (LDV) framework for ordinal tests or one can decide not to. We adopt this framework initially.

5.4.1 *The binormal latent variable framework*

Let L denote the underlying continuous decision variable for a single reader (multiple readers will be considered in the next chapter). Recall that the binormal model assumes that $\text{ROC}(t) = \Phi(a + b\Phi^{-1}(t))$ and in the LDV framework, by convention, we assume that $L \sim \text{N}(0,1)$ in the non-diseased population, although this imposes no real structure on the data. With this convention, the ROC curve form implies that in the diseased population $L \sim \text{N}(a/b, (1/b)^2)$. The unknown parameters to be estimated are (a, b) and the threshold values $c_1, \ldots, c_{P-1}$, which yield the ordinal test results, Y, through the relation

$$Y = y \quad \Longleftrightarrow \quad c_{y-1} < L < c_y.$$

Observe that the only real assumption made in this framework concerns the parametric form of the ROC curve. To estimate the parameters we have data $\{Y_{Di}, i = 1, \ldots, n_D; \ Y_{\bar{D}j}, j = 1, \ldots, n_{\bar{D}}\}$. The data give rise to a likelihood, assuming that observations are independent. (The independence assumption can be relaxed, as we have discussed.) The likelihood contribution for a non-disease observation with $Y_{\bar{D}j} = y$ is

$$P[Y_{\bar{D}} = y] = P[L_{\bar{D}} < c_y] - P[L_{\bar{D}} < c_{y-1}]$$
$$= \Phi(c_y) - \Phi(c_{y-1}).$$

For a disease observation with $Y_{Di} = y$ the likelihood is

$$P[Y_D = y] = P[L_D < c_y] - P[L_D < c_{y-1}]$$
$$= \Phi(bc_y - a) - \Phi(bc_{y-1} - a).$$

The log likelihood function is then constructed as

$$\sum_{i=1}^{n_D} \log P[Y_D = Y_{Di}] + \sum_{j=1}^{n_{\bar{D}}} \log P[Y_{\bar{D}} = Y_{\bar{D}j}] \qquad (5.14)$$

and is maximized with respect to the parameters $\{a, b, c_1, \ldots, c_{P-1}\}$. Standard theory for likelihood-based estimation implies that these estimates, $\{\hat{a}, \hat{b}, \hat{c}_1, \ldots, \hat{c}_{P-1}\}$, are asymptotically normally distributed and statistically efficient. The second derivative of the log likelihood is the variance–covariance matrix of the estimates if observations are independent. Otherwise, a robust variance–covariance matrix can be constructed.

The estimated ROC curve is $\text{ROC}(t) = \Phi(\hat{a} + \hat{b}\Phi^{-1}(t))$, a smooth binormal curve with domain $(0,1)$. The standard error for $\hat{a} + \hat{b}\Phi^{-1}(t)$ is

$$\text{se} = \left\{ \text{var}(\hat{a}) + \left(\Phi^{-1}(t)\right)^2 \text{var}(\hat{b}) + 2\Phi^{-1}(t)\,\text{cov}(\hat{a}, \hat{b}) \right\}^{1/2}. \qquad (5.15)$$

Corresponding confidence limits for $a + b\Phi^{-1}(t)$, written as

$$\hat{a} + \hat{b}\Phi^{-1}(t) \pm \Phi^{-1}(1 - \alpha)\,\text{se},$$

give rise to pointwise confidence limits for $\text{ROC}(t) = \Phi(a + b\Phi^{-1}(t))$. Ma and Hall (1993) discuss the construction of confidence bands for the ROC curve with the Working–Hotelling approach, which was developed originally for regression lines.

Example 5.5

Consider the rating data for the study of liver metastasis (Section 1.3.4) described by Tosteson and Begg (1988). The discriminatory capacity of ultrasound for detecting liver metastasis in colon cancer was studied by having a radiologist read 48 images from subjects without metastasis and 22 with metastasis. The numbers of images rated in each of five categories are displayed below.

		Rating				
Hepatic metastasis	1	2	3	4	5	Total
No	27	17	2	1	1	$n_{\bar{D}} = 48$
Yes	4	1	2	2	13	$n_D = 22$

The maximum likelihood fit of the binormal parameters are: $\hat{c}_1 = 0.17$, $\hat{c}_2 = 1.29$, $\hat{c}_3 = 1.76$, $\hat{c}_4 = 2.24$, with intercept $\hat{a} = 1.02$ (se $= 0.34$) and slope $\hat{b} = 0.35$ (se $= 0.16$). The fitted ROC curve is displayed in Fig. 5.6.

Also output from this analysis are the estimated AUC $= \Phi(\hat{a}/\sqrt{\{1 + \hat{b}^2\}}) = 0.83$ and its standard error, se $= 0.074$, calculated with the delta method. ∎

Dorfman and Alf (1969) are generally cited for developing the maximum likelihood algorithm for fitting the binormal LDV model to rating data. Ogilvie

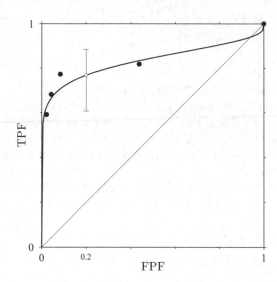

FIG. 5.6. Binormal ROC curve fitted using maximum likelihood methods to the liver metastasis ultrasound data (Tosteson and Begg, 1988). Also shown is a 90% confidence interval for ROC(0.2)

and Creelman (1968) developed the same algorithm but using a logistic form for the ROC, namely $\mathrm{logit\,ROC}(t) = a + b\,\mathrm{logit}(t)$, and assuming that $L_{\bar{D}}$ has a mean 0 and variance 1, logistic distribution. The Dorfman and Alf algorithm is by far the most popular way of approximating an ROC curve with rating data.

5.4.2 *Fitting the discrete binormal ROC function*

Suppose now that we consider the ROC for ordinal data as a discrete function. A parametric relationship between the $P - 1$ ROC points can be assumed, for example,
$$\mathrm{ROC}(t) = \Phi(a + b\Phi^{-1}(t)), \quad t \in \{t_2, \ldots, t_P\}.$$

It turns out that the Dorfman and Alf (1969) algorithm also yields the maximum likelihood parameter estimates in this case. Let us revisit the development of Section 5.4.1 but without the latent decision variable L.

In the discrete ROC function framework, the parameters to be estimated are the attainable false positive fractions $\{t_2, \ldots, t_P\}$ and $\{a, b\}$. We order the false positive fractions from largest to smallest so that $t_2 > \cdots > t_P$. Let us reparameterize t_k as $c_{k-1} = \Phi^{-1}(1 - t_k)$, that is $c_{k-1} = -\Phi^{-1}(t_k)$. For a non-disease observation with $Y_{\bar{D}j} = y$ we have

$$\mathrm{P}[Y_{\bar{D}} = y] = t_y - t_{y+1} = \Phi(c_y) - \Phi(c_{y-1}).$$

For a disease observation with $Y_{Di} = y$ we have

$$\begin{aligned}
\mathrm{P}[Y_D = y] &= \mathrm{ROC}(t_y) - \mathrm{ROC}(t_{y+1}) \\
&= \Phi\left(a + b\Phi^{-1}(t_y)\right) - \Phi\left(a + b\Phi^{-1}(t_{y+1})\right) \\
&= \Phi\left(a - bc_{y-1}\right) - \Phi\left(a - bc_y\right) \\
&= \Phi\left(-a + bc_y\right) - \Phi\left(-a + bc_{y-1}\right).
\end{aligned}$$

The likelihood $\prod_i \mathrm{P}[Y_D = Y_{Di}] \prod_j \mathrm{P}[Y_{\bar{D}} = Y_{\bar{D}j}]$ can be maximized in order to estimate the parameters.

Observe that the likelihood contributions, $\mathrm{P}[Y_{\bar{D}} = y]$ and $\mathrm{P}[Y_D = y]$ in the discrete ROC framework, are exactly the same as those developed in the LDV model. Hence the estimation of parameters and inference follows in the same way for both approaches. We summarize this in the next result.

Result 5.7

The likelihood-based ROC curve parameter estimates derived from the latent decision variable framework are the same as those derived from the discrete ROC function framework for ordinal tests.   ∎

The difference with the LDV analysis is only in how the parameters are interpreted. The fitted discrete ROC function consists of a finite number of points, whereas in the LDV framework the whole curve with domain $(0, 1)$ is considered as the output of the analysis.

The fitted discrete ROC function for the liver metastasis data is displayed in Fig. 5.7. In this discrete ROC setting the values of $\{c_1, \ldots, c_{P-1}\}$ are interpreted simply as transformations of the attainable false positive fractions, not as threshold values associated with a latent decision variable. Moreover, the fitted values, though related by the parametric form $\text{ROC}(t_k) = \Phi(\hat{a} + \hat{b}\Phi^{-1}(t_k))$, are not considered to be points on an ROC curve.

5.4.3 *Generalizations and comparisons*

Although the binormal form is the classic parametric form for ROC curves, other parametric forms can be adopted. We mentioned the logistic form above (Ogilvie and Creelman, 1968). Any parametric form adopted can be fitted using ordinal data likelihood methods in exactly the same fashion as described in the previous section.

One can fit two (or more) ROC curves (or functions), such as $\text{ROC}_1(t) = \Phi(a_1 + b_1\Phi^{-1}(t))$ and $\text{ROC}_2(t) = \Phi(a_2 + b_2\Phi^{-1}(t))$, by solving the corresponding estimating equations simultaneously. If individuals contribute several observations, as in a paired design of two tests, say, then the parameter estimates for the different curves will be correlated. The robust variance–covariance for $(\hat{a}_1, \hat{b}_1, \hat{a}_2, \hat{b}_2)$ will account for the clustering.

Traditionally, AUC summary indices are used as the basis for comparing binormal ROC curves. The standard error of the difference

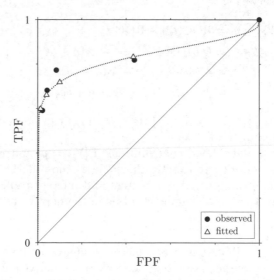

FIG. 5.7. The discrete ROC function of binormal form fitted using maximum likelihood methods to the liver metastasis study data (open triangles). Also shown is the empirical discrete ROC function (solid circles)

$$\hat{\mathrm{AUC}}_1 - \hat{\mathrm{AUC}}_2 = \Phi\left(\frac{\hat{a}_1}{\sqrt{1 + \hat{b}_1^2}}\right) - \Phi\left(\frac{\hat{a}_2}{\sqrt{1 + \hat{b}_2^2}}\right)$$

is calculated with the delta method. Alternative summary indices can likewise be used. Metz and Kronman (1980) suggest that instead of comparing summary indices (which in fact compare summary indices rather than ROC curves), the fitted ROC parameters can be compared. A chi-squared test statistic with two degrees of freedom under the null hypothesis, $H_0: a_1 = a_2,\ b_1 = b_2$, is

$$\begin{pmatrix} \hat{a}_1 - \hat{a}_2 \\ \hat{b}_1 - \hat{b}_2 \end{pmatrix}' \sum{}^{-1} \begin{pmatrix} \hat{a}_1 - \hat{a}_2 \\ \hat{b}_1 - \hat{b}_2 \end{pmatrix}, \tag{5.16}$$

where $\sum$ is the variance–covariance matrix for $(\hat{a}_1 - \hat{a}_2, \hat{b}_1 - \hat{b}_2)$ and the prime denotes vector transpose.

5.5 Parametric distribution-free methods: continuous tests

We return now to tests with results on a continuous scale. Earlier in this chapter we discussed nonparametric empirical methods for making statistical inferences. We then discussed an approach that modeled the distributions of test results in order to arrive at the induced estimator of the ROC curve. We now consider a strategy that is intermediate between these two. In particular, we will parameterize the form of the ROC curve but we will not make any additional assumptions about the distributions of test results. It is similar to the methods described for ordinal tests in these regards.

5.5.1 *LABROC*

Metz *et al.* (1998*b*) described a parametric distribution-free approach that is an extension of that described in Section 5.4 for ordinal data. They note that one way to deal with continuous data is to categorize them into a finite number of pre-defined categories and to apply methods for fitting parametric ROC curves to ordinal data. Observe that the ordinal data methods only make assumptions about the parametric form for the ROC curve. No assumptions are made about the false positive fractions $t_2, \ldots, t_P$. In other words, no assumptions are made about $S_{\bar{D}}$, the survivor function for the discrete test result $Y_{\bar{D}}$.

The theoretical asymptotic properties of the estimator require that the categories are pre-defined. Nevertheless, Metz *et al.* (1998*b*) proposed that one could define the categories using the observed data, and still apply the ordinal data estimating procedures to calculate slope and intercept parameters for the binormal curve. In particular, all test result values that correspond to vertical or horizontal jumps in the empirical ROC are used to define categories. As an illustration, consider 4 disease and 6 non-disease observations

$$\{Y_{\bar{D}1}, Y_{\bar{D}2}, Y_{\bar{D}3}, Y_{\bar{D}4}, Y_{\bar{D}5}, Y_{\bar{D}6}, Y_{D1}, Y_{D2}, Y_{D3}, Y_{D4}\}.$$

If the data are pooled and arranged in increasing order while maintaining their disease/non-disease labels, say

$$Y_{\bar{D}1}, Y_{\bar{D}2}, Y_{\bar{D}3}, Y_{D1}, Y_{D2}, Y_{\bar{D}4}, Y_{\bar{D}5}, Y_{D3}, Y_{D4}, Y_{\bar{D}6},$$

then the values $Y_{\bar{D}6}, Y_{D3}, Y_{\bar{D}4}, Y_{D1}, Y_{\bar{D}1}$ provide threshold values for defining categories. Having defined categories, the data are categorized accordingly and the Dorfman and Alf (1969) algorithm is applied. The procedure, originally called LABROC, is publicly available as a Fortran program, which implements it for the conventional binormal models. It is part of the ROCKIT set of procedures developed at the University of Chicago by Metz and colleagues.

The maximum likelihood method of LABROC is not completely rigorous from a theoretical point of view because the number of parameters, notably the category defining cut-points, increases with the sample size. Metz *et al.* (1998*b*) provide results of simulation studies that support the validity of the methods (however, see also Example 5.6). Moreover, relative to a procedure that modeled the test result distributions, the LABROC procedure was highly efficient. This is encouraging. However, computationally the LABROC approach can be demanding. The procedure must estimate the false positive fractions corresponding to each threshold simultaneously with the binormal ROC intercept and slope parameters. This entails inversion of a $(P + 1) \times (P + 1)$ matrix which will be large if P is large. Since P increases with the sample size, this can quickly become a problem. To reduce this computational burden, adjacent categories can, if necessary, be combined. Metz *et al.* (1998*b*) present an *ad hoc* but satisfactory algorithm. Interestingly, although collapsing categories amounts to a loss of information, the reduction in efficiency appears to be small.

The most appealing feature of LABROC is that it is distribution free. It requires modeling only the ROC curve and no other assumptions. The estimation only involves the ranks of the test results. Therefore, the LABROC estimator of the ROC curve is invariant to monotone increasing data transformations, and in that sense it reflects a fundamental property of true ROC curves. Another rank-based estimator is described in the next section.

5.5.2 *The ROC–GLM estimator*

Recall the concept of the placement value defined in Section 5.2.5, and that one representation of the ROC curve is as the distribution of placement values:

$$\begin{aligned}
\text{ROC}(t) &= \text{P}[Y_D > S_{\bar{D}}^{-1}(t)] \\
&= \text{P}[S_{\bar{D}}(Y_D) \leqslant t].
\end{aligned} \tag{5.17}$$

Writing $U_{it} = I[S_{\bar{D}}(Y_{Di}) \leqslant t]$, the binary variable denoting whether or not the placement value exceeds t, we see that

$$\text{E}(U_{it}) = \text{P}[S_{\bar{D}}(Y_{\bar{D}}) \leqslant t] = \text{ROC}(t). \tag{5.18}$$

Suppose now that we adopt a parametric form for the ROC curve:

$$g\left(\text{ROC}(t)\right) = \sum_s \alpha_s h_s(t),\qquad\qquad(5.19)$$

where g is a link function and $h = \{h_1, \ldots, h_S\}$ are specified functions. As a special case, the binormal model is specified by (5.19) when $g = \Phi^{-1}$, $h_1(t) = 1$ and $h_2(t) = \Phi^{-1}(t)$. The ROC model in (5.19) defines a generalized linear model for U_{it} with link function g and covariates $\{h_s(t), s = 1, \ldots, S\}$. The ROC–GLM approach (Pepe, 2000; Alonzo and Pepe, 2002) is to use procedures for fitting generalized linear models to binary data in order to estimate the parameters α.

In particular, pick a set $T = \{t \in T\}$ over which the model is to be fitted, and calculate the empirical placement values $\{\hat{S}_{\bar{D}}(Y_{Di}), i = 1, \ldots, n_D\}$. Putting these two together we calculate, for each $t \in T$, the binary indicators based on the empirical placement values:

$$\hat{U}_{it} = I[\hat{S}_{\bar{D}}(Y_{Di}) \leqslant t],$$

for $i = 1, \ldots, n_D$. Binary regression methods with link function g and covariates $h(t) = \{h_1(t), \ldots, h_S(t)\}$ provide estimates of $\{\alpha_1, \ldots, \alpha_S\}$ from the data

$$\left\{ \left(\hat{U}_{it}, h_1(t), \ldots, h_S(t)\right),\ t \in T,\ i = 1, \ldots, n_D \right\}\qquad(5.20)$$

arranged as $n_D \times n_T$ records, where n_T is the number of points in T. The ROC–GLM procedure is based again only on the ranks of the data, and requires a model only for the ROC curve, not for the distributions of test results. Hence it is a parametric rank-based distribution-free method.

How do we choose the set T of false positive fractions for fitting the model? If there are no ties in the non-disease set of observations, T can include $n_{\bar{D}} - 1$ equally-spaced values without redundance: $T = \{1/n_{\bar{D}}, \ldots, (n_{\bar{D}} - 1)/n_{\bar{D}}\}$. In this case

$$\left\{\hat{U}_{it},\ t \in T,\ i = 1, \ldots, n_D\right\} = \left\{I[Y_{Di} \geqslant Y_{\bar{D}j}],\ j = 1, \ldots, n_{\bar{D}},\ i = 1, \ldots, n_D\right\},$$

see Pepe (2000). Such a large set for T can produce a very large unwieldy 'dataset', (5.20), with $n_D \times n_{\bar{D}}$ observations to which the binary regression techniques are applied. Preliminary results from Alonzo and Pepe (2002) show that a relatively small set T can be used without much loss of efficiency. This result is similar in spirit to that of Metz et al. (1998b) regarding the collapsing of adjacent small categories without sacrificing efficiency in the LABROC algorithm.

Example 5.6

As an illustration, we use audiology data (not described in Chapters 1 or 4) from a study of the distortion product otoacoustic emissions (DPOAE) test for hearing impairment reported by Stover et al. (1996). The test result is the negative signal-to-noise ratio, $-\text{SNR}$, at the 1001 Hz frequency when the test was performed with input stimulus at a level of 65 dB. The gold standard behavioral test yields an audiometric threshold at the same frequency and we define $D = 1$ if the audiometric threshold is greater than 20 dB HL. A total of 107 hearing-impaired subjects were tested and 103 normally-hearing subjects. Each subject was tested in only one ear. These data were analyzed in some detail in Pepe (1998). The empirical ROC curve for the data is shown in Fig. 5.8.

In the general model (5.19) let $g = \Phi^{-1}$, $h_1(t) = 1$ and $h_2(t) = \Phi^{-1}(t)$, so that the ROC curve model is binormal $\mathrm{ROC}(t) = \Phi(\alpha_1 + \alpha_2 \Phi^{-1}(t))$. Thus binary probit regression, with $\hat{U}_{it}$ as the binary dependent variable and $\Phi^{-1}(t)$ as the covariate, provides ROC–GLM estimators of (α_1, α_2).

Using $T = \{1/n_{\bar{D}}, \ldots, (n_{\bar{D}} - 1)/n_{\bar{D}}\}$ we calculate $\hat{\alpha}_1 = 1.37$ (se = 0.36) and $\hat{\alpha}_2 = 0.73$ (se = 0.23), where se denotes bootstrap standard errors. The fitted curve is shown in Fig. 5.8. It follows the empirical curve reasonably well, although less so in the midrange of FPF values. The binormal curve fitted with the LABROC algorithm is also shown. The LABROC estimates are $\hat{\alpha}_1 = 1.43$ and $\hat{\alpha}_2 = 0.81$. The curve is very close, but not identical, to the ROC–GLM estimator.

Bootstrap estimates of standard errors for the LABROC parameters, se$(\hat{\alpha}_1) = 0.35$ and se$(\hat{\alpha}_2) = 0.20$, are similar to those found for the ROC–GLM estimates. However, the bootstrapped standard errors are substantially larger than those calculated using the inverse information values, se$(\hat{\alpha}_1) = 0.27$ and se$(\hat{\alpha}_2) = 0.14$. The asymptotic and small sample properties of LABROC need further investigation. At this point we recommend bootstrap resampling for calculating standard errors over the application of maximum likelihood asymptotic theory.   ■

We note that ROC–GLM can also be used with discrete ordinal test result

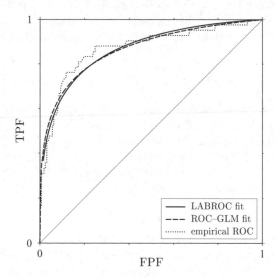

FIG. 5.8. The DPOAE test for hearing impairment (Stover *et al.*, 1996). The empirical ROC curve and two binormal ROC curves fitted to the data with LABROC and ROC–GLM are shown

data. The observed false positive fractions would be the natural choice for T in this case. Alonzo and Pepe (2002) investigated the efficiency of ROC–GLM for estimating a binormal ROC curve with ordinal data. They found that its performance was close to that of LABROC, which is the Dorfman and Alf maximum likelihood method for ordinal data. The main advantage of ROC–GLM over the LABROC approach is that it is easier and faster computationally when data are continuous. It appears to have a somewhat different conceptual basis, although conceptual links between the two will undoubtedly be uncovered with time.

We close this section with a statement of some theoretical results for the ROC–GLM estimator. A proof is outlined in Pepe (2000).

Result 5.8

The ROC–GLM estimator $\hat{\alpha} = \{\hat{\alpha}_1, \ldots, \hat{\alpha}_S\}$ for the model $g\{\text{ROC}(t)\} = \sum \alpha_s h_s(t)$ is the solution to the equation

$$\sum_{i=1}^{n_D} \sum_{t \in T} h'(t) w(t) \{\hat{U}_{it} - \text{ROC}(t)\} = 0,$$

where

$$\text{ROC}(t) = g^{-1}\left\{\sum \alpha_s h_s(t)\right\},$$

$$w(t) = \left(\frac{\partial}{\partial \mu} g^{-1}(\mu)\right) \{\text{ROC}(t)(1 - \text{ROC}(t))\}^{-1},$$

$$\mu = \sum \alpha_s h_s(t).$$

and $h'(t)$ is the transpose of $h(t)$.

If the observations $\{Y_{Di}, i = 1, \ldots, n_D; Y_{\bar{D}j}, j = 1, \ldots, n_{\bar{D}}\}$ are independent and $T = \{1/n_{\bar{D}}, \ldots, (n_{\bar{D}} - 1)/n_{\bar{D}}\}$, then $\hat{\alpha}$ is consistent and asymptotically normal with variance–covariance matrix approximated by

$$\text{var}(\hat{\alpha}) = \frac{1}{(n_D + n_{\bar{D}})^2} I^{-1}(\alpha) V(\alpha) I^{-1}(\alpha),$$

where

$$I(\alpha) = \sum_{t \in T} h'(t) h(t) w^2(t) \text{ROC}(t)(1 - \text{ROC}(t)),$$

$$V(\alpha) = \frac{1}{n_D} V_1 + \frac{1}{n_{\bar{D}}} V_2,$$

$$V_1 = \sum_{t \in T} \sum_{s \in T} h'(t) h(s) w(t) w(s) \text{ROC}(\min(t,s)) [1 - \text{ROC}(\max(t,s))],$$

$$V_2 = \sum_{t \in T} \sum_{s \in T} h'(t) h(s) w(t) w(s) \text{ROC}'(t) \text{ROC}'(s) (\min(t,s) - ts),$$

h' denotes the transpose of h and $\text{ROC}'(t)$ denotes the derivative of $\text{ROC}(t)$. ∎

We note that in the sandwich variance expression, var($\hat{\alpha}$), there are two components to $V(\alpha)$. The first is derived from variability in the disease observations and the second from variability in the non-disease set. Interestingly, the additive components are reminiscent of a similar additive form for the variance of the empirical ROC derived in Result 5.1 and of the empirical AUC given in Result 5.5. Further discussion about the form of var($\hat{\alpha}$) can be found in Pepe (2000).

5.5.3 *Inference with parametric distribution-free methods*

The LABROC and ROC–GLM methods provide estimates of parameters and an estimate of the variance–covariance matrix (either analytic or more usually calculated via resampling). Pointwise confidence intervals for ROC(t) can therefore be constructed, as can Working–Hotelling confidence bands (Ma and Hall, 1993).

Models can be fitted simultaneously for multiple curves, and hypothesis tests for equality can be based either on a comparison of summary indices or of the parameter estimates themselves (if the same model forms are used). These procedures were described in Section 5.4.3 as they pertain to the LDV framework for ordinal tests, but they apply equally well to the parametric distribution-free framework for continuous tests. We will elaborate on this in the next chapter where we extend the ROC–GLM methodology to a regression analysis technique.

Example 5.7

Let us reconsider the pancreatic cancer data set of Wieand *et al.* (1989). Binormal

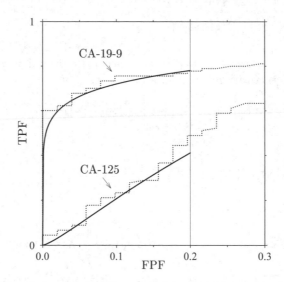

FIG. 5.9. Binormal curves fitted to the pancreatic cancer data using the ROC–GLM algorithm (solid lines). The analysis is restricted to FPF $\leqslant$ 20%. The empirical ROC curves are also displayed (dotted lines)

curves $ROC(t) = \Phi(a + b\,\Phi^{-1}(t))$ fitted to these data yielded intercept and slope parameters $(\hat{a}_1, \hat{b}_1) = (1.18, 0.47)$ for CA-19-9 and $(\hat{a}_2, \hat{b}_2) = (0.74, 1.07)$ for CA-125. Formal comparisons based on the chi-squared statistic of (5.16) yield $p = 0.001$ using 5000 bootstrap samples.

Recall that in this study interest was focused on low false positive fractions. We ran the ROC–GLM analysis again, but restricting the fitting to FPF $\leqslant$ 20%. In this range the binormal parameter estimates are $(\hat{a}_1, \hat{b}_1) = (1.14, 0.44)$ and $(\hat{a}_2, \hat{b}_2) = (0.91, 1.35)$. The associated chi-squared statistic (5.16) is highly significant ($p < 0.001$).

The empirical and ROC–GLM fitted curves are shown in Fig. 5.9. The smooth binormal curves seem to fit the raw data well in this range of FPFs. Recall from Example 5.2 that a comparison of the markers based on the difference in empirical partial AUC statistics, $\Delta pAUC(0.2) = 0.14 - 0.05 = 0.09$, is highly significant ($p < 0.01$ using 5000 bootstrap samples). This agrees with the conclusion based on the chi-squared statistic. ∎

5.6   Concluding remarks

This chapter considered the estimation of the ROC curve. Three approaches were described that apply to quantitative tests: empirical methods (Section 5.2), distribution-free parametric methods (Section 5.5) and distribution modeling methods (Section 5.3). Observe that the empirical and distribution-free methods are based only on the ranks of the data, while the latter is not. Even when a semiparametric model is used for the test results (Section 5.3.2), the ROC curve is seen to depend on the means and variances of the test results and is therefore not invariant to monotone increasing data transformations. As discussed in Section 5.3.3, I prefer rank-based methods on the philosophical grounds that the ROC curve is invariant to monotone increasing data transformations and therefore so should its estimator.

The distinction between the empirical (Section 5.2) and distribution-free methods (Section 5.5) is that the former places no structure on the ROC curve while the latter assumes a parametric form for it. Two distribution-free approaches were described here for estimating the parametric ROC curve, namely LABROC and ROC–GLM. Zou and Hall (2000) developed the maximum likelihood rank-based estimator of the ROC curve. This is fully efficient but unfortunately computationally difficult. Simulations indicated that parameter values from the LABROC approach were similar to those from the maximum likelihood approach.

The second issue discussed in this chapter was the comparison of two ROC curves. When a parametric form is assumed for the ROC curves, they can be compared on the basis of estimated parameters. This approach is extended in the next chapter, where it is embedded in a regression modeling framework for ROC curves in much the same way as binary covariates were employed in Chapter 3 to compare TPFs (or FPFs).

The traditional approach for comparing ROC curves, however, is to compare summary indices, in particular the AUC index. Differences in AUCs are typically calculated using the empirical or parametric distribution-free methods. Explicit variance expressions were provided here for the empirical $\Delta A\hat{U}C_e$ when simple paired or unpaired designs are employed. For more complex studies, where data are clustered in more general ways, the bootstrap can be employed to make inferences. Resampling is done using 'cluster' as the unit for resampling. It is possible to derive explicit analytic variance expressions for $\Delta A\hat{U}C_e$ with some clustered data designs (see Obuchowski, 1997a and Metz et al., 1998a). Jack-knifing has also been used to calculate variances of estimated AUC and $\Delta A\hat{U}C_e$ values (Hajian-Tilaki et al., 1997; Song, 1997) with clustered data. Radiology experiments, however, often give rise to correlated data in which there are no independent cluster units. A typical experiment might involve a set of readers from a population *each* reading the same sets of images generated with two modalities, say. This gives rise to a crossed-correlation structure. Dorfman et al. (1992) use a method that generates jack-knife pseudovalues for the AUC, and employs random effects for readers and images in models for the pseudovalues to account for the crossed correlation while comparing modalities. The idea appears to be promising (Dorfman et al., 1995), although theoretical justification for using random effects models in this way would benefit from further research.

All of these procedures can be used with summary indices other than the AUC. Wieand et al. (1989) base comparisons on differences in weighted AUCs. In Example 5.2 we used the partial AUC and the $ROC(t_0)$ indices to compare markers. Venkatraman and Begg (1996) introduce a distribution-free procedure for comparing ROC curves that is not explicitly based on a summary index. A permutation test is proposed and further developed in Venkatraman (2000).

Statistical procedures that were described here for inference are justified for large samples. The validity of confidence intervals, hypothesis tests and so forth in small samples should be investigated further. Table 5.1 shows results of simulation studies for AUC confidence intervals. Small sample inference for the AUC is discussed further by Mee (1990), Obuchowski and Lieber (1998, 2002) and Tsimikas et al. (2002). The latter two papers focus on inference for accurate tests whose AUCs are close to 1.0, where inference based on asymptotic results is seen to be less reliable.

Software for ROC analysis has not traditionally been a part of standard statistical packages. Data analysts have been indebted for many years to Charles Metz and colleagues at the University of Chicago, who have made freely available their programs, currently called ROCKIT. Recently, packages such as STATA have included procedures for empirical and distribution-free estimation and comparison of ROC curves. Programs written with STATA code to implement the analyses in each of the examples of this chapter are available at the website http://www.fhcrc.org/labs/pepe/book. These are written in a modular fashion and may be adapted relatively easily for other applications. See the website for details.

5.7   Exercises

1. Write the following two-sample rank test statistics as functions of the empirical ROC curve and the sample prevalence $n_D/(n_D + n_{\bar{D}})$ (if necessary):

   (a) the Wilcoxon statistic;
   (b) the Cramer von Mises statistic;
   (c) the logrank statistic.

2. The empirical ROC curve can be written in terms of the empirical distribution of the empirical placement values. Show this formally (i) for the non-disease placement values, and (ii) for the disease placement values.

3. Prove Result 5.4 which gives the exact variance of the empirical AUC.

4. The $\Delta A\hat{U}C_e$ statistic can be interpreted as a paired comparison of the placement values based on their mean difference, similar to the numerator of a paired t-test. Discuss the use of the other paired test statistics, such as the rank-sum test, for comparing the empirical placement values for two tests, and if procedures for comparing ROC curves might be based on them.

5. Show that when there are no tied data points, the empirical partial AUC statistic can be written as

$$\mathrm{pA\hat{U}C}_e(0, t_0) = \sum_i \sum_j I\left[Y_{Di} > Y_{\bar{D}j},\ \hat{S}_{\bar{D}}\left(Y_{\bar{D}j}\right) \leqslant t_0\right]/n_D n_{\bar{D}},$$

   at least if t_0 is an attained empirical FPF, i.e. a multiple of $1/n_{\bar{D}}$.

6. Fit a binormal model to the data of Exercise 9 in Chapter 4, assuming that the frequencies represent data for $n_D = 100$ diseased and $n_{\bar{D}} = 100$ non-diseased subjects. Use the maximum likelihood Dorfman and Alf algorithm and the ROC–GLM approach, and compare both the parameter estimates and their standard errors. How do the estimates compare with those from the simple linear fit to the empirical values of $(\Phi^{-1}(\mathrm{F\hat{P}F}), \Phi^{-1}(\mathrm{T\hat{P}F}))$, as suggested in Chapter 4?

7. Consider the ROC–GLM model for a discrete test:

$$g(\mathrm{ROC}(t_y)) = \sum \alpha_s h_s(t_y), \quad y = 2, \ldots, P.$$

   Write down the likelihood-based score equations for the parameters $\{\alpha_1, \ldots, \alpha_S, t_2, \ldots, t_P\}$. Contrast these with the estimating equations for the ROC–GLM procedure as given in Result 5.8.

5.8   Proofs of theoretical results

Proof of Result 5.1   We have

$$\hat{\text{ROC}}_e(t) - \text{ROC}(t)$$

$$= \hat{S}_D\big(\hat{S}_{\bar{D}}^{-1}(t)\big) - S_D\big(S_{\bar{D}}^{-1}(t)\big)$$

$$= \Big\{\hat{S}_D\big(\hat{S}_{\bar{D}}^{-1}(t)\big) - S_D\big(\hat{S}_{\bar{D}}^{-1}(t)\big)\Big\} + \Big\{S_D\big(\hat{S}_{\bar{D}}^{-1}(t)\big) - S_D\big(S_{\bar{D}}^{-1}(t)\big)\Big\}$$

$$= \{A\} + \{B\}.$$

Given $\{B\}$, or equivalently $\hat{S}_{\bar{D}}^{-1}(t)$, the first term $\{A\}$ is derived from a proportion among the n_D diseased observations. Therefore conditioning on B we have that A has mean 0 and binomial variance

$$\text{var}(A|B) = S_D\big(\hat{S}_{\bar{D}}^{-1}(t)\big)\Big\{1 - S_D\big(\hat{S}_{\bar{D}}^{-1}(t)\big)\Big\}\Big/n_D,$$

which is approximately $\text{ROC}(t)\,(1 - \text{ROC}(t))\,/n_D$ in large samples. Moreover, because $\text{E}\{A|B\} = 0$, we have that A and B are uncorrelated. Hence,

$$\text{var}\big\{\hat{\text{ROC}}_e(t) - \text{ROC}(t)\big\} = \text{var}(A) + \text{var}(B).$$

Observe that $\text{E}\{A|B\} = 0$ also implies that $\text{var}(A) = \text{E}\{\text{var}(A|B)\}$. Turning to $\text{var}(B)$ we note that the asymptotic variance of the quantile $\hat{S}_{\bar{D}}^{-1}(t)$ is such that, approximately,

$$\text{var}\big\{\hat{S}_{\bar{D}}^{-1}(t) - S_{\bar{D}}^{-1}(t)\big\} = \frac{t(1-t)}{n_{\bar{D}}\big\{f_{\bar{D}}\big(S_{\bar{D}}^{-1}(t)\big)\big\}^2}.$$

Recognizing that S_D is a continuous function with derivative $-f_D(\cdot)$, the delta method implies that

$$\text{var}(B) = \frac{\big\{f_D\big(S_{\bar{D}}^{-1}(t)\big)\big\}^2\,t(1-t)}{n_{\bar{D}}\big\{f_{\bar{D}}\big(S_{\bar{D}}^{-1}(t)\big)\big\}^2}.$$

Putting $\text{var}(A)$ and $\text{var}(B)$ together, we obtain the result. ∎

Proof of Result 5.5   Noting that $\text{AUC} = \text{E}(S_D(Y_{\bar{D}}))$ and using (5.9), we write

$$\hat{\text{AUC}}_e - \text{AUC} = \sum_{j=1}^{n_{\bar{D}}} \left(\frac{\hat{S}_D(Y_{\bar{D}j})}{n_{\bar{D}}}\right) - \text{E}(S_D(Y_{\bar{D}}))$$

$$= \sum_{j=1}^{n_{\bar{D}}} \frac{\hat{S}_D(Y_{\bar{D}j}) - S_D(Y_{\bar{D}j})}{n_{\bar{D}}} + \sum_{j=1}^{n_{\bar{D}}} \frac{S_D(Y_{\bar{D}j}) - \text{E}(S_D(Y_{\bar{D}}))}{n_{\bar{D}}}.$$

These two terms are uncorrelated since, conditional on the random variables in the second component, $\{Y_{\bar{D}j}, j = 1, \ldots, n_{\bar{D}}\}$, the first has mean 0. The second component has variance equal to $\mathrm{var}(S_D(Y_{\bar{D}j}))/n_{\bar{D}}$. The first term can be rewritten as

$$1 - \sum_{i=1}^{n_D} \frac{\hat{S}_{\bar{D}}(Y_{Di})}{n_D} - \sum_{j=1}^{n_{\bar{D}}} \frac{S_D(Y_{\bar{D}j})}{n_{\bar{D}}}.$$

Conditional on $\{Y_{\bar{D}j}, j = 1, \ldots, n_{\bar{D}}\}$, it has variance $\mathrm{var}(\hat{S}_{\bar{D}}(Y_{Di}))/n_D$ and we noted earlier that it has conditional mean 0. Hence, unconditionally it has variance $\mathrm{E}\{\mathrm{var}(\hat{S}_{\bar{D}}(Y_{Di}))\}/n_D$. In large samples this is approximated by $\mathrm{var}(S_{\bar{D}}(Y_{Di}))/n_D$. The result then follows. ∎

6

COVARIATE EFFECTS ON CONTINUOUS AND ORDINAL TESTS

6.1 How and why?

In Chapter 3 we discussed factors that can affect the result of a diagnostic test beyond disease status. The need to identify such factors is as relevant for continuous and ordinal tests as it is for binary tests. However, as we will see in this chapter, conceptual and technical approaches are more complex.

6.1.1 *Notation*

We use the notation established in Chapter 3 and the distinction made between covariates and covariables. Covariates, denoted by Z, are the factors whose effects we wish to model. Covariables, denoted by X, are the specific mathematical variables that enter into the statistical model. In other words, X is how we choose to code and model the covariate Z.

We write $S_{D,Z}$ and $S_{\bar{D},Z}$ for the survivor functions of the test result Y in the diseased and non-diseased populations, respectively, with covariate value Z. We allow these covariates to be different in the two populations, and on occasion write Z_D $(Z_{\bar{D}})$ for covariates that are specific to the diseased (non-diseased) population, while Z denotes covariates that are in common. The ROC curve that describes the separation between S_{D,Z,Z_D} and $S_{\bar{D},Z,Z_{\bar{D}}}$ is denoted by $\mathrm{ROC}_{Z,Z_D,Z_{\bar{D}}}$. To ease notation we drop the subscripts for disease- and non-disease-specific covariates in discussions where the meaning is not obscured. To fix ideas consider an example.

Example 6.1

Consider the hearing test study of Stover *et al.* (1996). A subset of the study data was analyzed in Example 5.6. For each ear the DPOAE test was applied under nine different settings for the input stimulus. Each setting is defined by a particular frequency (f) and intensity (L) of the auditory stimulus. The response of the ear to the stimulus could be affected by the stimulus parameters, as well as by the hearing status of the ear. In addition, among hearing-impaired ears the severity of hearing impairment, as measured by the true hearing threshold, would be expected to affect the result of the DPOAE test.

Recall that the test result Y is the negative signal-to-noise ratio response, $-\mathrm{SNR}$, to coincide with our convention that higher values are associated with hearing impairment. The disease variable, D, is hearing impairment of $20\,\mathrm{dB\,HL}$ or more. Covariates, Z, are the frequency and intensity levels of the stimulus.

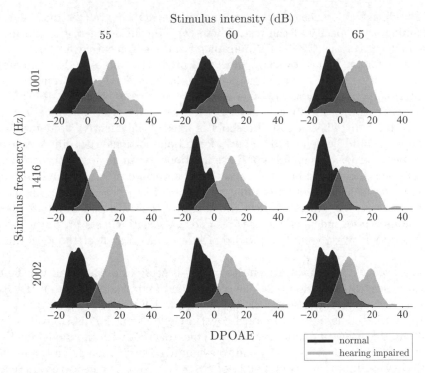

Stimulus intensity (dB)

DPOAE

F IG. 6.1. Probability distributions of DPOAE test results among hearing-impaired and normally-hearing ears at different stimulus frequencies and
intensities

Figure 6.1 displays the distributions of test results for normally-hearing and
impaired ears at each set of stimulus levels.

We use both covariates on their original scales (although they only take three
values each) with X_f = frequency/100, which is measured in Hertz (Hz), and
X_L = intensity/10, which is measured in decibels (dB). Finally, degree of hearing
loss, a disease-specific covariate, Z_D, is coded as

$$X_D = (\text{hearing threshold} - 20\,\text{dB})/10\,.$$

This is measured in decibels and takes values which are greater than 0 dB for
hearing-impaired ears, while it is undefined for normally-hearing ears. ■

6.1.2 Aspects to model

We have observed that there are two dimensions to describing test accuracy,
and that we need to evaluate covariate effects on both. In Chapter 3 we modeled
covariate effects on both the FPF and the TPF. Here, the two primary dimensions
we consider are $S_{\bar{D}}$ and the ROC curve. That is, we evaluate covariate effects on

the non-disease reference distribution and on the ROC curve that quantifies the discriminatory capacity of the test. These can be considered as the continuous data analogues of the (FPF, TPF) parameterizations of accuracy for binary tests. Analogues for modeling covariate effects on predictive values and on diagnostic likelihood ratios have not yet been developed for non-binary tests, and so we do not discuss their extensions.

By evaluating covariate effects on $S_{\bar{D}}$ we determine what factors affect false positive fractions when a test threshold is fixed. Equivalently, we determine if thresholds should be defined differently for subpopulations with different covariate values in order to keep false positive fractions the same across those subpopulations. On the other hand, the evaluation of covariate effects on the ROC curve is geared towards an essentially different aspect of test performance, namely on whether or not the covariates affect the ability of the test to discriminate disease from non-disease, independent of threshold. Covariate effects on both $S_{\bar{D}}$ and ROC together give a complete picture of how covariates affect the performance of the test.

The evaluation of covariate effects on $S_{\bar{D}}$ is straightforward and will be discussed at length in Section 6.2. The evaluation of covariate effects on the ROC curve is a non-standard statistical problem for which there are currently two basic approaches. The first is to model covariate effects on the distribution of test results in the diseased population, $S_{D,Z}$. This, together with the model for $S_{\bar{D},Z}$, allows one to calculate $\mathrm{ROC}_Z(\cdot)$ and to evaluate covariate effects on the induced ROC curves. Simultaneous modeling of $S_{D,Z}$ and $S_{\bar{D},Z}$ is considered in Section 6.3. The second approach directly models covariate effects on the ROC curve. It adapts some GLM model fitting algorithms to estimate parameters. This approach is described in Section 6.4. The two approaches parallel those discussed in Chapter 5 for estimating ROC curves by modeling the test results (Section 5.3) and by distribution-free modeling of a parametric form for the ROC curve (Section 5.5).

6.1.3 *Omitting covariates/pooling data*

The consequences of neglecting to evaluate covariate effects are several. We have briefly mentioned above (and will discuss further in Section 6.2) the importance of modeling the test result, Y, in the non-diseased population in order to appropriately set thresholds in subpopulations and to understand the sources of false positive results. In addition, inference about the accuracy of the test for distinguishing between diseased and non-diseased subjects can be biased by neglecting covariate effects. Classic confounding of the association between disease and test results due to covariates occurs if test results are related to covariates and distributions of covariates are different for disease and non-disease study groups. We now show that inference about test accuracy can be biased even if covariate distributions are the same in both populations.

In particular, the next result shows that if a covariate affects the distribution of $Y_{\bar{D}}$, but not the ROC curve, then the pooled ROC curve that ignores the

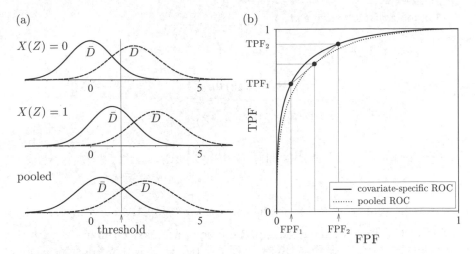

FIG. 6.2. Illustration of a setting where the ROC curve that ignores dependence of $Y_{\bar{D}}$ on a covariate is attenuated relative to the covariate-specific ROC curve. The threshold that yields the three ROC points
in (b) is indicated with a vertical line in (a). The covariate distribution is
$P[X(Z) = 1|D = 1] = P[X(Z) = 1|D = 0] = 0.5$

covariate effect on $Y_{\bar{D}}$ is attenuated. Figure 6.2 shows an illustration of this
phenomenon. In order to state and prove the general result formally we use the
notation $\mathrm{ROC}^P(t) = S_D(S_{\bar{D}}^{-1}(t))$ for the pooled ROC curve and the constituent
marginal survivor functions, $S_D(\cdot)$ and $S_{\bar{D}}(\cdot)$, which ignore covariates, while
$\mathrm{ROC}_Z(t) = S_{D,Z}(S_{\bar{D},Z}^{-1}(t))$ denotes the covariate-specific ROC curve.

Result 6.1

Suppose that

$$\mathrm{ROC}_Z(t) = \mathrm{ROC}(t) \quad \forall Z,$$

then

$$\mathrm{ROC}^P(t) \leqslant \mathrm{ROC}(t), \tag{6.1}$$

under the (reasonable) assumptions that the common covariate-specific ROC
curve is concave, and that covariate distributions are the same for diseased and
non-diseased subjects.

Proof For a threshold c, let t_Z and t denote the corresponding covariate-
specific and marginal false positive fractions, respectively. Observe that

$$t = P[Y_{\bar{D}} \geqslant c] = \int P[Y_{\bar{D}} \geqslant c|Z]\,d\mu(Z) = \int t_Z\,d\mu(Z),$$

where $\mu(Z)$ is the probability distribution of the covariate.

The pooled ROC curve at t is

$$
\begin{aligned}
\mathrm{ROC}^P(t) = \mathrm{P}[Y_D \geqslant c] &= \int \mathrm{P}[Y_D \geqslant c|Z]\,\mathrm{d}\mu(Z) \\
&= \int \mathrm{ROC}_Z(t_Z)\,\mathrm{d}\mu(Z) \\
&= \int \mathrm{ROC}(t_Z)\,\mathrm{d}\mu(Z) \\
&\leqslant \mathrm{ROC}\left(\int t_Z\,\mathrm{d}\mu(Z)\right) \\
&= \mathrm{ROC}(t)\,,
\end{aligned}
$$

where the inequality follows from the concavity of the ROC curve.   ∎

The plot in Fig. 6.2 shows the special case of a binary covariate Z with the probability $\mathrm{P}[X(Z) = 1|D = 1] = \mathrm{P}[X(Z) = 1|D = 0] = 0.5$. Consider a point $(\mathrm{FPF}, \mathrm{TPF})$ on the pooled ROC curve. The threshold c that gives rise to that point, gives rise to a point $(\mathrm{FPF}_1, \mathrm{TPF}_1)$ on the ROC curve for $X = 0$ and another point $(\mathrm{FPF}_2, \mathrm{TPF}_2)$ on the ROC curve for $X = 1$. We have

$$
\begin{aligned}
\mathrm{FPF} &= \mathrm{P}[Y \geqslant c|D = 0] \\
&= 0.5\,\mathrm{P}[Y \geqslant c|D = 0, X = 0] + 0.5\,\mathrm{P}[Y \geqslant c|D = 0, X = 1] \\
&= (\mathrm{FPF}_1 + \mathrm{FPF}_2)/2\,.
\end{aligned}
$$

Similarly $\mathrm{TPF} = (\mathrm{TPF}_1 + \mathrm{TPF}_2)/2$. Therefore each $(\mathrm{FPF}, \mathrm{TPF})$ point on the pooled ROC curve is derived by vertical and horizontal averages of two points on the covariate-specific curve.

Attenuation of the ROC curve by ignoring covariates that affect the distribution of $Y_{\bar{D}}$ has long been appreciated in radiology applications (Swets and Pickett, 1982, p. 65; Hanley, 1989; Rutter and Gatsonis, 2001). Pooling data from multiple readers that use the rating scales differently results in an ROC curve that is attenuated relative to the reader-specific ROC curves (see Section 4.5.4 and Fig. 4.11). Identifying 'reader' in this case as the covariate, we see that this follows from Result 6.1.

Which ROC curve is of more practical interest: pooled or covariate specific? Clearly, in the radiology setting, the radiologist-specific one is most relevant because in practice radiologists use their own inherent rating scales for both diseased and non-diseased images, and the discrimination that he/she sees between disease and non-disease images is shown by the radiologist-specific ROC. The ROC curve that pools data across radiologists, does not reflect the separation of actual rating distributions for any radiologist. Similarly, if the covariate is 'site' in a multicenter study, the site-specific rather than pooled-data ROC is the practically relevant entity. In PSA screening the age-specific ROC curve would be most relevant if age-specific thresholds are to be used for defining screen positivity criteria. However, if a common threshold is to be used across all ages, then the pooled-data ROC curve reflects the actual use of the test in practice and hence is of more importance. In general, if the use of a test result, Y, in practice depends on a covariate, Z, in the sense that at covariate level Z the threshold corresponding to t for a positive test is $S_{\bar{D},Z}^{-1}(t)$, then the covariate-specific ROC should be reported. However, if the threshold does not depend on Z, then the pooled ROC should be reported. In data analysis it might be of interest to calculate both the pooled and covariate-specific ROC curves in order to ascertain the gains in accuracy that can be achieved by using covariate-specific thresholds. With age as a covariate, this could be of interest for prostate cancer screening with PSA, for example.

We turn now to the case where a covariate does not affect the distribution of $Y_{\bar{D}}$, but it does affect the ROC curve. That is, in contrast to the setting of Result 6.1, it affects the distribution of Y_D only. One example of such a covariate is disease severity, but non-disease-specific covariates may also have this attribute. In this case, the pooled-data ROC curve is a weighted average of the covariate-specific ROC curves.

Result 6.2

Suppose that $S_{\bar{D},Z}(\cdot) = S_{\bar{D}}$. Then

$$\mathrm{ROC}^P(t) = \int \mathrm{ROC}_Z(t)\,\mathrm{d}\mu(Z) \qquad (6.2)$$

at each $t \in (0,1)$, where μ is the distribution of Z in the diseased population.

Proof We have

$$\mathrm{ROC}^P(t) = \mathrm{P}[Y_D \geqslant S_{\bar{D}}^{-1}(t)]$$

$$= \int \mathrm{P}[Y_D \geqslant S_{\bar{D}}^{-1}(t)|Z]\,\mathrm{d}\mu(Z)$$

$$= \int \mathrm{P}[Y_D \geqslant S_{\bar{D},Z}^{-1}(t)|Z]\,\mathrm{d}\mu(Z)$$

$$= \int \mathrm{ROC}_Z(t)\,\mathrm{d}\mu(Z). \qquad \blacksquare$$

That is, the pooled-data ROC curve is a simply interpreted summary of the covariate-specific ROC curves when the distribution of $Y_{\bar{D}}$ does not depend on Z. In the special case displayed in Fig. 6.3, each point on the pooled-data ROC is an average of the two corresponding points from the covariate-specific ROC curves:

$$\mathrm{ROC}^P(t) = \{\mathrm{ROC}_0(t) + \mathrm{ROC}_1(t)\}/2.$$

Although the pooled ROC curve is meaningful and reflects the average performance of the test in practice, it is often of interest to evaluate covariate-specific ROC curves. This can highlight populations or test operating parameters where

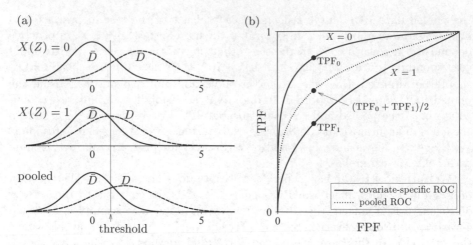

F$_{\text{IG}}$. 6.3. Illustration of a setting where $S_{\bar{D},Z}$ does not depend on the binary covariate. The threshold that yields the three ROC points in (b) is indicated with a vertical line in (a)

the test performs particularly well or particularly poorly. If disease-specific covariates are evaluated, these can indicate characteristics of disease that lead to worse or better test performance.

When covariates affect both $S_{\bar{D}}$ and the ROC curve, general statements about pooled versus covariate-specific ROC curves are harder to make. Recommendations for analysis are easier to make, namely:

(i) One should report ROC curves that reflect $S_{\bar{D},Z}$ if thresholds for test positivity (implicit or explicit) will be covariate specific in practice. Otherwise, the marginal distribution $S_{\bar{D}}$ should be used for calculating ROC curves.

(ii) Covariate-specific ROC curves should be examined in the analysis and summarized with the average ROC curve if deemed appropriate.

(iii) Most importantly, the interpretation of the ROC curve should be made clear when reporting results.

6.2   Reference distributions

6.2.1   *Non-diseased as the reference population*

It is important to understand how the test result varies in the non-diseased population and what factors influence it. For example, serum levels of PSA tend to be higher in older men than in younger men. In addition, levels tend to be high in men with enlarged (but not cancerous) prostate glands. In audiology, it is likely that the SNR response from normally-hearing ears depends on the parameters of the auditory stimulus.

There are two possible implications from the knowledge that covariates affect the distribution of $Y_{\bar{D}}$. First, if the values of covariates are available at the time a subject is tested, then thresholds for defining test positivity can be chosen to vary with covariate values. As mentioned earlier, it has been proposed that criteria for a positive PSA test should be more stringent in older men. In audiology, the thresholds for the DPOAE test can be chosen differently, depending on the parameters of the input stimulus. Formally, if a false positive fraction t_0 is deemed acceptable, $S_{\bar{D},Z}^{-1}(t_0)$ is the corresponding covariate-specific threshold for the test.

A covariate, such as benign hyperplasia of the prostate (BPH), will not be available when interpreting the results of the PSA test. Therefore, one cannot choose positivity criteria to depend on this sort of covariate. Nevertheless, knowledge about the existence of an effect of this sort of covariate can be used to direct research into technical modifications of the test that specifically seek to distinguish BPH from prostate cancer.

Our discussion uses the motivating context of estimating covariate-specific quantiles $S_{\bar{D},Z}^{-1}(t)$ of the distribution of $Y_{\bar{D}}$. As mentioned previously, this may be important to operationalize the test in practice. Moreover, we will see that quantile estimates are necessary as a precursor to fitting ROC regression models (Section 6.4). However, note that these procedures also allow one to simply evaluate whether covariates affect the distribution of $Y_{\bar{D}}$, as would be the primary purpose in determining BPH effects on the PSA test, for example.

Estimation of quantiles of $Y_{\bar{D}}$ can be viewed as estimation of the non-disease reference distribution, $S_{\bar{D},Z}$. Estimation of reference distributions is common in laboratory medicine, where sometimes only a range of values that constitute the normal reference range is of interest, such as the 1st to the 99th percentiles. Reference distributions for anthropometric measurements (head circumference, height and weight) and other clinical parameters have been established from the National Health and Nutrition Surveys (NHANES), which survey normal healthy populations in the United States. Indeed, measurements of height and weight are generally converted from their raw values to their percentile scores in the healthy reference population, in order to be interpreted for clinical purposes. Statistical methods for establishing reference distributions and for determining if reference distributions vary with covariates is the topic of this section. We provide a summary of the main approaches and refer to the literature for details of the more complex methods that have been developed for large datasets.

6.2.2 *The homogenous population*

First, suppose that there are no covariates and that data on $n_{\bar{D}}$ non-diseased test units are available $\{Y_{j\bar{D}}, j = 1, \ldots, n_{\bar{D}}\}$. There are basically two options for estimating the $(1-t)$th quantile of $Y_{\bar{D}}$ that we denote by $q(1-t) = S_{\bar{D}}^{-1}(t)$, either a nonparametric approach or a parametric approach.

The empirical nonparametric quantile can be used. This is

$$\hat{q}(1-t) = \min\{y : \hat{S}_{\bar{D}}(y) \leqslant t\},$$

where $\hat{S}_{\bar{D}}$ is the empirical survivor function. We have already used the empirical quantiles in Chapter 5, and their statistical properties are well established

(Shorack and Wellner, 1986). We denote the empirical $1 - t$ quantile as $\hat{S}_{\bar{D}}^{-1}(t)$ in the next result, which applies to continuous tests only. Its proof is straight-forward.

Result 6.3

In large samples $\sqrt{n_{\bar{D}}}(\hat{S}_{\bar{D}}^{-1}(t) - S_{\bar{D}}^{-1}(t))$ has a mean zero normal distribution with variance $\sigma^2(t) = t(1 - t)/\{f_{\bar{D}}(S_{\bar{D}}^{-1}(t))\}^2$, where $f_{\bar{D}}(y)$ is the probability density of $Y_{\bar{D}}$ at y. ∎

We see that the quantile can be very variable in the tail of the distribution if the probability density is low there. This makes sense because with sparse data in the tail of the distribution it will be hard to pin down the location of $S_{\bar{D}}^{-1}(t)$.

Parametric estimates are based on an assumption that the distribution of $Y_{\bar{D}}$ follows a parametric form, $S_{\bar{D},\alpha}$. The parameters, denoted by α, are estimated from the data and the quantiles are calculated using the fitted survivor function, $S_{\bar{D},\hat{\alpha}}$:

$$\hat{q}_\alpha(1 - t) = \min\{y : S_{\bar{D},\hat{\alpha}}(y) \leqslant t\}. \tag{6.3}$$

The variance of the quantile will depend on the parametric form assumed and on the distribution of $Y_{\bar{D}}$. A more flexible form will presumably yield a more variable estimator. A confidence interval can be based on the variance–covariance of $\hat{\alpha}$ using the delta method.

Example 6.2

We generated data, $Y_{\bar{D}}$, from a standard normal distribution and estimated quantiles of $S_{\bar{D}}$ using (i) the nonparametric empirical method, and (ii) the assumption that $S_{\bar{D}}$ is normal with unknown mean (μ) and variance (σ). The parameters, denoted above in (6.3) by α, are (μ, σ). The parametric quantile estimator is then $\hat{q}_\alpha(1 - t) = \hat{\mu} + \hat{\sigma}\Phi^{-1}(1 - t)$, where the sample mean and sample variance are used as estimates of the parameters. Table 6.1 shows the relative efficiency of the quantile estimates. The variance of the parametric estimator appears to be between 50% and 80% of that for the nonparametric estimator. The gains in efficiency seem to be greater further out in the tail of the distribution, i.e. for smaller t, as one would expect. ∎

Table 6.1 *Estimating the quantile of a normal distribution: efficiency of the nonparametric relative to the parametric estimators*

Sample size	$t = 0.05$	$t = 0.10$	$t = 0.20$
20	64%	73%	77%
50	54%	63%	68%
100	59%	64%	72%
200	58%	63%	65%
500	52%	63%	67%

Can we recommend parametric versus nonparametric estimates for use in practice? The usual dilemma between bias and variance arises here for estimates of $q(1-t)$, especially for small (or large) t. Specifying a parametric distribution that is valid in the tails of $S_{\bar{D}}$ is hard because, by definition, there is little data to model the distribution in the tail. On the other hand, the nonparametric estimates will be variable in the tail of the distribution because there may be little data to estimate it there. We recommend the use of the nonparametric approach when possible, because of its robustness. Moreover, efforts should be made to design studies with sample sizes that are adequate to allow sufficiently precise estimation with nonparametric estimates.

We next turn to estimation of covariate-specific quantiles. Again, nonparametric and parametric methods exist that generalize those for homogeneous populations. We also present a semiparametric method that can be considered as a compromise between the two.

6.2.3 Nonparametric regression quantiles

If the covariate is discrete and sufficient numbers of observations exist at each distinct level, then the empirical quantiles can be calculated at each level to yield a nonparametric estimate of $q_Z(1-t)$. If the covariate or some components of it are continuous, it can be categorized (or 'binned') and empirical quantiles calculated within each bin. A smooth function of covariables can then be fitted to these empirical quantiles to yield a nonparametric regression quantile function estimate, $\hat{q}_Z(1-t)$. This 'bin and smooth' approach has been applied to data from the NHANES surveys to calculate reference percentiles of anthropometric measures (Hamill et al., 1977).

An alternative approach is to model the regression quantile as a parametric function of covariables $X(Z)$:

$$q_Z(1-t) = h(\alpha, X),$$

where h is a specified function and α denotes parameters to be estimated. This approach is parametric in the sense that $h(\alpha, X)$ is a parametric function, but nonparametric in that the distribution function for $Y_{\bar{D}}$ is not specified. Koenker and Bassett (1978) base estimation of α on minimizing the function

$$\sum_j \rho_{1-t}(Y_{\bar{D}j} - h(\alpha, X)),$$

where $\rho_{1-t}(u) = (1-t)\max(u,0) + t\max(-u,0)$. Efron (1991) uses a different objective function. The estimates from these approaches, like those from the bin and smooth approach, reduce to the usual empirical quantiles when no covariates are included in the analysis.

The main disadvantage of these approaches is that they estimate each regression quantile function separately. That is, $q_Z(1-t_1)$ is estimated separately from $q_Z(1-t_2)$ for $t_1 \neq t_2$. Not only is this computationally inefficient when quantiles at multiple levels of t are required (or when the whole distribution, $S_{\bar{D},Z}$, is of interest, as in Sections 6.3 and 6.4), but neither is there any acknowledgment in the estimation that the regression quantile functions are, by definition, ordered in t:

$$q_Z(1 - t_1) \geqslant q_Z(1 - t_2) \quad \text{if} \quad t_1 < t_2 \,.$$

In finite samples the procedures can yield estimates that do not satisfy this constraint (He, 1997). Procedures that incorporate this constraint are likely to be more statistically efficient and less susceptible to illogical results.

6.2.4   Parametric estimation of $S_{\bar{D},Z}$

Parametric methods simultaneously estimate regression quantiles for all t by specifying a parametric form for $S_{\bar{D},Z}$. The simplest example is where a normal linear model is assumed:

$$Y_{\bar{D}} = \alpha_0 + \alpha_1 X + \varepsilon \,, \quad \varepsilon \sim \mathrm{N}(0, \sigma^2) \,.$$

Once the parameters α and σ^2 are estimated with the usual linear modeling methods, the regression quantile is estimated with

$$\hat{q}_Z(1 - t) = \hat{\alpha}_0 + \hat{\alpha}_1 X + \hat{\sigma}\Phi^{-1}(1 - t) \,.$$

Much more flexible models have been used. Cole (1990) introduced the 'LMS' method, where it is assumed that for a transformation W_Z we have

$$W_Z(Y) \sim \mathrm{N}(0, 1) \,.$$

The transformation involves three parametric functions of covariates: $M(Z)$, which denotes the median of Y; $V(Z)$, which is the (approximate) coefficient of variation; and $L(Z)$, the Box–Cox power transform, which is required to achieve normality. Specifically, the LMS model assumes that

$$W_Z(Y) = \frac{\{Y/M(Z)\}^{L(Z)} - 1}{L(Z)V(Z)} \sim \mathrm{N}(0, 1) \,.$$

Cole and Green (1992) suggest that smoothing splines be used to model $L(Z)$, $M(Z)$ and $V(Z)$, and base estimation on penalized likelihood. This parametric method is extremely flexible and yields the entire set of regression quantiles as

$$\hat{q}_Z(1 - t) = \hat{M}(Z)\{1 + \Phi^{-1}(1 - t)\hat{L}(Z)\hat{V}(Z)\}^{1/\hat{L}(Z)} \,.$$

An unsatisfactory aspect of the parametric approach is that data used to estimate $q_Z(1 - t)$ is not necessarily local to the quantile. For instance, data in the middle of the distribution, say at $t = 0.5$, affects the estimated quantile at $t = 0.01$ because it is used to estimate parameters and the parameters dictate the entire distribution for $t \in (0, 1)$. Indeed, the parametric approach even yields quantile estimates outside of the range of data. One must be cognizant of the inherent extrapolation in the parametric method. Some checking for goodness of fit in the tail of the distribution seems prudent, and caution needs to be exercised in making inferences outside of the observed data.

6.2.5 Semiparametric models

Intermediate between the fully parametric and nonparametric methods is an approach suggested by Heagerty and Pepe (1999) (see also He, 1997). The basic idea is to model covariate effects on some attributes of the distribution of $Y_{\bar{D}}$ but without specifying the distribution itself. In particular, they assume that

$$Y_{\bar{D}} = \mu(Z) + \sigma(Z)\varepsilon\,,$$

where $\mu(Z) = \mathrm{E}(Y_{\bar{D}}|Z)$ and $\sigma(Z) = \sqrt{\{\mathrm{var}(Y_{\bar{D}}|Z)\}}$ are specified as parametric functions of Z, but the distribution of ε, denoted by F_0, is completely unspecified except that it has mean 0 and variance 1. Quasilikelihood methods yield estimates of the parameters in the functions μ and σ, while the empirical distribution of the standardized residuals, $\{(Y_{\bar{D},j} - \hat{\mu}(Z_j))/\hat{\sigma}(Z_j)\}$, yields a nonparametric estimate of F_0 (see also Section 6.3.3).

He (1997) considers this to be a modification of the Koenker and Bassett (1978) approach to nonparametric regression quantile estimation, a modification that ensures estimated quantiles do not cross. Moreover, it reduces to the empirical quantiles in the absence of covariates. One models only covariate effects, not the distribution itself. However, with the above specification one does assume that covariates influence all quantiles similarly. We refer to Heagerty and Pepe (1999) for a relaxation of this assumption that allows the distribution of ε to also depend on covariates.

6.2.6 Application

Example 6.3

The data in Fig. 6.4 shows body mass index (BMI, defined as weight/height^2) for female children between 0 and 36 months of age. These data were derived from measurements taken on healthy children at clinic visits to a health maintenance organization in Seattle, USA (Whitaker et al., 1997). BMI varies substantially with age in young children, increasing rapidly during the first 9 months or so of life and decreasing slowly thereafter. When assessing the nutritional status of a child from her BMI, it is important to know both upper and lower quantiles of BMI in healthy children of the same age. We estimated quantiles using nonparametric, parametric and semiparametric methods. For details see a full description of these analyses in Heagerty and Pepe (1999). Briefly, the nonparametric method of Koenker and Bassett (1978) was applied separately for each of the nine quantile functions at $t = 0.01, 0.05, 0.10, 0.25, 0.50, 0.75, 0.90, 0.95$ and 0.99. Each was modeled as a natural cubic spline:

$$q_{\mathrm{age}}(1-t) = \sum_{k=1}^{K} \alpha_k^{1-t} R_k(\mathrm{age})\,,$$

where $\{R_k(\cdot),\ k = 1, \ldots, K\}$ is a set of natural spline basis functions with knots at 2, 4, 9, 15 and 25 months. Observe from Fig. 6.4(a) that the estimated quantiles almost cross at the upper end of the age range. Cole's parametric LMS

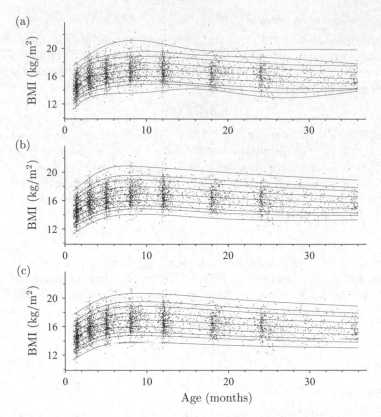

FIG. 6.4. Estimated quantiles of BMI for children aged between 0 and 36 months: (a) nonparametric (Koenker and Bassett, 1978), (b) LMS parametric (Cole, 1990) and (c) semiparametric (Heagerty and Pepe, 1999)

method was applied with $M(\text{age}) = \sum_k M_k R_k^C(\text{age})$, $L(\text{age}) = \sum_k L_k R_k^C(\text{age})$ and $S(\text{age}) = \sum_k S_k R_k^C(\text{age})$, where the basis $\{R_k^C, k = 1, \ldots, K\}$ had knots at 4, 9 and 18 months. Since this fully parameterizes the distribution of BMI, likelihood equations are used to estimate the parameters. The estimated quantile functions are shown in Fig. 6.4(b). Finally, quantile estimates were produced by the semiparametric method. Here we modeled mean and variance functions as

$$\mu(\text{age}) = \sum \mu_k R_k^{\mu}(\text{age}), \quad \log \sigma(\text{age}) = \sum \sigma_k R_k^{\sigma}(\text{age}),$$

where the natural spline basis had knots at 4, 9 and 18 months for $\mu(\cdot)$ and at 6 and 18 months for $\log \sigma(\cdot)$. Heagerty and Pepe (1999) found that the location-scale model fitted the data rather well. Thus the semiparametric and nonparametric functions are reasonably close. Increased variability in nonparametric estimates for high and low values of t is apparent, however. The parametric estimator is also reasonably close to the other two.   ∎

For the most part we use empirical quantiles when feasible. In this way assumptions about covariate effects on distributions are avoided. When this is not feasible, such as when covariates are continuous and/or there are many levels of distinct covariate values, we tend to use the semiparametric approach. It is easy to implement and only requires assumptions about covariate effects on means and variances that are reasonably easy to check with graphical methods. The assumption that the distribution of ε is the same across covariate values can be checked and relaxed, as described in Heagerty and Pepe (1999). We also refer the interested reader to that paper for discussion about modeling multiple covariates that are highly correlated, as often arises, and which introduces interesting challenges to the analysis.

6.2.7 Ordinal test results

The discussion thus far has implicitly assumed that Y is measured on a continuous scale. It is, of course, just as important to determine for ordinal tests if the distribution of $Y_{\bar{D}}$ depends on covariates. The empirical distribution can be calculated if the covariates are sufficiently few and discrete. Otherwise, ordinal regression models can be used to evaluate covariate effects (McCullagh and Nelder, 1999).

Generalized linear models of the form

$$g(\mathrm{P}[Y_{\bar{D}} \leqslant y | Z]) = c_y + \beta X \,,$$

where the c_y are category-specific constants and g^{-1} is a monotone increasing cumulative distribution function, can be fitted in most statistical packages. Logistic or probit link functions are popular choices for g. The category-specific constants are defined by the category cumulative probabilities when the covariables are $X = 0$. More complex models that incorporate multiplicative effects on the category-specific parameters are of the form

$$g(\mathrm{P}[Y_{\bar{D}} \leqslant y | Z]) = \sigma(Z)c_y + \mu(Z) \,,$$

and will be discussed later. For identifiability of c_y we set $\sigma(Z_0) = 1$ and $\mu(Z_0) = 0$ at the baseline covariate level Z_0 corresponding to the covariable $X = 0$. With μ and σ parameterized, likelihood methods analogous to those described previously in Section 5.4.2 can be used to estimate parameters.

Ordinal regression models typically make no assumptions about the threshold parameters, c_y. In essence, they are nonparametric with respect to the baseline distribution function:

$$\mathrm{P}[Y_{\bar{D}} \leqslant y | Z_0] = g^{-1}(c_y) \,.$$

We therefore consider them to be semiparametric, and indeed there is an obvious correspondence with the semiparametric model forms for continuous tests described in Section 6.2.5.

6.3 Modeling covariate effects on test results

6.3.1 *The basic idea*

We now return to the consideration of tests for distinguishing between diseased and non-diseased subjects, and how covariates can influence their discriminatory capacity. In particular, since we have addressed evaluation of covariates on the first dimension of accuracy, $S_{\bar{D}}$, we now consider the evaluation of covariate effects on the second dimension, namely on the ROC curve.

The first approach for evaluating covariate effects on the ROC curve was proposed by Tosteson and Begg (1988) in a seminal and very widely cited paper that was later expanded upon by Toledano and Gatsonis (1995). Their development was geared specifically towards ordinal data, but it actually applies more generally (Pepe, 1998). The basic idea is to model $S_{D,Z}$ in addition to $S_{\bar{D},Z}$ and to then calculate the induced covariate-specific ROC curve, $\mathrm{ROC}_Z(t) = S_{D,Z}(S_{\bar{D},Z}^{-1}(t))$, for any particular covariate values of interest. A comprehensive model is possible that includes both Y_D and $Y_{\bar{D}}$ in one model by incorporating disease status as a covariate. We present both fully parametric and semiparametric models in Sections 6.3.2 and 6.3.3, respectively, that are analogous to those described earlier in Sections 5.3.1 and 5.3.2 for the ROC curve estimation problem.

The strategy of modeling the test result distributions and calculating induced ROC curves is the longest established approach for evaluating covariate effects on the ROC. It is popular in part because modeling distributions is a familiar task for statisticians. Unfortunately, in general, it does not yield simple ways of summarizing covariate effects on the ROC curve. We will see, however, that under certain parameterizations for the distributions, $S_{D,Z}$ and $S_{\bar{D},Z}$, a simple correspondence between covariate effects on the test results and on the ROC curve can be established. Much of our discussion here concerns this correspondence.

6.3.2 *Induced ROC curves for continuous tests*

We begin with some examples.

Example 6.4

Suppose that
$$Y = \alpha_0 + \alpha_1 D + \alpha_2 X + \alpha_3 XD + \sigma(D)\varepsilon\,,$$

where $\varepsilon \sim \mathrm{N}(0,1)$ and $\sigma(D) = \sigma_D I[D = 1] + \sigma_{\bar{D}} I[D = 0]$. This allows the variance of Y to differ for disease versus non-disease observations. Then some algebra, similar to that in Result 4.7, yields that the ROC curve is

$$\mathrm{ROC}_Z(t) = \Phi\left(\frac{\alpha_1}{\sigma_D} + \frac{\alpha_3}{\sigma_D}X + \frac{\sigma_{\bar{D}}}{\sigma_D}\Phi^{-1}(1-t)\right).$$

This is a binormal curve with intercept $a = (\alpha_1 + \alpha_3 X)/\sigma_D$ and slope $b = \sigma_{\bar{D}}/\sigma_D$. Observe that, if a covariate has only a main effect in the regression model for the test result, i.e. $\alpha_3 = 0$, then it does not influence the separation between S_D

and $S_{\bar{D}}$, that is it does not affect the ROC curve. A covariate affects the ROC curve only if there is an interaction between X and D in the linear model for the test result. In particular, if the effect of X on Y is larger in diseased than in non-diseased subjects, then the ROC will increase with increasing values of X. ∎

Example 6.5

Suppose now that Z_D is a covariate specific to diseased subjects, such as disease severity or some subtype classification of disease. A model like that in Example 6.4, but without main effects, might be stipulated, since X_D does not apply to non-diseased subjects. The comprehensive model

$$Y = \alpha_0 + \alpha_1 D + \alpha_3 X_D D + \sigma(D)\varepsilon$$

is another way of writing the following constituent models for diseased and non-diseased subjects:

$$Y_D = \gamma_{0D} + \gamma_{1D} X_D + \sigma_D \varepsilon ,$$
$$Y_{\bar{D}} = \gamma_{0\bar{D}} + \sigma_{\bar{D}} \varepsilon .$$

Assuming again that $\varepsilon \sim N(0,1)$, the induced ROC curve model is

$$\mathrm{ROC}_{Z_D}(t) = \Phi \left(\frac{\alpha_1}{\sigma_D} + \frac{\alpha_3}{\sigma_D} X_D + \frac{\sigma_{\bar{D}}}{\sigma_D} \Phi^{-1}(1-t) \right) . \qquad ∎$$

The results in the above examples follow from the next general result for location-scale families of test result distributions.

Result 6.4

If the distribution function for Y conditional on disease status D and covariates Z follows a location-scale model:

$$Y = \mu(D, Z) + \sigma(D, Z)\varepsilon , \qquad (6.4)$$

where ε has survivor function S_0 with mean 0 and variance 1, then the corresponding covariate-specific ROC curve is

$$\mathrm{ROC}_Z(t) = S_0 \left(-a(Z) + b(Z) S_0^{-1}(t) \right) , \qquad (6.5)$$

where

$$a(Z) = (\mu(1, Z) - \mu(0, Z)) / \sigma(1, Z) ,$$
$$b(Z) = \sigma(0, Z)/\sigma(1, Z) .$$

Proof The threshold for Y that corresponds to a false positive fraction t is

$$q_Z(1-t) = \mu(0, Z) + \sigma(0, Z) S_0^{-1}(t) .$$

Therefore,

$$\mathrm{ROC}_Z(t) = \mathrm{P}[Y_D \geqslant q_Z(1-t)] = S_0 \left(\frac{q_Z(1-t) - \mu(1,Z)}{\sigma(1,Z)} \right)$$
$$= S_0 \left(\frac{\mu(0,Z) - \mu(1,Z)}{\sigma(1,Z)} + \frac{\sigma(0,Z)}{\sigma(1,Z)} S_0^{-1}(t) \right).$$ ∎

In our earlier examples S_0 is the standard normal survivor function, $S_0(y) = 1 - \Phi(y)$. Other natural choices might be logistic or exponential. Also, in our examples the variance parameters are not allowed to depend on covariates, although they do depend on disease status. In such cases, when $\sigma(0,Z) = \sigma(0)$ and $\sigma(1,Z) = \sigma(1)$, the covariate effect on the ROC curve is contained in the covariate effect on the difference in means between diseased and non-diseased subjects, $\mu(0,Z) - \mu(1,Z)$.

If the test results do not follow a location-scale family, we can still derive covariate-specific ROC curves as $\mathrm{ROC}_Z(t) = S_{D,Z}(S_{\bar{D},Z}^{-1}(t))$, where $S_{D,Z}$ and $S_{\bar{D},Z}$ are estimated either separately (Section 6.2) or in some comprehensive fashion. Simple analytic expressions that summarize covariate effects on the induced ROC curves are, however, generally not feasible. This is a drawback because it does not allow one to make general statements about the effect of a covariate on the discriminatory capacity of the test. With a location-scale structure, on the other hand, we are in the fortunate situation that parameters relating to covariate effects on test results translate directly into parameters that quantify covariate effects on the ROC curve.

With regards to techniques for estimation, parameters in fully parameterized models can be estimated using the usual likelihood or GEE techniques. The delta method yields standard errors for induced ROC parameters and confidence bands for induced ROC curves. Bootstrapping techniques may also be applied, and these are often easier to implement.

Example 6.6

Consider again the DPOAE audiology data described in Example 6.1. Recall that the covariables X_f, X_L and X_D code for stimulus frequency, stimulus intensity and severity of hearing impairment, respectively. We fit normal linear models to Y in the disease (hearing-impaired) and non-disease samples, written in a comprehensive form as

$$Y = \alpha_0 + \alpha_1 X_f + \alpha_2 X_L + \alpha_3 D$$
$$+ \alpha_4 D X_f + \alpha_5 D X_L + \alpha_6 D X_D + \sigma(D)\varepsilon, \qquad (6.6)$$

where $\sigma(D) = I[D=1]\sigma_D + I[D=0]\sigma_{\bar{D}}$. The parameter estimates are shown in Table 6.2. A p–p plot of the residuals suggests that the normal model holds reasonably well over the bulk of the data (Fig. 6.5).

Table 6.2 *Estimated parameters for the normal linear model for results of the DPOAE test*

Covariate	Parameter	Estimate
Constant	α_0	1.11
X_f	α_1	−0.14
X_L	α_2	−0.86
D	α_3	23.48
DX_f	α_4	0.47
DX_L	α_5	−4.91
DX_D	α_6	3.04
Scale $(D = 1)$	σ_D	8.01
Scale $(D = 0)$	$\sigma_{\bar{D}}$	7.74

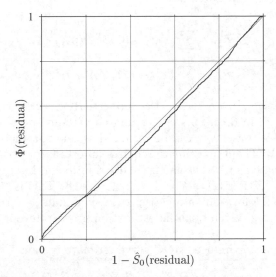

FIG. 6.5. Standardized residuals after fitting model (6.6). Shown is a normal probability plot, the standard normal cumulative distribution function versus the empirical distribution function of the residuals

The induced covariate-specific ROC curves are therefore

$$
\begin{aligned}
\mathrm{ROC}_Z(t) &= \Phi\left(\sigma_D^{-1}\{\alpha_3 + \alpha_4 X_f + \alpha_5 X_L + \alpha_6 X_D + \sigma_{\bar{D}}\Phi^{-1}(1-t)\}\right) \\
&= \Phi\left(2.93 + 0.06\,X_f - 0.61\,X_L + 0.38\,X_D + 0.97\,\Phi^{-1}(1-t)\right).
\end{aligned}
$$

The results suggest that increasing the intensity of the input stimulus yields a less accurate test. However, the test appears to be more accurate at higher frequencies. As expected, the coefficient for X_D is positive, implying that it is easier to distinguish more severely hearing-impaired ears from normal ears than it is to distinguish mildly-impaired ears from normally-hearing ears.   ∎

6.3.3 *Semiparametric location-scale families*

A location-scale model, as defined in Result 6.4, can be fitted using quasilikelihood methods without specifying S_0, the distribution of ε. In the special case where $\mu(D, Z)$ is parameterized by a vector of parameters α and the scale function $\sigma(D, Z)$ does not depend on the covariates, $\sigma(D, Z) = I[D = 1]\sigma_D + I[D = 0]\sigma_{\bar{D}}$, the estimator for α satisfies the estimating equation

$$\sum \left\{ \left(\frac{\partial}{\partial \alpha}\right) \mu(D, Z) \right\} \left(\frac{Y - \mu(D, Z)}{\sigma(D)}\right) = 0, \qquad (6.7)$$

while $\sigma_{\bar{D}}$ and σ_D are estimated as

$$\hat{\sigma}_{\bar{D}} = \sum_{}^{n_{\bar{D}}} (Y_{\bar{D}} - \hat{\mu}(0, Z))^2 / n_{\bar{D}},$$
$$\hat{\sigma}_D = \sum_{}^{n_D} (Y_D - \hat{\mu}(1, Z))^2 / n_D. \qquad (6.8)$$

Observe that the parameters of the induced ROC curve that quantify covariate effects, $a(Z)$ in Result 6.4, are estimated without specifying the survivor function S_0. In this sense they can be regarded as semiparametric estimates.

The induced ROC curve estimate requires an estimator for S_0. Pepe (1998) proposed to estimate S_0 with the empirical distribution of the standardized residuals $\{(Y_k - \hat{\mu}(D_k, Z_k))/\hat{\sigma}(D_k), k = 1, \ldots, n_D + n_{\bar{D}}\}$. This is the same idea as used in Section 6.2.5 for semiparametric regression quantile estimation. Indeed, that approach to regression quantile estimation grew from our earlier work on ROC analysis.

The semiparametric induced ROC curve estimate is then

$$\hat{\mathrm{ROC}}_Z(t) = \hat{S}_0 \left(\frac{\hat{\mu}(0, Z) - \hat{\mu}(1, Z)}{\hat{\sigma}(1, Z)} + \frac{\hat{\sigma}(0, Z)}{\hat{\sigma}(1, Z)} \hat{S}_0^{-1}(t) \right).$$

Example 6.6 (continued)

Consider (yet again!) the audiology data and the linear model specified in Example 6.6. The parameter estimates calculated with quasilikelihood are the same as those calculated with maximum likelihood. The only change is that here we estimate S_0, whereas in Section 6.3.2 we assume that S_0 is standard normal. Figure 6.5 is a plot of the standard normal cumulative distribution function versus $1 - \hat{S}_0$. It suggests that S_0 is indeed approximately standard normal.   ∎

Example 6.7

A reduced linear model that omits the disease severity covariate is

$$Y = \alpha_0 + \alpha_1 X_f + \alpha_2 X_L + \alpha_3 D + \alpha_4 D X_f + \alpha_5 D X_L + \sigma(D)\varepsilon.$$

The induced ROC curve at each frequency and intensity level from this model is

$$\mathrm{ROC}_Z(t) = S_0 \left(\sigma_D^{-1}\{-\alpha_3 - \alpha_4 X_f - \alpha_5 X_L + \sigma_{\bar{D}} S_0^{-1}(t)\}\right),$$

where S_0 is the survivor function for ε. These curves are compared with the corresponding empirical nonparametric ROC curves in Fig. 6.6 for three different settings. Curves that assume a normally distributed error are shown as well as the semiparametric estimator that estimates S_0 nonparametrically from the residuals.

It appears that the curves based on the normal linear model follow the empirical data rather well at the 1001 Hz stimulus frequency level. ∎

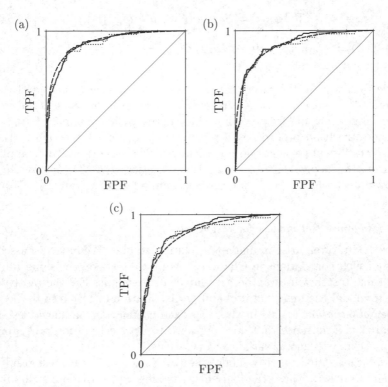

FIG. 6.6. ROC curves estimated with DPOAE test data using the normal linear model (dashed lines), the semiparametric linear model (solid lines) and the nonparametric method (dotted lines). Results are shown for the stimulus frequency of 1001 Hz and stimulus intensities of (a) 55 dB, (b) 60 dB and (c) 65 dB

6.3.4 *Induced ROC curves for ordinal tests*

For ordinal tests too, covariate-specific ROC curves can be calculated from fitted models for $S_{\bar{D},Z}$ and $S_{D,Z}$. Tosteson and Begg (1988) propose a location-scale-type ordinal regression model for ordinal test results. In our notation they postulate that

$$P[Y \geqslant y | Z, D] = S_0 \left(\frac{c_y - \mu(D, Z)}{\sigma(D, Z)} \right),$$ (6.9)

with particular specifications for μ, σ and S_0. For identifiability of c_y, we take $\mu(0, Z_0) = 0$ and $\sigma(0, Z_0) = 1$ at a baseline covariate value Z_0. The ordinal data location-scale model also yields the induced ROC curve form (6.5) that we found previously in the case of continuous data. We summarize this in the next result.

Result 6.5

Under the ordinal regression model (6.9), the induced ROC function at Z is

$$\mathrm{ROC}_Z(t) = S_0 \left(-a(Z) + b(Z) S_0^{-1}(t) \right)$$

for $t \in T(Z) = \{S_0([c_y - \mu(0, Z)]/\sigma(0, Z)), y = 1, \ldots, P - 1\}$, where $a(Z)$ and $b(Z)$ are given in Result 6.4.   ∎

Note that we use the discrete ROC function framework here and that the domain for the ROC curve, $T(Z)$, in general varies with the value of the covariate Z. The latent variable framework yields curves with domain $t \in (0, 1)$ using the same estimation procedures. Unfortunately, ordinal regression methods in standard statistical packages do not readily fit these models. The complication arises from the dependence of the scale parameter, $\sigma(D, Z)$, on disease status and covariates, which is generally not accommodated in standard software at present.

6.3.5 *Random effect models for test results*

Clustered data often arise in diagnostic testing studies. We have discussed some sources of such correlations in Chapter 3. Multiple tests on the same subject or by the same tester will often be correlated, for example. For the most part we choose to model the marginal probability distribution of test results (i.e. model on a *per observation basis*). In this approach correlations amongst test results are treated as a nuisance that does not need to alter estimation procedures but is simply acknowledged in variance calculations.

Approaches that explicitly model the correlations between test results have also been proposed. These random effects models can provide insights into the variability in test results. Etzioni *et al.* (1999*b*) propose such models for a continuous test outcome, namely multiple longitudinally-collected serum PSA measurements on subjects for prostate cancer detection. They are considered for binary tests in the context of meta-analysis by Rutter and Gatsonis (2001) (see Section 9.1). The issue has received most attention perhaps in the radiology literature, where multiple readings of different images by the same radiologist are common. In addition, multiple readings of the same image by different radiologists are likely to be correlated. We refer to Ishwaran and Gatsonis (2000) for a thorough and technically sophisticated treatment of the topic. See Gatsonis (1995) for an earlier discussion.

Location-scale models that incorporate random effects into the location and/or scale parameters are used universally. Let us briefly consider the radiology setting where Y_{kr} is an ordinal reading of the kth image by reader r. A relatively simple model formulation that incorporates between-reader variability is

$$\mathrm{P}[Y_{kr} \geqslant y] = S_0\left((c_y - \gamma_r - \alpha_{1r}D_k - \alpha_{2r}X_{kr} - \alpha_{3r}D_kX_{kr})/\sigma(D_k)\right),$$

where $(\gamma_r, \alpha_{1r}, \alpha_{2r}, \alpha_{3r})$ are parameters that are allowed to vary randomly with radiologist, and by convention $\sigma(D_k) = 1$ when $D_k = 0$. This model allows readers to vary in their baseline threshold values (at $X_{kr} = 0$) through the terms γ_r. The varying effects of X_{kr} on their thresholds is quantified through variability in α_{2r}. The induced radiologist-specific ROC curves are

$$\mathrm{ROC}(t) = S_0\left(\frac{1}{\sigma_D}\{-\alpha_{1r} - \alpha_{3r}X_{kr} + S_0^{-1}(t)\}\right).$$

Thus, the α_{1r} parameters quantify the variability across readers in their baseline ROC curves (at $X_{kr} = 0$) and α_{3r} accounts for covariate effects. It is interesting to decompose the variability in test results across readers into two components, which describe their varying use of thresholds and their varying inherent accuracies (or ROC curves). When only a few readers are involved explicit fixed-effect covariates can be included for each reader (see Example 6.12). However, when there are many readers and inference is sought that applies to the population of readers from which they are drawn, then random effects models are appropriate.

The fitting of random effects models in diagnostic testing applications is not different from that in other contexts. We do not discuss the technical implementation here but refer to the extensive literature on the topic (Diggle *et al.*, 2002). The one aspect that is particular to diagnostic testing is the decomposition of variability into that affecting $S_{\bar{D}}$ and that affecting the separation between S_D and $S_{\bar{D}}$, i.e. the ROC curves. Again we refer to Ishwaran and Gatsonis (2000) for extensive illustrations.

6.4 Modeling covariate effects on ROC curves

Covariate effects on ROC curves can be quantified directly by modeling the ROC curve itself. This contrasts with the approach set forth in the previous section, where covariate effects on test results were quantified and their effects on the ROC curves were calculated indirectly. There are several advantages to the direct modeling approach. Foremost amongst them is that the interpretation of model parameters pertains directly to the ROC curves. In addition, multiple tests can be accommodated simultaneously, providing a mechanism for comparing tests even when their results are quantified in different units, with or without adjustment for other covariates. This cannot be achieved by modeling test results. The relative merits of directly modeling ROC curves versus test results are discussed in detail later in Section 6.5.2. First we introduce the approach.

6.4.1   The ROC–GLM regression model

An ROC regression model to quantify covariate effects on the ROC curves has two components. These are, firstly, the covariables X which are the chosen numerical characterizations of Z and, secondly, a formulation for the ROC curve as a function of t. The following defines the class of ROC–GLMs.

Definition

Let $h_0(\cdot)$ and $g(\cdot)$ denote monotone increasing (or decreasing) functions on $(0,1)$. Then the equation

$$g(\text{ROC}_Z(t)) = h_0(t) + \beta X , \qquad (6.10)$$

with $t \in T_Z \subset (0,1)$ is an ROC–GLM regression model.   ∎

The link function g is specified as part of the model. Examples might be probit with $g(t) = \Phi^{-1}(t)$, or logistic with $g(t) = \text{logit}\, t = \log(t/(1 - t))$ or logarithmic with $g(t) = \log t$. The baseline function $h_0(t)$ is unknown. A parametric form for it can be specified (Alonzo and Pepe, 2002), or it can remain completely unspecified (Cai and Pepe, 2002).

The restrictions on h_0 and on g are meant to ensure that $\text{ROC}_Z(t)$ is an ROC curve in the sense that its domain and range are in $(0,1)$ and that it is increasing in t. Note, however, that the model need not be defined for the entire interval $t \in (0,1)$ but possibly only on a proper subset, and that the subset can vary with Z. Thus, these models are applicable to ordinal tests where T_Z could denote the attainable false positive fractions for the test operating at covariate value Z. In some cases one is only interested in modeling the ROC over a proper subset of $(0,1)$, so that again $T_Z \neq (0,1)$. In particular, for population screening tests one might only model ROC curves over $T = (0, t_0)$ for some small value t_0.

The covariable vector X can have components that depend on t. For example, if G is a binary variable denoting gender, then by including in the model the components $X_1 = G \times I[t \in (0, 0.5)]$ and $X_2 = G \times I[t \in (0.5, 1)]$ we allow the effect of gender on the ROC curve to differ over the false positive ranges $(0, 0.5)$ and $(0.5, 1)$. The general formulation therefore does not necessarily stipulate that the covariate effect is constant over $t \in (0, 1)$, although a conscious effort to model the varying effect will be necessary in practice. This is similar to relaxing the proportional hazards assumption in the Cox regression model for failure time data by modeling the time-varying effect (Collett, 1994).

Examples 6.8

1. Consider a dichotomous covariate, Z, indicating group membership, say, with covariable $X = 0$ or 1 and the model

$$\Phi^{-1}\{\mathrm{ROC}_Z(t)\} = \alpha_0 + \alpha_1 \Phi^{-1}(t) + \beta X \,.$$

Then $g = \Phi^{-1}$, and $h(t) = \alpha_0 + \alpha_1 \Phi^{-1}(t)$ is a parametric function. The model stipulates that for both groups the ROC curve is binormal with the same slope parameter α_1. The intercepts may differ. If $\beta > 0$ then the ROC curve for the group with $X = 1$ is higher than that for the group coded as $X = 0$.

2. Consider the same context as above, but a model with different link function and unspecified baseline ROC function:

$$\mathrm{logit}\,\mathrm{ROC}_Z(t) = h_0(t) + \beta X \,.$$

The parameter β can be interpreted as the odds ratio of correctly classifying a diseased subject in the two groups when the thresholds for the test are chosen, possibly differently in each group, but so that the false positive fractions of the test are equal in the two groups. The model stipulates that the odds ratio of TPFs is the same, no matter at what common false positive fraction the tests are operating.

3. Again with a dichotomous covariate consider

$$\log \mathrm{ROC}_Z(t) = h_0(t) + \beta_1 X + \beta_2 (t - 0.1) I[t \in (0.1, 0.2)] X$$

for $t \leqslant 0.20$. This model uses a log link, so that β_1 and β_2 pertain to relative true positive fractions when false positive fractions are set equal for $X = 1$ and $X = 0$. Suppose that there are two tests and X denotes the test type covariable, $X = 1$ for test A. Then one can interpret $\exp(\beta_1 + \beta_2(t - 0.1)I[t > 0.1])$ as the relative true positive fraction, $\mathrm{rTPF}(A, B)$, when thresholds are chosen for the two tests so that they both have false positive fractions equal to t. The $\log \mathrm{rTPF}(A, B)$ is constant for $t \in (0, 0.1)$ and increases (or decreases) linearly thereafter. The model is specified only for $t \in (0, 0.2)$.

4. Consider the DPOAE hearing test study (Example 6.1) and the following model:

$$\log \mathrm{ROC}_{Z,Z_D}(t) = \alpha_0 + \alpha_1 \Phi^{-1}(t) + \beta_1 X_f + \beta_2 X_L + \beta_3 X_D \,.$$

This model quantifies the increase in the TPF of the DPOAE test for a 100 Hz increase in frequency as $\exp \beta_1$, when the FPF and all other covariates are held constant. Similarly, $\exp \beta_2$ quantifies the increase in the TPF with a 10 dB increase in intensity of the stimulus. Finally, $\exp \beta_3$ is the increase in the TPF for every 10 dB of hearing loss. The form of the ROC curve in this model is fully parameterized with $h_0(t) = \alpha_0 + \alpha_1 \Phi^{-1}(t)$. ∎

The form of the ROC–GLM is general and flexible. We also note that special cases of it arise from models for test result distributions that were employed in the previous section.

Result 6.6

If the test result distribution follows a linear model

$$Y = \gamma_0 + \gamma_1 D + \gamma_2 X + \gamma_3 XD + \sigma(D)\varepsilon,$$

where ε has mean 0 and variance 1, then the induced ROC model is an ROC–GLM.

Proof   Writing the survivor function for ε as $S_0(\cdot)$, from Result 6.4 we see that

$$S_0^{-1}\left(\mathrm{ROC}_Z(t)\right) = \frac{\sigma(0)}{\sigma(1)}S_0^{-1}(t) - \frac{\gamma_1}{\sigma(1)} - \frac{\gamma_3 X}{\sigma(1)}.$$

This is of the ROC–GLM form with

$$g = S_0^{-1}, \quad h_0(t) = -\frac{\gamma_1}{\sigma(1)} + \frac{\sigma(0)}{\sigma(1)}S_0^{-1}(t) \quad \text{and} \quad \beta = -\frac{\gamma_3}{\sigma(1)}. \quad \blacksquare$$

In a similar fashion, Result 6.5 indicates that the Tosteson and Begg model for ordinal test results (6.9) gives rise to an ROC–GLM if the covariates do not affect the scale function $\sigma(D, Z)$ and affect the location function $\mu(D, Z)$ through a linear function of covariables and disease status.

Although models for test result distributions induce models for ROC curves, the reverse is not true. The ROC–GLM in and of itself does not imply models for test results. It only specifies how the distributions of Y_D and $Y_{\bar{D}}$ are related to each other. In this sense the approach in this Section 6.4 makes less assumptions than the approach presented in Section 6.3. Indeed, when no covariates are included the distinctions already made between the two approaches in Sections 5.3 and 5.5 are equally relevant here.

6.4.2   *Fitting the model to data*

Suppose that we parameterize $h_0(t) = \sum \alpha_s h_s(t)$, as in Section 5.5.2. The ROC is then fully parameterized. The techniques we describe here for fitting this parametric ROC–GLM regression model are similar to those described in Section 5.5 for calculating the ROC–GLM estimator of the ROC curve. There are two key concepts. The first is that the test result from each diseased unit is transformed to its *placement value* in the relevant non-diseased distribution. Recall that in Section 5.2.5 the placement value was defined in the setting where no covariates were involved. Here we generalize the notion. Thus, if (Y_{Di}, Z_i, Z_{Di}) denotes the test result and covariates for the ith diseased observation, then we write its placement value as

$$\text{placement value} = S_{\bar{D}, Z_i}(Y_{Di}).$$

The appropriate non-disease reference distribution depends on the covariates, Z_i. Only the covariates in common with those for non-diseased subjects are relevant, not Z_{Di}. Recall that the distribution of the placement values is the ROC curve, i.e.

$$\mathrm{P}[S_{\bar{D},Z_i}(Y_{Di}) \leqslant t | Z_i, Z_{Di}] = \mathrm{ROC}_{Z_i, Z_{Di}}(t). \qquad (6.11)$$

The second key concept is that, for any t, the binary random variable

$$U_{it} = I[S_{\bar{D},Z_i}(Y_{Di}) \leqslant t] \qquad (6.12)$$

follows a generalized linear model, because according to (6.11) and the form of the ROC–GLM (6.10) we have

$$\begin{aligned} g\left(\mathrm{E}[U_{it}|Z_i, Z_{Di}]\right) &= g\left(\mathrm{ROC}_{Z_i, Z_{Di}}(t)\right) \\ &= h_0(t) + \beta X_i. \end{aligned}$$

Then an algorithm for fitting the ROC–GLM is given in Table 6.3.

The algorithm requires making several choices: the estimator for the reference distribution $S_{\bar{D},Z}$; the domain of false positive fractions at which the ROC model is to be fitted, which we denote by T; and the working covariance matrix for fitting the marginal model in step 5. With respect to the last point, we use independence working covariance matrices primarily because we then do not need to worry about the validity of the Pepe–Anderson condition (Pepe and Anderson, 1994) for generalized estimating equations. With regards to the estimator for $S_{\bar{D},Z}$, any of those described in Section 6.2 could be used.

The choice for T depends of course on the subinterval of $(0, 1)$ over which the model is stipulated to hold. In addition, in order to use standard packages for fitting the model in step 5, the number of observations $n_T \times n_D$ must be finite, where n_T denotes the number of points in T. One could fix n_T at some reasonable (finite) value and choose equally-spaced values in the domain of interest (Alonzo and Pepe, 2002). How to choose values in the domain in order to achieve optimal

Table 6.3 *An algorithm for fitting the parametric ROC–GLM regression model*

Step	Procedure
1	Estimate the non-disease reference distributions, $\hat{S}_{\bar{D},Z}$, using test results for non-disease observations
2	Calculate estimated placement values for each disease observation $\hat{S}_{\bar{D},Z_i}(Y_{Di})$, $i = 1, \ldots, n_D$
3	For each $t \in T$, calculate the binary placement value indicators $\{\hat{U}_{it}, t \in T, i = 1, \ldots, n_D\}$, where $\hat{U}_{it} = I[\hat{S}_{\bar{D},Z_i}(Y_{Di}) \leqslant t]$
4	For each $t \in T$, calculate $\{h_s(t), s = 1, \ldots, S\}$
5	Fit the marginal generalized linear binary regression model to the data $\{(\hat{U}_{it}, h_1(t), \ldots, h_S(t), Z_{Di}, Z_i), i = 1, \ldots, n_D, t \in T\}$

efficiency is an open question at this time. Alonzo and Pepe (2002) did investigate efficiency gains by using larger numbers of observations, i.e. by increasing n_T. Their results suggest that efficiency is high with reasonably small values for n_T. In practice one could estimate parameters with increasing values for n_T and quit when the decrease in parameter standard errors is adequately small. Observe that, if n_T is very large, the computational effort with standard algorithms can be very large because in effect the fitting algorithm must deal with $n_T \times n_D$ observations. With finite n_T, these estimating equations for α and β are of the form

$$\sum_{k=1}^{n_T} \sum_{i=1}^{n_D} (X_i, h(t_k))' \, w\, (X_i, t_k) \, (\hat{U}_{it_k} - g^{-1}(h_0(t_k) + \beta X_i)) = 0 \,, \qquad (6.13)$$

where $(X_i, h(t))'$ denotes the transpose of $\{X_i, h_1(t), \dots, h_S(t)\}$ and $w(X_i, t)$ is a weight function that may depend on α and β.

Alternatively, one can solve the limiting estimating equations as $n_T \to \infty$ (Pepe, 1997; Cai and Pepe, 2002). If we seek to fit over an interval, $T = (t_1, t_2)$ say, with uniform distribution of t in T, then the limiting estimating equation as $n_T \to \infty$ is

$$\sum_{i=1}^{n_D} \int_{t_1}^{t_2} (X_i, h(t))' \, w(X_i, t)(\hat{U}_{it} - g^{-1}(h_0(t) + \beta X_i)) \, \mathrm{d}\mu(t) = 0 \,, \qquad (6.14)$$

where μ is the Lebesgue measure. Other measures can be used in (6.14), and indeed by using a counting measure on $\{t_1, \dots, t_{n_T}\}$ eqn (6.14) reduces to (6.13), so (6.14) is just a more general formulation. Similarly, for ordinal data the measure μ will be discrete and could be chosen as the observed probability measure for $Y_{\bar{D}}$.

The semiparametric ROC–GLM, in which the baseline function $h_0(t)$ is not parameterized, can also be fitted with some modifications to the algorithm of Table 6.3. In particular, we drop step 4, and in step 5 we iterate between solving

$$\sum_{k=1}^{n_T} \sum_{i=1}^{n_D} X_i' \, w(X_i, t_k)(\hat{U}_{it_k} - g^{-1}(\hat{h}_0(t_k) + \beta X_i)) = 0$$

for β given $\{\hat{h}_0(t_k), k = 1, \dots, n_T\}$ and

$$\sum_{i=1}^{n_D} (\hat{U}_{it_k} - g^{-1}(h_0(t_k) + \hat{\beta} X_i)) = 0$$

for $h_0(t_k)$ given $\beta = \hat{\beta}$, $k = 1, \dots, n_T$. We refer to Cai and Pepe (2002) for details.

Asymptotic distribution theory for the parametric approach is similar to that given in Result 5.8 for the parameters of the parametric distribution-free estimator of the ROC curve. Cai and Pepe (2002) derive distribution theory for the semiparametric approach and allow data to be clustered. For inference in practice, however, we use bootstrap procedures to evaluate sampling variability. The relative merits of bootstrapping versus asymptotic theory for inference remains to be explored.

6.4.3   Comparing ROC curves

We used the regression framework in Chapter 3 to compare binary tests with regards to their true and false positive fractions, their predictive values and their diagnostic likelihood ratios. Here we use the regression framework to compare tests with regards to their ROC curves. We write 'Test' for the covariate denoting test type, A or B, and define the covariable $X_{\text{Test}} = 1$ for test type A and $X_{\text{Test}} = 0$ for test type B.

Consider the model

$$g(\text{ROC}_{\text{Test}}(t)) = h_0(t) + \beta X_{\text{Test}} \qquad (6.15)$$

on the domain $t \in T$. This model stipulates that, for test type B, its ROC curve is $\text{ROC}(t) = g^{-1}(h_0(t))$, while that for test A is $\text{ROC}(t) = g^{-1}(h_0(t) + \beta)$. If the two tests have the same ROC curve over T, then $\beta = 0$.

Example 6.9

The data in Fig. 6.7 pertain to the ovarian cancer gene expression study, described in Section 1.3.6, that includes $n_{\bar{D}} = 23$ normal ovarian tissues and $n_D = 30$ cancerous ovarian tissues. The empirical ROC curves for genes 1 and 2 in this dataset suggest that gene 2 is the better biomarker for cancer.

We first fit a parametric ROC–GLM of the form (6.15), with g being the logit function $\Psi(u) = \log(u/(1-u))$, $h_0(t) = \alpha_0 + \alpha_1 \Psi^{-1}(t)$ and X_{Test} denoting the two genes ($X_{\text{Test}} = 1$ for gene 2). We chose to estimate $S_{\bar{D},\text{Test}}$ separately for the two biomarkers using the empirical survivor functions. Each subject has two data records, one for each biomarker. Non-diseased subjects contribute one each to the estimation of $\hat{S}_{\bar{D},0}$ and $\hat{S}_{\bar{D},1}$. For subjects with cancer, two placement values are calculated from the pair of biomarker values measured on them. We set $T = \{1/n_{\bar{D}}, \ldots, (n_{\bar{D}}-1)/n_{\bar{D}}\}$, the maximal set of unique empirical false positive fractions, and fit a probit regression model to the binary variables $\{\hat{U}_{it_k}\}$ with 'covariates' $\{(\Psi^{-1}(t_k), X_{\text{Test}_i}), i = 1, \ldots, 2n_D, k = 1, \ldots, n_{\bar{D}} - 1\}$.

We find $\hat{\beta} = 0.933$ with standard error 0.332 (estimated with the bootstrap). The semiparametric approach yields $\hat{\beta} = 0.938$ with a somewhat larger standard error of 0.416. Both approaches yield quantitatively similar results with p values for the hypothesis $\beta = 0$ being less than 0.05 for both approaches ($p = 0.02$ for the semiparametric model and $p = 0.005$ for the parametric model). The two curves can also be compared using the classic nonparametric AUC statistic (Section 5.2.6). We calculate estimated AUCs of 0.839 (gene 2) and 0.625 (gene 1), with p value for equality of AUCs equal to 0.027.   ■

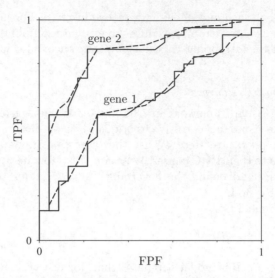

FIG. 6.7. Estimated ROC curves for gene expression relative intensities at two genes in ovarian cancer and non-cancer tissue. Estimates are based on a semi-parametric ROC–GLM approach (dashed lines). Shown also are empirical ROC curves (solid lines)

Example 6.10

We return now to the pancreatic cancer data of Wieand *et al.* (1989). In Example 5.7 we estimated binormal ROC curves for the two biomarkers, CA-19-9 and CA-125, and compared the intercept and slope parameters of the curves. Here we will do essentially the same thing, but set the analysis within the ROC regression framework. Write the comprehensive model as

$$\text{ROC}_{\text{Test}}(t) = \Phi(\alpha_0 + \alpha_1 \Phi^{-1}(t) + \beta_1 X_{\text{Test}} + \beta_2 X_{\text{Test}} \Phi^{-1}(t)),$$

where $X_{\text{Test}} = 1$ for CA-19-9 and $X_{\text{Test}} = 0$ for CA-125. This is an ROC–GLM with $h_0(t) = \alpha_0 + \alpha_1 \Phi^{-1}(t)$, $g = \Phi^{-1}$ and covariables $(X_{\text{Test}}, X_{\text{Test}} \Phi^{-1}(t))$. We fit this model over the interval of false positive fractions $(0, 0.2)$ using the empirical survivor functions for CA-19-9 and for CA-125 in non-diseased subjects as estimates of $S_{\bar{D},1}$ and $S_{\bar{D},0}$, respectively. Again, all observed empirical false positive fractions in $(0, 0.2)$ define T. The results are shown in Table 6.4.

The statistically significant estimate of β_2 indicates that the difference between the ROC curves is not constant on the probit scale, but decreases with increasing false positive fractions (Fig. 5.5). An overall test for equality of the curves using the Wald test based on $(\hat{\beta}_1, \hat{\beta}_2)$ yields a conclusive p value which is less than 0.001, identical to our previous analysis. ∎

Table 6.4 *ROC–GLM fit to the pancreatic cancer biomarker data to compare CA-125 and CA-19-9*

Parameter	Estimate	Standard error
α_0	0.91	0.66
α_1	1.35	0.44
β_1	0.23	0.71
β_2	-0.91	0.46

6.4.4   Three examples

We now apply the ROC–GLM methodology to three different datasets. The first is the audiology dataset that we previously analyzed by modeling test results. It will give us an opportunity to compare the two approaches. The second is a multireader radiology study comparing two imaging modalities. The last is a longitudinal dataset involving PSA trajectories for men with prostate cancer prior to their diagnosis and for controls that did not develop cancer. These examples are meant in part to convey the breadth of questions that can be asked within the ROC–GLM framework.

Example 6.11

Let us model the ROC curves for the DPOAE test as a function of the covariates, stimulus frequency (f), stimulus intensity (L) and degree of hearing loss. The corresponding covariables X_f, X_L and X_D were defined at the beginning of this chapter in Example 6.1. We write the ROC–GLM model as

$$\Phi^{-1}(\text{ROC}(t)) = \alpha_0 + \alpha_1\Phi^{-1}(t) + \beta_1 X_f + \beta_2 X_L + \beta_3 X_D.$$

Results of an analysis using this model, but a slightly different fitting algorithm, are reported in Pepe (1998) and are quantitatively similar to those found earlier in Examples 6.6 and 6.7. The model is fitted over the entire $(0,1)$ interval. In particular, at each distinct covariate level, $Z = (f, L)$, i.e. for each unique combination of frequency and stimulus intensity, we set T_Z to be the observed false positive fractions $\{1/n_{\bar{D},Z}, \ldots, (n_{\bar{D},Z}-1)/n_{\bar{D},Z}\}$, where $n_{\bar{D},Z}$ is the number of normally-hearing ears tested with that stimulus setting. We choose $\hat{S}_{\bar{D},Z}$ to be the empirical survivor function for $Y_{\bar{D}}$ at covariate level $Z = (f, L)$.

Estimates calculated with the algorithm of Table 6.3 are $\hat{\beta}_1 = 0.050$ (se $=$ 0.031), $\hat{\beta}_2 = -0.433$ (se $= 0.118$) and $\hat{\beta}_3 = 0.443$ (se $= 0.089$). The standard errors, shown in parentheses, are calculated with the bootstrap. The test appears to perform better when the stimulus used has a lower intensity. The p value associated with β_2 is conclusive. There is some evidence that performance is better at higher frequencies ($\hat{\beta}_1 > 0$), but this result is not conclusive.

The estimate of β_3 clearly indicates that more severe hearing impairment is easier to detect than is mild impairment. Moreover, adjustment for degree of hearing impairment is important. The estimates of the parameters pertaining to the stimulus settings, β_1 and β_2, are both larger in the above model that includes degree of impairment than in a model that excludes it:

$$\Phi^{-1}(\text{ROC}(t)) = \alpha_0 + \alpha_1\Phi^{-1}(t) + \beta_1 X_f + \beta_2 X_L ,$$

where we calculate $\hat{\beta}_1 = 0.041$ (se $= 0.028$) and $\hat{\beta}_2 = -0.395$ (se $= 0.108$).   ∎

Example 6.12

Consider the radiology reading study described in Muller *et al.* (1989) and Thompson and Zucchini (1989) and analyzed with the ROC–GLM model in Pepe (1997). This experiment was conducted to compare two different modalities of constructing scintigraphic images. Fifty plates had a copper disc placed in a random position on one half of the plate. The copper disc simulated a lesion. The plates were processed with two different imaging modalities. Three readers read each half-plate (i.e. 200 images) in random order and classified it into one of five categories according to their degree of suspicion that a lesion was present. Category 1 indicated that a lesion was definitely not present, while category 5 indicated that a lesion was definitely present. The 4th and 5th categories were combined because of the rarity of evaluations in category 5. Thus Y takes the values $\{1, 2, 3, 4\}$. The reading process was repeated one week after the initial evaluations.

In this example, the covariates are readers (1, 2 and 3) and modalities (A and B). We define covariables for the readers, $X_2 = I[\text{reader 2}]$ and $X_3 = I[\text{reader 3}]$, and for the modality, $X_{\text{Test}} = I[\text{modality B}]$, and use the ROC–GLM

$$\text{logit ROC}(t) = \alpha_0 + \alpha_1 \text{logit} t + \beta_1 X_{\text{Test}} + \beta_2 X_2 + \beta_3 X_3 .$$

In this model, $\exp \beta_1$ is the odds of correctly classifying a disease image with modality B versus A when the false positive fractions are set equal. The odds ratio is assumed to be constant across t and across readers.

To fit the model we proceed as follows. For each modality we fit an ordinal regression model to test results from non-disease images in order to estimate $S_{\bar{D},Z}$. In particular, we fit models

$$\text{logit } S_{\bar{D},Z}(y) = c_y^{X_{\text{Test}}} + \gamma_2^{X_{\text{Test}}} X_2 + \gamma_3^{X_{\text{Test}}} X_3 ,$$

where the parameters γ_2, γ_3 and the c_y are estimated separately for the two modalities ($X_{\text{Test}} = 0$ and $X_{\text{Test}} = 1$). The ROC–GLM fitting algorithm is then applied with $T_Z = \{\hat{P}[Y_{\bar{D},Z} \geqslant y], y = 2, 3, 4\}$, where $\hat{P}[Y_{\bar{D},Z} \geqslant y]$ are the fitted values from the ordinal regression models. Results are displayed in Table 6.5.

It appears that modality B is better than A. The detection odds ratio is estimated as $\exp \hat{\beta}_1 = 1.55$ ($p < 0.05$). Figure 6.8 displays ROC curves for the two modalities when reader 1 reads images.

Turning now to the readers, we see that they are similar in their abilities to discriminate between images with and without lesions. Confidence intervals for β_2

Table 6.5 *Parameter estimates calculated for radiology data*

Parameter	Estimate	95% confidence interval
β_1	0.44	$(0.15, 0.83)$
β_2	0.12	$(-0.28, 0.50)$
β_3	-0.13	$(-0.65, 0.36)$
α_0	1.56	$(1.02, 2.19)$
α_1	0.71	$(0.57, 0.87)$

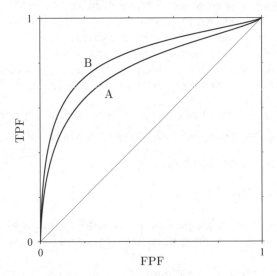

FIG. 6.8. Estimated ROC curves for reader 1 with two different imaging modalities. Here $X_2 = X_3 = 0$, $X_{\text{Test}} = 0$ in the lower curve and $X_{\text{Test}} = 1$ in the upper curve

and β_3 contain 0 well within their boundaries. Note that this comparison adjusts for differences amongst the readers in their uses of the rating scale because it is based on their ROC curves. Interestingly, the readers differ in their uses of the rating scale. With modality B we estimate $\hat{\gamma}_2^1 = 1.89$ $(1.32, 2.47)$ and $\hat{\gamma}_3^1 = 2.21$ $(1.61, 2.82)$, where 95% confidence intervals are shown in parentheses. With modality A we calculate $\hat{\gamma}_2^0 = 1.56$ $(1.01, 2.12)$ and $\hat{\gamma}_3^0 = 1.78$ $(1.21, 2.34)$. Thus readers 2 and 3 tend to use higher categories more often than does reader 1. ∎

Example 6.13

Our last example concerns the analysis of serum PSA levels for detecting subclinical prostate cancer. The study was described in Section 1.3.5. Briefly, 71 subjects enrolled in the CARET study that developed prostate cancer were identified, as were 70 age-matched controls. Serum samples that were stored as part of the CARET study were analyzed for total and free (unbound) PSA. Only samples taken prior to diagnosis were considered for the cases. At least three prediagnosis samples were available for 50 of the cases.

The focus of this study was to compare the standard PSA measure (total PSA) with an alternative, the negative ratio of free to total PSA measured in serum. We consider the type of PSA measure, total or ratio, as a covariate and define the corresponding covariable $X_{\text{type}} = 0$ if the PSA measure is the ratio and $X_{\text{type}} = 1$ for the total PSA concentration.

Two other covariates must be considered in the analysis. The first is age, because PSA levels are known to vary with age, even in subjects without cancer, and might do so differently in cases versus controls. The second has to do with the timing of the serum samples from cases in relation to their diagnosis. Samples taken shortly before diagnosis of clinical cancer are more likely to contain high levels of PSA compared with samples taken years before. Let

$$X_{\text{time}} = \text{time of diagnosis} - \text{time of serum sampling},$$
$$X_{\text{age}} = \text{age of the study subject in years} - 50.$$

We write the ROC–GLM model as

$$\Phi^{-1}\{\text{ROC}(t)\} = \alpha_0 + \alpha_1\Phi^{-1}(t) + \beta_1 X_{\text{type}} + \beta_2 X_{\text{time}} + \beta_3 X_{\text{type}} X_{\text{time}} + \beta_4 X_{\text{age}}.$$

This model allows the difference in discriminatory capacities of the two PSA measures to vary with the time at which the serum specimen was sampled relative to diagnosis.

To fit this model we first estimate $S_{\bar{D},Z}$, where $Z = (\text{age}, \text{PSA type})$ are the covariates that are not disease specific. We model age effects on the two biomarkers separately with semiparametric linear models

$$\log Y_{\bar{D}} = \gamma_0 + \gamma_1 X_{\text{age}} + \varepsilon_{\bar{D}},$$

where the distribution of $\varepsilon_{\bar{D}}$ is unspecified.

Results of fitting the ROC–GLM to data are shown in Table 6.6. Observe the negative coefficient associated with time. As expected, we see that the discriminatory capacities of both markers diminish with longer time-lags between serum sampling and clinical diagnosis. Total PSA appears to be the better biomarker for prostate cancer, the estimated coefficient for β_1 being 0.58 which is positive ($p < 0.01$). The difference between the biomarkers on the probit scale, however, decreases as the time of sampling prior to diagnosis lengthens ($\beta_3 < 0$). It appears that by about 7 years prior to diagnosis the two biomarkers are equivalent. Figure 6.9 displays fitted ROC curves for 65 year old men at various times prior to clinical diagnosis. For total PSA we see that by using a threshold that yields a 10% false positive fraction we will identify 64% of cancers 2 years before their clinical diagnosis, 51% at 4 years before diagnosis, but only 25% at 8 years prior

Table 6.6 *Estimated parameters for the ROC analysis of the PSA biomarker data*

Factor	Parameter	Estimate	95% confidence interval
Type	β_1	0.58	$(0.21, 1.08)$
Time (per year)	β_2	-0.09	$(-0.17, -0.01)$
Type $\times$ time	β_3	-0.08	$(-0.15, -0.02)$
Age (per decade)	β_4	-0.13	$(-0.06, 0.03)$
ROC intercept	α_0	1.30	$(0.53, 2.26)$
ROC slope	α_1	0.77	$(0.63, 0.93)$

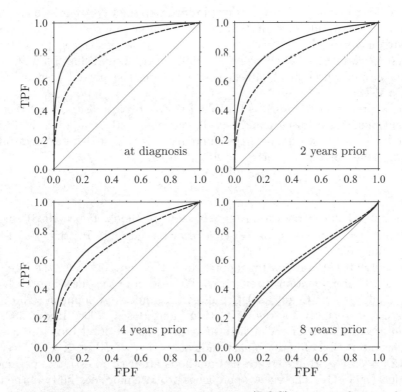

FIG. 6.9. Receiver operating characteristic (ROC) curves for total PSA (prostate-specific antigen) (solid lines) and the ratio of free to total PSA (dashed lines) at various times prior to diagnosis for a man 65 years old at serum sampling

to clinical diagnosis. For the ratio PSA measure the corresponding TPFs are 48%, 40% and 27%, respectively.

Etzioni *et al.* (1999*b*) used growth curves to model the test results, total PSA and ratio PSA for cases and controls. Induced ROC curves were then calculated. Fitted ROC curves were similar to those fitted using the ROC–GLM methodology, although the model and fitting method applied there was somewhat different from that used here. Formal comparisons between the two biomarkers are not possible with the growth curves, however, highlighting an important attribute of the ROC–GLM approach for addressing the main research question of this study.   ∎

6.5   Approaches to ROC regression

6.5.1   *Modeling ROC summary indices*

We have described in some detail two approaches to the ROC regression problem: modeling $(S_{\bar{D}}, S_D)$ and modeling $(S_{\bar{D}}, \mathrm{ROC})$. Another approach is to model some summary index of the ROC curve as a function of covariates. In particular, Dorfman *et al.* (1992) and Obuchowski (1995) suggest modeling the AUC, while Thompson and Zucchini (1989) suggest modeling the partial area under the curve, pAUC.

The approach as proposed is feasible if covariates are discrete and there are sufficient numbers of disease and non-disease observations at each distinct covariate level in order to estimate the summary index. If we denote the estimated summary index by $\hat{\theta}_Z$, the idea is to fit the model

$$\mathrm{E}\{g(\hat{\theta}_Z)\} = \beta_0 + \beta_1 X \qquad (6.16)$$

using standard linear regression (or ANOVA) methods. Pepe (1998) suggests modeling a transformation of $\hat{\theta}_Z$ while previous authors restrict g to be the identity function.

We will not elaborate on this approach further here but refer the interested reader to the aforementioned references. We also note that new approaches for fitting models to AUC and pAUC indices are under development. The methods described recently for the AUC (Fine and Bosch, 2000; Dodd, 2001) do not require estimates of the indices at each covariate level but are based on the observation that for the binary indicators, $U_{ij} = I[Y_{Di} \geqslant Y_{\bar{D}j}]$, we have $\mathrm{E}(U_{ij}|Z) = \mathrm{AUC}_Z$. Binary regression methods are used to estimate parameters in models for AUC_Z. These new approaches promise more flexibility in the types of covariates that can be accommodated and easy implementation.

6.5.2   *A qualitative comparison*

Let us now consider the relative merits of the two main approaches to regression discussed in this chapter. The first approach models covariate effects on $(S_{\bar{D}}, S_D)$. The second models covariate effects on $(S_{\bar{D}}, \mathrm{ROC})$. On the one hand, these approaches are equivalent in that for any particular covariate values the pair $(S_{\bar{D},Z}, \mathrm{ROC}_Z)$ can be derived from $(S_{\bar{D},Z}, S_{D,Z})$, and vice versa. However, the parameterization of covariate effects is different. An advantage of the ROC modeling approach is that it parameterizes covariate effects directly on the entities of interest for evaluating a test, which we contend are $S_{\bar{D}}$ and the ROC curve.

We have previously (Pepe, 1998) compared the two approaches with each other (and with the modeling of ROC summary measures). Table 6.7 summarizes advantages and disadvantages of the methods and updates the previous exposition. The second major advantage of the direct ROC modeling approach is that multiple tests can be evaluated and compared with each other within the regression framework, even if the test results are measured in different units or on different scales. Clearly this is not possible when modeling covariate effects on test results. It does not make sense to write a single regression model with test result as the outcome variable when some results are measured in one unit and some are measured in another.

Less fundamental, but nevertheless of practical import, is the ease with which practitioners can implement the approaches. Since fitting models to test result data is already a standard statistical task, its familiarity to statisticians makes it attractive. On the other hand, implementing the direct ROC modeling approach is now relatively easy too. Indeed, the steps in the parametric algorithm are all simple and/or familiar, and its implementation is only slightly more complex than the test result modeling approach. (This point (number 4 in Table 6.7) has changed since our earlier exposition (Pepe, 1998).)

The direct ROC modeling method naturally allows one to focus the analysis on ranges of FPFs that may be subsets of $(0, 1)$. This can also be done, albeit less naturally, with the other approaches. For example, if one wants to restrict attention to regions of data where $FPF < t_0$, say, then one calculates the $1 - t_0$ regression quantile for $Y_{\bar{D}}$ and drops from the analysis all test results from diseased and non-diseased subjects with values below it. The direct ROC modeling method also provides a natural way for determining if covariate effects on the ROC curve change with its domain. That is, interactions between X and functions of t are accommodated. This feature cannot easily be accommodated with test result models.

Table 6.7 *A qualitative comparison of two approaches to ROC regression*

Attribute	Modeling test results	Modeling ROC curves
(1) Model accuracy parameters directly	No	Yes
(2) Accommodates comparison between tests	No	Yes
(3) Familiar statistical task	Yes	No
(4) Easy to implement	Yes	Yes
(5) Can focus on subintervals of the FPF axis	Yes	Yes
(6) Allows interactions between covariates and FPFs	No	Yes
(7) Statistically efficient	Yes, usually	Unknown

An important issue that has not been adequately addressed concerns statistical efficiency. If likelihood-based methods are used to estimate parameters in models for test results, then the estimates and those of induced ROC model parameters make the best possible use of the data for estimating those quantities. On the other hand, the efficiency of the algorithm in Table 6.4 for estimating model parameters is unknown. It is possible that other more efficient algorithms could be developed in the future.

6.6   Concluding remarks

This chapter discussed statistical inference about covariate effects on tests with non-binary outputs. This complements the material in Chapter 3 that considered only binary tests. The notion of modeling the raw outputs, i.e. the test results, fits with well-established techniques in biostatistical practice. For binary tests, models for Y correspond to models for FPF and TPF, and so are the same as models for test accuracy parameters. This is not the case for continuous tests, however.

Modeling test accuracy through regression models for ROC curves is a relatively new notion (Section 6.4). At this time the ROC–GLM method seems to be the only approach available for directly modeling covariate effects on ROC curves. I hope that more and better techniques will be developed for this problem. In addition, improvements to the ROC–GLM method are warranted. For example, techniques must be developed for assessing model fit and for model building in this context. Statistically efficient procedures for estimating parameters need to be determined. Most importantly, we need to make these techniques available to practitioners, and for this software must be developed. Our STATA code for the data analyses in this chapter provides one starting point for implementation at this time.

ROC regression provides a new tool for addressing a wide range of questions in the evaluation of diagnostic tests. In Section 6.4.3 we have shown how it can be used to simply compare ROC curves. In Section 6.4.4 we demonstrated its application to the assessment of multiple factors affecting an audiology test, to a radiology reading study including multiple readers and modalities and to a longitudinal biomarker study. We return to the latter example in Chapter 9 when we consider notions of time-dependent ROC curves.

The idea that factors can affect the area under the ROC curve was recognized a long time ago by the early proponents of ROC analysis. The text by Swets and Pickett (1982) discusses components of the variance of the AUC in radiology reading studies as being due to variation between readers, variation among images and variation between imaging modalities. See Hanley (1989) and Roe and Metz (1997) for related discussions. Although we focus here on regression methods for the ROC curve, methods for regression analysis of AUCs and other summary indices deserve attention too. Existing methods mentioned in Section 6.5.1 are limited at present, but new promising approaches are under development. It may in fact turn out that regression analyses for summary indices are superior in some ways. For example, fewer modeling assumptions are required for summary indices than for ROC curves.

6.7   Exercises

1. (a) In Section 6.2.5 we discussed fitting semiparametric location-scale models to estimate regression quantiles of a reference distribution. Other semiparametric models could be used. Discuss estimation using the proportional hazards model, $S_{\bar{D},Z}(y) = (S_0(y))^{\beta X}$.

   (b) Suppose that a proportional hazards model also holds for the disease test results with $S_{D,Z}(y) = (S_0(y))^{\alpha+\beta^* X}$. Write down an expression for the induced ROC curve. Can a comprehensive model be written for both the disease and non-disease test result distributions and how would model parameters be estimated together?

2. Consider a clinical trial to compare a new treatment and placebo with regards to an outcome measure Y. Let D denote the treatment arm, with $D = 0$ for placebo and $D = 1$ for the new treatment, and consider the diagnostic testing framework to describe the separation between the distributions of Y in the two study arms (see Example 4.2). Describe how the evaluation of covariate effects on $S_{\bar{D},Z}$ and ROC_Z can be interpreted in this context.

3. Suppose that there are two natural non-disease control groups. In cancer research one could consider subjects with benign tumors as a control group or subjects without any tumor as a control group. Discuss how you would define an ROC–GLM regression model that incorporates comparisons between diseased subjects and each of the control groups. Technically, how would the model be fitted to the data?

4. When multiple tests are measured in different units they cannot be included as outcome measures in the same regression model. However, transforming the raw test results to their placement values puts them on a single scale. Does this provide another avenue for regression analysis?

7

INCOMPLETE DATA AND IMPERFECT REFERENCE TESTS

The inferential procedures developed in the previous chapters rely on several assumptions concerning study design. Foremost amongst these is that the reference or gold standard measure of disease, namely D, accurately reflects true disease status. In practice, the best available reference tests are often subject to error. The impact of such error, and methods to accommodate it, will be dealt with in Section 7.3. Even when a gold standard test is available, it may be invasive and/or costly. This means that in practice it cannot be applied to all study subjects. Subjects who appear to be at high risk of disease may very likely be offered the gold standard test, whereas subjects at lower risk may be less likely. This sort of selective testing can cause bias in estimated accuracies of tests unless properly accommodated in the estimation. We discuss appropriate statistical methods in Section 7.1. Finally, in some settings the reference test is very invasive and for ethical reasons can *only* be applied to subjects who are considered at high risk of disease based on a positive screening test result. In such cases, the error probabilities associated with the screening test are non-identifiable. However, it turns out that in such settings screening tests can still be compared, and we discuss this in Section 7.2.

The methodological developments in these areas apply at present primarily to binary screening tests. Thus we focus here on binary tests and mention briefly extensions to continuous and ordinal tests.

7.1 Verification biased sampling

7.1.1 *Context and definition*

Verification bias is an issue that occurs primarily in cohort screening studies. The screening test is applied to all subjects, yielding a test result Y for all study units. If the screening test is positive this suggests the presence of disease and subjects are appropriately sent for definitive diagnosis with the gold standard, D. If the screening test is negative, some subjects may forego definitive diagnosis. As an example, consider audiology screening in newborns with DPOAE. If the test suggests that a child is hearing impaired, then follow-up testing with the gold standard visual reinforcement audiometry (VRA) behavioral test is clinically indicated and is performed. However, if the DPOAE test suggests that the child's ears are responding to sound stimuli, then there are no clinical reasons to perform the VRA test. Moreover, the VRA test requires a second clinical appointment, is time consuming and costs money. Although for research purposes it is necessary to perform the VRA test on some subjects who screen negative, one might decide that only a fraction of the negatively-screening subjects should be selected for VRA testing in order to reduce study costs. In practice, even when the protocol specifies that definitive testing is supposed to occur for all subjects, subjects who screen negative may be less compliant about returning for follow-up. Some adjustment for loss to follow-up should also be attempted in this setting.

Definition

In a cohort screening study, if determination of D depends on the result of the screening test Y, then naive estimates of sensitivity and specificity based on disease-verified subjects are biased. This is called *verification bias*. Other terms for verification bias are work-up bias, referral bias, selection bias and ascertainment bias.   ∎

Example 7.1

Consider the following illustration, where on the left-hand side we display data assuming that all 1000 subjects in the cohort are tested for true disease status and on the right-hand side we display data if all screen positives are verified and a 10% sample of screen negatives are assessed with the gold standard. Naive estimates of TPF and FPF are clearly biased.

	Fully observed		Selected data	
	$D=1$	$D=0$	$D=1$	$D=0$
$Y=1$	40	95	40	95
$Y=0$	10	855	1	85
	50	950	41	180

We see that the actual TPF = 80% and the actual FPF = 10%. However, using the selected data the naive estimates of TPF and FPF are: naive TPF = 40/41 = 97.6% and naive FPF = 95/180 = 53%.   ∎

We define a variable V which indicates disease verification status as

$$V = \begin{cases} 1 & \text{if } D \text{ is ascertained}; \\ 0 & \text{if } D \text{ is not ascertained}. \end{cases}$$

Result 7.1

When screen positives are more likely to be verified for disease than screen negatives, the bias in naive estimates is always to increase sensitivity and to decrease specificity from their true values. Formally, if

$$P[V = 1|Y = 1, D] > P[V = 1|Y = 0, D], \tag{7.1}$$

then the naively estimated sensitivity is

$$P[Y = 1|D = 1, V = 1] > P[Y = 1|D = 1] = \text{TPF}$$

and the naively estimated specificity is

$$P[Y = 0|D = 0, V = 0] < P[Y = 0|D = 0] = 1 - \text{FPF}.$$ ∎

The proof of this result and of many others in this chapter are given together in Section 7.6.

7.1.2 *The missing at random assumption*

The key condition for identifiability of the true and false positive fractions when the sampling involves selection bias is that the decision to ascertain D cannot depend on any information related to true disease status other than the observed test result, Y. This is called the missing at random (MAR) assumption, in the language of Little and Rubin (1987). Formally we require

$$P[V = 1|D, Y] = P[V = 1|Y]. \qquad (7.2)$$

This condition could be violated, for example, if those with symptoms of the disease or with a family history of the disease were routinely referred for ascertainment of D.

Result 7.2

The MAR assumption (7.2) is equivalently written as

$$P[D = 1|V = 1, Y] = P[D = 1|Y]. \qquad (7.3)$$
∎

Equation (7.3) is interpreted to mean that, given the observed screening test result, the expected prevalence of disease amongst those who are verified is the same as the prevalence in the population from which the cohort is drawn. If the MAR assumption is violated, for example by referring for definitive diagnosis those with symptoms of disease or family history of disease, then one would expect that the prevalence of disease would be higher among those verified than in the general population. That is, violation of (7.2) would imply violation of (7.3). As another example, suppose that referral rates vary among clinics, with lower referral rates in clinics with higher prevalence. Then the prevalence in the study cohort (given Y) may be lower than in the general population. Thus (7.3) would be violated and hence also the MAR assumption, (7.2). We assume that the MAR assumption holds in the remainder of Section 7.1, although a somewhat relaxed version is introduced in Section 7.1.6.

7.1.3 *Correcting for bias with Bayes' theorem*

Under the MAR mechanism, (7.3) implies that the predictive values, PPV $=$ $P[D = 1|Y = 1]$ and NPV $= P[D = 0|Y = 0]$, are estimated directly from the observed data. The sample values are unbiased estimates of $P[D|Y, V = 1]$ which, by (7.3), are equal to $P[D|Y]$, the true population values. Observe, however, that the sampling variability of the estimates depends on the number of subjects verified, and hence variability can be large if only a small proportion of the study cohort is selected for ascertainment of D.

On the other hand, we have seen that naive sample estimates of TPF and FPF are biased. We can use Bayes' theorem and unbiased estimation of predictive values to derive valid estimates of TPF and FPF. Recall from Result 2.1 that

$$\mathrm{TPF} = \mathrm{P}[Y = 1|D = 1] = \frac{\mathrm{P}[D = 1|Y = 1]\mathrm{P}[Y = 1]}{\mathrm{P}[D = 1]}$$

$$= \frac{\mathrm{P}[D = 1|Y = 1]\mathrm{P}[Y = 1]}{\mathrm{P}[D = 1|Y = 1]\mathrm{P}[Y = 1] + \mathrm{P}[D = 1|Y = 0]\mathrm{P}[Y = 0]},$$

$$\mathrm{FPF} = \mathrm{P}[Y = 1|D = 0] = \frac{\mathrm{P}[D = 0|Y = 1]\mathrm{P}[Y = 1]}{\mathrm{P}[D = 0]}$$

$$= \frac{\mathrm{P}[D = 0|Y = 1]\mathrm{P}[Y = 1]}{\mathrm{P}[D = 0|Y = 1]\mathrm{P}[Y = 1] + \mathrm{P}[D = 0|Y = 0]\mathrm{P}[Y = 0]}.$$

Observe that $\mathrm{P}[Y = 1]$ can be estimated based on data from the entire study cohort. The remaining components can be estimated using empirical estimates of PPV and NPV. By substituting these into the above expressions for TPF and FPF, estimates of TPF and FPF that adjust for verification bias are derived. We call these estimates the Begg and Greenes bias adjusted estimates, due to their seminal paper (Begg and Greenes, 1983), and denote them by $\hat{\mathrm{TPF}}_{\mathrm{BG}}$ and $\hat{\mathrm{FPF}}_{\mathrm{BG}}$, respectively.

Example 7.1 (continued)

In the illustration one observes $40 + 95 = 135$ positive screens. Thus $\hat{\mathrm{P}}[Y = 1] = 13.5\%$. Also, based on the selected data, $\hat{\mathrm{P}}[D = 1|Y = 1] = 40/135 = 29.63\%$ and $\hat{\mathrm{P}}[D = 1|Y = 0] = 1/86 = 1.16\%$. Hence,

$$\hat{\mathrm{TPF}}_{\mathrm{BG}} = \frac{0.2963 \times 0.135}{0.2963 \times 0.135 + 0.0116 \times 0.865} = 0.80.$$

This is the same as the fully-observed data value. ∎

7.1.4 *Inverse probability weighting/imputation*

An intuitive way of adjusting for verification bias is to try to recreate the original fully-observed data table from the selected data. Thus, we multiply each cell in the selected data table by $1/\hat{\mathrm{P}}[V = 1|Y]$, i.e. the inverse of the (estimated) selection probability, in order to, in a sense, reverse the selection process. Having created an unbiased table, the usual empirical estimates of the TPF and FPF are calculated. We call the table the *inverse probability weighted table* or the *imputed data table*. The former name fits for obvious reasons and we denote the adjusted estimators by $\hat{\mathrm{TPF}}_{\mathrm{IPW}}$ and $\hat{\mathrm{FPF}}_{\mathrm{IPW}}$. The latter name is appropriate because, in a sense, we impute complete data (D, Y) for observations that have only partial information $(\cdot, Y)$, and do the usual simple analysis with imputed data.

Example 7.1 (continued)

In the illustration, $P[V = 1|Y = 1] = 1.0$ and $P[V = 1|Y = 0] = 0.1$. The selected data table (left) becomes the imputed data table (right), and the naive estimators calculated with the imputed data are

$$\hat{\text{TPF}}_{\text{IPW}} = 40/50 = 80\%$$

and

$$\hat{\text{FPF}}_{\text{IPW}} = 95/945 = 10\%.$$

These are exactly the same as the fully-observed data values.

	Selected data $D = 1$	$D = 0$		Imputed data $D = 1$	$D = 0$
$Y = 1$	40	95	$\times 1/1.0$	40	95
$Y = 0$	1	85	$\times 1/0.1$	10	850
	41	180		50	945

Interestingly, it turns out that the Begg and Greenes and the inverse probability weighted estimates of TPF and FPF are the same. Thus one can use either approach to calculate the bias-corrected classification probabilities. The result, proved in Section 7.6, is stated formally next.

Result 7.3

The following expressions hold:

$$\hat{\text{TPF}}_{\text{BG}} = \hat{\text{TPF}}_{\text{IPW}},$$

$$\hat{\text{FPF}}_{\text{BG}} = \hat{\text{FPF}}_{\text{IPW}}.$$

7.1.5 *Sampling variability of corrected estimates*

The Begg and Greenes estimators are the maximum likelihood estimates when observations are independent (Zhou, 1993). Begg and Greenes (1983) derived the variance formula given in the next result.

Result 7.4

If observations are independent, then, in large samples,

$$\text{var}\left(\log\frac{\hat{\text{TPF}}_{\text{BG}}}{1 - \hat{\text{TPF}}_{\text{BG}}}\right) = \frac{1}{N}\left(\frac{1}{\tau(1-\tau)} + \frac{1 - \text{PPV}}{\text{PPV}\,P_1^V\tau} + \frac{\text{NPV}}{(1 - \text{NPV})P_0^V(1-\tau)}\right),$$

where $\tau = P[Y = 1]$, N is the study cohort sample size and P_y^V is the proportion of subjects for whom $Y = y$ that are verified for disease status. Similarly,

$$\text{var}\left(\log\frac{\hat{\text{FPF}}_{\text{BG}}}{1 - \hat{\text{FPF}}_{\text{BG}}}\right) = \frac{1}{N}\left(\frac{1}{\tau(1-\tau)} + \frac{\text{PPV}}{(1 - \text{PPV})P_1^V\tau} + \frac{1 - \text{NPV}}{\text{NPV}\,P_0^V(1-\tau)}\right).$$

A confidence interval for TPF can be based on approximate confidence limits for $\log(\text{TPF}/(1 - \text{TPF}))$, using the above asymptotic distribution theory. Similarly for FPF.

Observe that there are three additive components to variability which are derived from estimating $P[Y = 1]$, PPV and NPV. In a low prevalence study the NPV is likely to be very large and hence $1 - \text{NPV}$ may be very small. The third component of variance for $\text{T\hat{P}F}_{\text{BG}}$ is derived from $\text{var}(\log(1 - \text{N\hat{P}V}))$, and therefore may be very large indeed. We see in the next example that it tends to dominate the variance and leads to instability in $\text{T\hat{P}F}_{\text{BG}}$. On the other hand, the asymptotic variance for $\text{F\hat{P}F}_{\text{BG}}$ appears to be more stable.

Example 7.1 (continued)

Recall that $\tau = 0.135$, $\text{P\hat{P}V} = 0.296$, $\text{N\hat{P}V} = 0.9884$, $P_1^V = 1.0$ and $P_0^V = 0.10$. Therefore,

$$
\text{var}\left(\log \frac{\text{T\"PF}_{\text{BG}}}{1 - \text{T\hat{P}F}_{\text{BG}}} \right) = \frac{1}{1000} \left(\frac{1}{0.135(1 - 0.135)} + \frac{1 - 0.296}{0.296 \times 0.135 \times 1} \right.
$$
$$
\left. + \frac{0.9884}{0.0116 \times (1 - 0.135) \times 0.10} \right)
$$
$$
= \frac{1}{1000}(8.56 + 17.62 + 985.05)
$$
$$
= 1.011 = (1.0056)^2 .
$$

This translates into a 95% confidence interval for $\log(\text{TPF}/(1 - \text{TPF}))$ of $\log(0.8/0.2) \pm 1.96 \times 1.0056 = (-0.59, 3.36)$ or a 95% interval for TPF equal to $(0.36, 0.97)$. This is very wide indeed. The width derives largely from the third variance component which reflects uncertainty in estimating $\log(1 - \text{NPV})$.

∎

Although asymptotically valid (consistent) estimates of TPF and FPF can be calculated from studies with verification biased sampling, the above illustration suggests that variability in estimates of TPF can be hugely compromised by such sampling. In particular, it raises the question of whether or not small verification sample sizes are at all useful when an accurate estimate of the TPF is sought. The variability of $\text{T\hat{P}F}_{\text{BG}}$ that derives to a large extent from the uncertainty in $\log(1 - \text{NPV})$ is only exacerbated by incomplete ascertainment of D among screen negatives.

Example 7.1 (continued)

To illustrate this in the context of our example, observe first that the estimate $\text{T\hat{P}F}_{\text{BG}}$ is dominated by the false negatives. The selected data was configured as follows:

	$D = 1$	$D = 0$
$Y = 1$	40	95
$Y = 0$	1	85

This yields $\hat{\text{TPF}}_{\text{BG}} = \hat{\text{TPF}}_{\text{IPW}} = 40/(40+1 \times 10) = 80\%$. If instead of observing *one* false negative, *two* had been observed, then $\hat{\text{TPF}}_{\text{BG}} = 40/(40 + 2 \times 10) = 67\%$. On the other hand, if the number in the lower left-hand corner were replaced by *zero*, then $\hat{\text{TPF}}_{\text{BG}} = 40/(40 + 0 \times 10) = 100\%$. That is, small changes in the number of false negatives have a large effect on the estimate of $\hat{\text{TPF}}_{\text{BG}}$. This is also borne out by the asymptotic variance calculation.

Suppose now that instead of sampling 10% of screen negative subjects, we choose to sample 50% or 100%. In this case the confidence intervals are $(0.61, 0.90)$ or $(0.67, 0.89)$, respectively, and these are much more acceptable than the uninformative interval $(0.36, 0.97)$ calculated from a 10% validation sample.   ∎

The data in the example raise one final point of concern. The applicability of large sample theory to inference in realistic sample sizes is called into question.

Example 7.1 (continued)

The large sample theory relies on approximating the distribution of $\log(1 - \hat{\text{NPV}}) = \log \hat{\psi} = \log \hat{P}[D = 1 | Y = 0, V = 1]$ with a normal distribution. However, the distribution of $1 - \hat{\text{NPV}}$ is decidedly discrete, concentrated on a few points and skewed. In particular, if we assume that the true NPV is equal to its observed value, $\text{NPV} = 855/865$, we have

$$P[1 - \hat{\text{NPV}} = 0/86] = 0.36\,,$$
$$P[1 - \hat{\text{NPV}} = 1/86] = 0.37\,,$$
$$P[1 - \hat{\text{NPV}} = 2/86] = 0.18\,,$$
$$P[1 - \hat{\text{NPV}} = 3/86] = 0.08\,,$$
$$\vdots$$

where probabilities are calculated from the binomial distribution with sample size 86 and probability of success parameter equal to $10/865$. This is very different from a normal distribution.

The 95% confidence interval for TPF calculated earlier with asymptotic theory is $(0.36, 0.97)$. We also calculated a confidence interval based on $\hat{\text{TPF}}_{\text{BG}}$ using 2.5 and 97.5 percentiles of its bootstrapped distribution. The bootstrap interval is $(0.54, 1.00)$. This is quite different from the asymptotic theory-based interval, again suggesting that normal theory may not be adequate in small samples.   ∎

Further work on inference with the Begg and Greenes corrected estimators is warranted. Although large sample variance expressions may be useful for initial sample size calculations and such in study design, resampling and/or simulation techniques may be better suited to inference with realistic sample sizes. In practice, one might at least compare results from asymptotic theory with those from resampling/simulation.

7.1.6   *Adjustments for other biasing factors*

If factors other than the test result Y are indicative of the risk for disease and are implicitly or explicitly used to select subjects for disease verification, this too can lead to biased estimates of TPF and FPF. We have already mentioned the possibility of such factors in Section 7.1.2 and the potential for violating the MAR assumptions in such cases. Examples of such factors are symptoms of disease and family history of disease. Another important example is when a second test is implemented and selection also depends on the results of that second test. In order for bias to occur, these factors must be associated with both disease status and the test result Y. We use the notation A to denote factors other than Y that may be related to the probability of verification and call A auxiliary variables.

Example 7.2

Consider the same data as in Example 7.1, but now suppose that verification depends on the presence or absence of symptoms of disease, denoted by A. Suppose symptoms are present in all diseased subjects that test positive and in half of diseased subjects that test negative. Symptoms also occur in 10% of non-diseased subjects with a positive test, but not in subjects with a negative test. Suppose that the definitive diagnostic test D is ascertained for all subjects with symptoms or with a positive test and for only 30% of the remaining subjects. The fully-observed and selected data are shown in the tables.

Fully-observed data

	Symptoms present $D = 1$	$D = 0$	Symptoms absent $D = 1$	$D = 0$
$Y = 1$	40	10	0	85
$Y = 0$	5	0	5	855

Selected data (stratified)

	Symptoms present $D = 1$	$D = 0$	Symptoms absent $D = 1$	$D = 0$
$Y = 1$	40	10	0	85
$Y = 0$	5	0	2	273

Selected data (combined)

	$D = 1$	$D = 0$
$Y = 1$	40	95
$Y = 0$	7	273

The naive estimates of accuracy parameters are TPF $= 40/47 = 85\%$, FPF $= 95/368 = 26\%$, PPV $= 40/135 = 29.6\%$ and NPV $= 273/280 = 97.5\%$, which contrast with the actual values of 80%, 10%, 29.6% and 99%, respectively.   ∎

Observe that, when verification depends on auxiliary variables, the predictive values can be biased. This was the case for NPV in the above illustration.

The missing at random assumption is again necessary in this setting in order to make inferences. When auxiliary variables are involved, it is stated as the following condition:

$$P[V = 1|D, Y, A] = P[V = 1|Y, A],\tag{7.4}$$

which is interpreted to mean that the decision to verify depends only on the observed data, (Y, A), and not on anything else related to the unobserved D. Similar to Result 7.2, the condition can be written equivalently as

$$P[D = 1|V, Y, A] = P[D = 1|Y, A].\tag{7.5}$$

If the auxiliary variables are discrete, unbiased estimates of the predictive values can be obtained as weighted averages of the stratum-specific values, where strata are defined by A:

$$PPV = P[D = 1|Y = 1] = \sum P[D = 1|Y = 1, A]P[A|Y = 1],$$
$$NPV = P[D = 0|Y = 0] = \sum P[D = 0|Y = 0, A]P[A|Y = 0].$$

Estimators for the TPF and FPF follow and were proposed by Begg and Greenes (1983). In particular, empirical quantities are substituted into the following expressions, with stratum-specific predictive values based on subsets for which D is observed and frequencies, $\hat{P}[Y, A]$, based on the entire cohort:

$$TPF = \frac{\sum_A P[D = 1|Y = 1, A]P[Y = 1, A]}{\sum_A \sum_Y P[D = 1|Y, A]P[Y, A]},\tag{7.6}$$

$$FPF = \frac{\sum_A P[D = 0|Y = 1, A]P[Y = 1, A]}{\sum_A \sum_Y P[D = 0|Y, A]P[Y, A]}.\tag{7.7}$$

Begg and Greenes also provide analytic expressions for asymptotic variances of the estimators, although, as we have seen, some caution is needed in applying such results to finite samples. If auxiliary variables are continuous, the above expressions are easily extended by replacing summations and probabilities with integrals and probability densities. Alonzo (2000) develops estimators for such settings.

Example 7.2 (continued)

Using the data shown in the tables above, we have

$$\hat{P}[Y = 1, A = 1] = 0.05, \qquad\qquad \hat{P}[Y = 0, A = 1] = 0.005,$$
$$\hat{P}[Y = 1, A = 0] = 0.085, \qquad\qquad \hat{P}[Y = 0, A = 0] = 0.86,$$
$$\hat{P}[D = 1|Y = 1, A = 1] = 0.8, \qquad \hat{P}[D = 1|Y = 0, A = 1] = 1.0,$$
$$\hat{P}[D = 1|Y = 1, A = 0] = 0.0, \qquad \hat{P}[D = 1|Y = 0, A = 0] = 0.0073,$$

where the stratum-specific predictive values are calculated from the 'Selected data (stratified)' table. The Begg and Greenes estimator of the TPF is then calculated as $0.04/(0.04 + 0.01128) = 0.78$.   ∎

It can be shown that, in the stratified case also, the Begg and Greenes estimator is equal to the naive estimator calculated on an imputed dataset. In this case each complete observation (D_i, Y_i, A_i) is replaced by $(P[V = 1|Y = Y_i, A = A_i])^{-1}$ observations, or equivalently each cell (D, Y, A) in the 'Selected data' table is inflated by a factor $(P[V = 1|Y, A])^{-1}$. The result follows from the observation that $P[D, Y, A] = P[D, Y, A, V = 1]/P[V = 1|Y, A]$ and arguments similar to Result 7.3.

In our example, $P[V = 1|Y = 1, A = 1] = 1.0$, $P[V = 1|Y = 1, A = 0] = 1.0$, $P[V = 1|Y = 0, A = 1] = 1.0$ and $P[V = 1|Y = 0, A = 0] = 0.3$. Thus the cells of the selected data table become approximately those of the complete data table when inflated by the inverse selection probabilities, and the empirical estimates of TPF and FPF based on the imputed data are 0.78 and 0.10, respectively.

7.1.7   A broader context

The problem of verification bias can be considered as a missing data problem. The disease status variable is missing for some subjects. The mechanism giving rise to 'missingness' leads to a study design that can be considered as 'two stage'. At the first stage, data on Y (and possibly A and covariates X) are obtained. At the second stage, the variable D is ascertained for some subjects, with the probability of ascertaining D potentially dependent on any or all data items collected at the first stage, (Y, A, X). Two-stage studies are especially common in survey sampling. Data analysis methodology for two-stage studies has received a lot of attention in the literature and many of the techniques will be directly applicable to studies of diagnostic tests with verification biased sampling. A review of methodology for two-stage studies can be found in Carroll et al. (1995). We mention here a few useful techniques but refer the interested reader to the literature for a more thorough description.

Inverse probability weighting is a broadly applicable approach. We have already applied it to the problem of estimating TPF and FPF. It is also known as the Horvitz–Thompson method (Horvitz and Thompson, 1952), particularly in the survey sampling literature. Consider a more involved statistical task, a regression analysis of TPF, say. An analysis based on only the complete observations that ignores the selection mechanism can yield biased estimates of covariate effects. If the data are missing at random, in the sense that

$$P[V = 1|Y, A, X, D] = P[V = 1|Y, A, X] \tag{7.8}$$

and the selection probabilities can be consistently estimated, then by weighting each complete data observation by the inverse selection probability, $(P[V = 1|Y, A, X])^{-1}$, and applying standard analyses to the data, consistent estimates of regression parameters can be calculated.

The intuitive justification for inverse probability weighting is the argument we used previously, namely that it seeks to impute the complete data by reversing the selection process that used probabilities $P[V = 1|Y, A, X]$. A more formal justification is provided by considering the estimating equations for parameters. Consider again a regression model for TPF, say, $g(\mathrm{TPF}(Z)) = \beta X$. The estimating equation for β using complete data is

$$\sum_{i=1}^{N} S_\beta(D_i, Y_i, X_i) = 0 \,, \tag{7.9}$$

where the binary GLM score function, $S_\beta(D, Y, X)$, is such that at the true value $\beta = \beta_*$, we have $E(S_{\beta_*}(D, Y, X)) = 0$. This latter condition is the key to valid estimation. With selection for verification of D, we use the inverse probability weighted estimating equation

$$\sum_{i=1}^{N} \frac{I[V_i = 1]}{P[V_i = 1|Y_i, A_i, X_i]} S_\beta(D_i, Y_i, X_i) = 0 \,. \tag{7.10}$$

Result 7.5

Under the missing at random assumption at $\beta = \beta_*$,

$$E \left\{ \frac{I[V = 1]}{P[V = 1|Y, A, X]} S_\beta(D, Y, X) \right\} = 0 \,. \qquad \blacksquare$$

This result, proven in Section 7.6, indicates that, in large samples, β_* is a solution to the IPW estimating equation although β_* is not a solution to the unweighted equation. The result, of course, applies to any analysis based on an estimating equation of the form (7.10). In particular, it applies to most of the regression analysis methods described in previous chapters, although extensions to the ROC–GLM methodology remain to be developed. We illustrate it with a regression model for the TPF previously considered in Chapter 3.

Example 7.3

Consider the CASS data (Section 1.3.2) and in particular the comparison of the two tests for coronary artery disease. Using the fully-observed dataset we calculate true positive fractions for the EST and CPH tests of

$$\hat{\mathrm{TPF}}_{\mathrm{EST}} = 80\% \,, \quad \hat{\mathrm{TPF}}_{\mathrm{CPH}} = 95\% \,,$$

which provide a log odds ratio of -1.52. Suppose now that all subjects were tested with the EST and CPH tests but that only a random 30% of those with a negative EST test were tested for coronary artery disease with the gold standard angiogram. The selected data indicates naive estimates $\hat{\mathrm{TPF}}_{\mathrm{EST}} = 92\%$ and $\hat{\mathrm{TPF}}_{\mathrm{CPH}} = 96\%$ and a log odds ratio of -0.78.

	Selected data	
	Diseased	Non-diseased
Number of subjects	886	204
Positive EST (%)	815	115
Positive CPH (%)	852	121

Let us compare the tests with a logistic regression model

$$\text{logit TPF} = \beta_0 + \beta_1 X_{\text{Test}},$$

where the test type covariate $X_{\text{Test}} = 1$ for records associated with the EST test and $X_{\text{Test}} = 0$ for those associated with the CPH test. We do so using the methods described in Chapter 3, but now using only the selected data, weighting the observations with $(0.30)^{-1}$ if $X_{\text{Test}} = 1$, and $Y = 0$. This yields a log odds ratio estimate of $\hat{\beta}_1 = 1.86$, which is much closer to the fully-observed data value of -1.52 than is the unadjusted estimate of -0.78.   ∎

If the selection probabilities are known constants, as in the above example, then standard inferential methods apply. Interestingly, it turns out that substantial efficiency can be gained by estimating selection probabilities from the data (Pepe et al., 1994; Alonzo et al., 2002a). Inference should acknowledge sampling variability in the weights. One way to accommodate this is to use resampling methods for inference. Since resampling must mimic the two-stage study design, simple resampling from the observed data is not appropriate. Instead, given fitted models for $P[V = 1|Y, A, X]$ and $P[D = 1|Y, A, X]$, one could resample from these distributions to generate bootstrapped datasets.

Although inverse probability weighting is easy to apply and has been used for a long time in sample surveys (Horvitz and Thompson, 1952), there is evidence that it is not a very efficient technique (Clayton et al., 1998; Alonzo et al., 2002a). Alternative techniques, such as the mean-score method (Reilly and Pepe, 1995; Clayton et al., 1998; Alonzo, 2000), appear to make more efficient use of data. Robins and colleagues (Robins et al., 1994; Robins and Rotnitzky, 1995) have proposed semiparametric efficient techniques which are more robust but are often technically difficult to implement. At this point, inverse probability weighting is the only technique that is straightforward to use with available software.

7.1.8   Non-binary tests

For non-binary tests, at each threshold for defining test positivity the corresponding FPF and TPF points can be biased by the verification selection process. This sometimes only shifts points along the ROC curve. More generally, however, it results in bias in the ROC curve (Hunink et al., 1993). There has been little discussion in the literature about verification bias for continuous tests. Some results concerning estimation of ROC curves in this setting can be found in a Ph.D. thesis (Alonzo, 2000). Further work is needed. For ordinal data more progress has been made.

Gray *et al.* (1984) consider estimating the discrete ROC curve with verification biased data. Since each operating point on the discrete ROC curve is defined by the binary test that dichotomizes with the corresponding threshold, the estimation proceeds essentially by applying the Begg and Greenes methods at each threshold. Zhou (1996) develops methods for making inferences about the AUC of the discrete ROC curve.

Gray *et al.* (1984) also consider estimation of the binormal ROC curve under verification biased sampling. Maximum likelihood methods are proposed and implemented with the expectation maximization (EM) algorithm (Dempster *et al.*, 1977). This extends the Dorfman and Alf procedure to settings where D is missing for some observations. Similarly, the ordinal regression models that Tosteson and Begg (1988) propose for evaluating covariate effects on ROC curves can be fitted using maximum likelihood methods with the EM algorithm (Rodenberg and Zhou, 2000).

In principle, inverse probability weighting (or equivalently imputation) can also be applied in all of these settings. See Hunink *et al.* (1990) for an example. It is a general method that is easy to implement and from that standpoint it is attractive. However, the maximum likelihood methods may be more efficient. We refer the reader to Zhou (1998), who provides a review of methods for ROC analysis of ordinal data subject to verification bias.

7.2   Verification restricted to screen positives

7.2.1   *Extreme verification bias*

There are many settings where the gold standard assessment of disease status is very invasive or costly. For example, definitive diagnosis of cancer usually requires that a sample of tissue be biopsied. In such settings, it is simply unethical to measure D on subjects that appear to be at low risk for having disease. Cohort studies for evaluating disease screening tests frequently employ a design where *only* subjects that screen positive on one or more screening tests are evaluated with the gold standard definitive diagnostic test when the gold standard assessment is invasive or dangerous. Ethical considerations demand the gold standard assessment for subjects screening positive and, conversely, prevent it for subjects screening negative.

Example 7.4

The St Louis prostate cancer screening study described in Section 1.3.8 is an example of such a study. Almost 20 000 men were screened with the digital rectal exam (DRE) and also with the serum prostate-specific antigen (PSA) test. The latter was dichotomized using the standard threshold, PSA > 4.0 ng/ml, defining a positive result. Most of the men in this cohort were negative according to both screening tests, and did not undergo prostate biopsy procedures. Men who were screen positive according to one or both tests did undergo biopsy and their true status is presented in Table 7.1.   ∎

Table 7.1 *Results of prostate cancer screening with PSA and DRE in white (N = 18 527) and black (N = 949) men. Only subjects screening positive with at least one test were referred for definitive testing*

		Without cancer ($D = 0$)		Prostate cancer ($D = 1$)	
		$Y_{\mathrm{DRE}} = 0$	$Y_{\mathrm{DRE}} = 1$	$Y_{\mathrm{DRE}} = 0$	$Y_{\mathrm{DRE}} = 1$
White men	$Y_{\mathrm{PSA}} = 0$	?	978	?	137
	$Y_{\mathrm{PSA}} = 1$	717	138	264	179
Black men	$Y_{\mathrm{PSA}} = 0$	?	26	?	8
	$Y_{\mathrm{PSA}} = 1$	38	3	28	10

This is an extreme form of verification biased sampling in that *only* subjects that screen positive are verified. We will see that true and false positive fractions are non-identifiable in such settings. All is not lost, however. In the next subsections we define measures of accuracy that can be estimated from such data and we show that tests can be compared with regards to their true and false positive fractions even though the absolute values of these parameters cannot be calculated.

7.2.2   Identifiable parameters for a single test

Table 7.2 displays the layout of data for a study of a single test with extreme verification bias. We use N to denote the total number of subjects tested, of whom n^+ screen positive. Of the screen positives n_D^+ are found to have disease. We see that the parameters which can be estimated are

$$\tau = \mathrm{P}[Y = 1],$$
$$\mathrm{PPV} = \mathrm{P}[D = 1 | Y = 1],$$

but the following simply cannot be estimated: NPV, $\rho = \mathrm{P}[D = 1]$, TPF and FPF. Indeed, if naive estimates of TPF and FPF are calculated, they are both equal to 1!

Equivalent to τ and PPV are the following two parameters, which are key to the methodology which we will describe for analyzing data from studies with extreme verification bias:

Table 7.2 *Layout of data for a cohort study of a single test subject to extreme verification bias*

	$D = 0$	$D = 1$	
$Y = 0$	?	?	n^-
$Y = 1$	$n_{\bar{D}}^+$	n_D^+	n^+
	?	?	N

$$\text{detection probability} = \text{DP} = P[D = 1, Y = 1], \qquad (7.11)$$
$$\text{false referral probability} = \text{FP} = P[D = 0, Y = 1]. \qquad (7.12)$$

The detection probability (DP) is the proportion of subjects that screen positive and have disease, while the false referral probability (FP) is the proportion that screen positive and do not have disease. The detection probability and false referral probability are estimated from a study with extreme verification bias as

$$\hat{\text{DP}} = n_D^+/N \quad \text{and} \quad \hat{\text{FP}} = n_{\bar{D}}^+/N.$$

Observe that the quantities DP and FP depend on both the prevalence of the disease in the population and on the capacity of the test to distinguish between diseased and non-diseased states. Formally,

$$\text{DP} = \rho\text{TPF} \quad \text{and} \quad \text{FP} = (1 - \rho)\text{FPF}. \qquad (7.13)$$

Although neither ρ, TPF or FPF are identifiable, the functions of them defined by DP and FP are. The detection probability will be low if either ρ or TPF are low, and similarly FP will be high if either the FPF is high or the prevalence is low. In a study with poor performance of the screening test as measured by DP and FP, one cannot determine if it is the poor operating characteristics of the test, the low prevalence or both that cause the poor performance.

For an ideal test, with TPF = 1 and FPF = 0, we have DP = ρ and FP = 0. That is, a proportion ρ of the population screen positive and all of them are diseased. We note the identities

$$\tau = \text{DP} + \text{FP} \quad \text{and} \quad \text{PPV} = \text{DP}/\tau.$$

Therefore, for an ideal test $\tau = \rho$ and PPV = 1.

The DP and FP parameters are of interest in their own right. They quantify, as a proportion of the total population, how many diseased subjects will be identified with the screening test and how many false referrals there will be. Ultimately these are important for measuring the value of applying the screening test in the population.

Example 7.4 (continued)

To fix ideas we calculate the DPs and FPs for the DRE and PSA tests among the 18 527 white men. For the DRE test, $179 + 137 = 316$ men screened positive and were found to have prostate cancer. Thus DP(DRE) = 1.7%. Similarly, we have FP(DRE) = 6.0%, DP(PSA) = 2.4% and FP(PSA) = 4.6%. Clearly PSA seems to be the better test. Its detection probability is higher and its false referral probability is lower than that of the DRE test. We consider the comparison more formally in the next section.   ∎

Table 7.3 *Layout of data for unpaired and paired designs subject to extreme verification bias*

	Unpaired design (total $= N_A + N_B$)			
	$Y = 1, D = 1$	$Y = 1, D = 0$	$Y = 0$	Total
Test A	$n_{D,A}^+$	$n_{\bar{D},A}^+$	n_A^-	N_A
Test B	$n_{D,B}^+$	$n_{\bar{D},B}^+$	n_B^-	N_B

	Paired design (total $= N$)			
	$D = 1$		$D = 0$	
	$Y_B = 0$	$Y_B = 1$	$Y_B = 0$	$Y_B = 1$
$Y_A = 0$	?	b	?	f
$Y_A = 1$	c	d	g	h

7.2.3 *Comparing tests*

As discussed in detail in Chapter 3, designs to compare two tests can generally be considered as paired or unpaired (although the marginal probability methods accommodate hybrids too). Table 7.3 lays out the data structure for both types of design. We assume that in the unpaired design each subject receives only one screening test, and if it is positive ($Y = 1$) the true disease status is ascertained. In the paired design each subject receives both tests and has D measured if either of the screening tests is positive. Observe the correspondence between cells in the paired and unpaired data layouts:

$$n_{D,A}^+ = c + d, \qquad\qquad n_{D,B}^+ = b + d,$$
$$n_{\bar{D},A}^+ = g + h, \qquad\qquad n_{\bar{D},B}^+ = f + h,$$
$$n_A^- = N - (c + d + g + h), \qquad n_B^- = N - (b + d + f + h).$$

The empirical estimates (ignoring subscripts for tests) are $\hat{DP} = n_D^+/N$, $\hat{FP} = n_{\bar{D}}^+/N$ and $\hat{\tau} = 1 - n^-/N$. These are binomial proportions allowing straightforward calculation of confidence intervals. Moreover, comparisons between tests with regards to DP, FP or τ are made with unpaired or paired designs using Pearson chi-squared or McNemar's tests, respectively. We turn next to inference about classification probabilities, FPF and TPF.

Recall the links established in eqn (7.13) between DPs and TPFs and between FPs and FPFs. We observe that the null hypothesis for equality of the DP (FP) parameters is the same as that for equality of the TPF (FPF) parameters, as long as prevalence of disease among populations tested with test A is the same as that tested with test B. This latter condition is trivially satisfied in a paired study. It will also be true in a well-designed unpaired study where it can be guaranteed by randomization.

Furthermore, we see that the relative detection probability is algebraically identical to the relative true positive fraction and the relative false referral probability is algebraically identical to the relative false positive fraction.

Result 7.6

In a paired study or a randomized unpaired study we have

$$rDP(A, B) \equiv DP_A/DP_B = rTPF(A, B) \tag{7.14}$$

and similarly

$$rFP(A, B) \equiv FP_A/FP_B = rFPF(A, B). \tag{7.15}$$

In a paired study these equalities also hold for the empirical sample values.   ∎

The result, usually attributed to Schatzkin *et al.* (1987), implies that we can quantify the relative classification probabilities by quantifying the relative detection and false referral probabilities. The latter are identifiable even under extreme verification biased sampling. This means, therefore, that we can make inferences about relative accuracies, $rTPF(A, B)$ and $rFPF(A, B)$. This is remarkable in light of the fact that the absolute values for the constituent TPF and FPF parameters themselves cannot be estimated.

Example 7.4 (continued)

The relative detection and false referral probabilities for the PSA test compared to the DRE test are

$$r\hat{D}P(PSA, DRE) = 2.4\%/1.7\% = 1.40,$$

$$r\hat{F}P(PSA, DRE) = 4.6\%/6.0\% = 0.77.$$

Therefore, the PSA test is both more sensitive and specific than the DRE test in white men, according to Smith's data.   ∎

It is important to recognize that it is only on the multiplicative scale that comparisons of detection probabilities are synonymous with those for true positive fractions, and similarly that comparisons of false referral probabilities are synonymous with those for false positive fractions. For example, odds ratios for detection rates are not equivalent to odds ratios for true positive fractions. Indeed, the latter cannot be estimated at all from studies with extreme verification bias. We now turn to the variability of estimated relative performance parameters.

Result 7.7

(a) For an unpaired study design we have

$$\operatorname{var}(\log r\hat{T}PF(A, B)) = \frac{1 - DP_A}{N_A DP_A} + \frac{1 - DP_B}{N_B DP_B},$$

$$\operatorname{var}(\log r\hat{F}PF(A, B)) = \frac{1 - FP_A}{N_A FP_A} + \frac{1 - FP_B}{N_B FP_B}.$$

(b) For a paired study design we have

$$\text{var}(\log \text{r}\hat{\text{T}}\text{PF}(A,B)) = \frac{\text{DP}_A + \text{DP}_B - 2\text{DDP}}{N\text{DP}_A\text{DP}_B},$$

$$\text{var}(\log \text{r}\hat{\text{F}}\text{PF}(A,B)) = \frac{\text{FP}_A + \text{FP}_B - 2\text{FFP}}{N\text{FP}_A\text{FP}_B},$$

where $\text{DDP} = P[Y_A = Y_B = 1, D = 1]$ and $\text{FFP} = P[Y_A = Y_B = 1, D = 0]$.

∎

Similar to the proof of Result 3.1, for unpaired studies with complete ascertainment of disease status, Result 7.7(a) follows using Simel's formula. The second result is due to Cheng and Macaluso (1997). Result 7.7(b) is in fact the same as Result 3.4 which concerns paired studies with complete disease ascertainment. This is reasonable because, as was pointed out in a seminal paper by Schatzkin *et al.* (1987), in a paired study $\text{r}\hat{\text{T}}\text{PF}(A,B) = n_{D,A}^+/n_{D,B}^+$ and $\text{r}\hat{\text{F}}\text{PF}(A,B) = n_{\bar{D},A}^+/n_{\bar{D},B}^+$ do not at all involve the disease status for subjects that screen negative on both tests. That is, in a paired study, it is irrelevant if one ascertains D given $Y_A = 0$ and $Y_B = 0$, for the purposes of estimating the relative classification probabilities (although such data must be ascertained if absolute classification probabilities are to be estimated for the tests).

Example 7.4 (continued)

Using the formulae above for $\text{var}(\log \text{r}\hat{\text{T}}\text{PF}(A,B))$ and $\text{var}(\log \text{r}\hat{\text{F}}\text{PF}(A,B))$, we find 90% confidence intervals for $\text{rTPF}(\text{PSA},\text{DRE}) = (1.28, 1.53)$ and for $\text{rFPF}(\text{PSA},\text{DRE}) = (0.76, 0.78)$. We can reject the null hypothesis H_0: $\text{rTPF}(\text{PSA},\text{DRE}) = 1$. The estimated $\log \text{r}\hat{\text{T}}\text{PF}(\text{PSA},\text{DRE})$ and its standard error yield a Z-statistic of 6.22. Equivalently, we can use McNemar's test because it is based on the discordant pairs, for which we have complete data (Schatzkin *et al.*, 1987). This yields almost the same p value. ∎

In summary, when only screen positives have true disease status ascertained, we can compare tests with regards to their detection rates and with regards to their false referral probabilities. When analyzed on a multiplicative scale, these are the same as comparisons based on relative true positive and relative false positive fractions. Note that the design also allows for estimation of PPVs and hence for comparisons of tests with regards to their positive predictive values. No modifications to the methods discussed in Chapter 3 are required. On the other hand, the study design precludes comparisons of negative predictive values.

7.2.4 *Evaluating covariate effects on* (DP, FP)

Let Z denote covariates and let $X = X(Z)$ be the corresponding vector of covariables. As in previous chapters, we continue to distinguish between Z, the qualitative description of factors to be modeled, and $X(Z)$, the numeric variables coding for Z that are included in the regression model. One can fit generalized linear models to detection probabilities and false referral probabilities. Consider the model

$$g(\mathrm{DP}(Z)) = g(\mathrm{P}[D = 1, Y = 1|Z]) = \beta_0 + \beta X . \tag{7.16}$$

Using the detection indicator variables, $\{I[D_i = 1, Y_i = 1], i = 1, \ldots, N\}$, this marginal probability model can be fitted to the data. Similarly, a marginal probability model can be fitted to the false referral indicator variables, $\{I[D_i = 0, Y_i = 1], i = 1, \ldots, N\}$, which we write as

$$g(\mathrm{FP}(Z)) = g(\mathrm{P}[D = 0, Y = 1|Z]) = \theta_0 + \theta X . \tag{7.17}$$

An alternative approach is to fit a polychotomous regression model (Hosmer and Lemeshow, 2000). That is, W, the outcome of the screening test and subsequent determination of disease status can be regarded as belonging to one of three categories:

$$W = \begin{cases} 1 & \text{if } Y = 0 ; \\ 2 & \text{if } Y = 1 \text{ and } D = 0 ; \\ 3 & \text{if } Y = 1 \text{ and } D = 1 . \end{cases}$$

The multinomial probabilities for W, $\mathrm{P}[W = w]$, are modeled in (7.16) and (7.17). Note that polychotomous regression models usually parameterize conditional probabilities relative to a baseline category (Begg and Gray, 1984; Agresti, 1990). In particular, with category 1 as a baseline category, one has for each $w \neq 1$ the model $g(\mathrm{P}[W = w|W = w \text{ or } W = 1])$ for the conditional probability that W is in category w given that W is either in category w or category 1. On the other hand, our models (7.16) and (7.17) parameterize $\mathrm{P}[W = w]$, the marginal probabilities. If most subjects screen negative then the difference should be minor. The polychotomous regression approach should be more efficient than fitting two separate binary models because it incorporates more structure into the analysis. In particular, it acknowledges that the probabilities, $\mathrm{P}[Y = 0]$, $\mathrm{P}[Y = 1, D = 0]$ and $\mathrm{P}[Y = 1, D = 1]$, add up to 1. Interestingly, when Begg and Gray (1984) evaluated the relative efficiency they found the gains to be minor.

Example 7.4 (continued)

Consider the results of the DRE test only, for whites and for blacks. We can examine the effect of race on the DP and FP parameters (see Table 7.4). Define the indicator variable for race to be $X_R = 1$ for blacks and $X_R = 0$ for whites. The logistic regression models

$$\mathrm{logit}\,\mathrm{P}[D = 1, Y = 1|X_R] = \beta_0 + \beta_1 X_R ,$$
$$\mathrm{logit}\,\mathrm{P}[D = 0, Y = 1|X_R] = \theta_0 + \theta_1 X_R$$

fitted to the data yield $\hat{\beta}_0 = -4.1$ (0.06), $\hat{\beta}_1 = 0.11$ (0.24), $\hat{\theta}_0 = -2.7$ (0.03) and $\hat{\theta}_1 = -0.71$ (0.19), where the numbers in parentheses are standard errors. The higher false referral probability in whites, as indicated by $\hat{\theta}_1 = -0.71$, is statistically significant, while the detection probabilities seem to be similar in whites and in blacks. ∎

Table 7.4 *Calculation of detection and false referral probabilities for prostate cancer screening tests*

Race	$Y = 0$	$Y = 1, D = 0$	$Y = 1, D = 1$	N
White	17 094 92%	1114 6%	316 2%	18 524
Black	902 95%	29 3%	18 2%	949

Inference about detection probabilities and false referral probabilities does not, in general, translate into inference about test accuracy parameters. As mentioned earlier, factors that affect either disease prevalence or test accuracy can affect the DP and FP parameters. Conversely, if a factor affects the DP (FP) say, we cannot tell if it is the prevalence, the true positive fraction (false positive fraction) or both that are associated with the factor. In Example 7.4, the higher false referral probability in whites may be due to a higher false positive fraction in whites or due to a lower prevalence of prostate cancer in whites. We simply cannot tell.

7.2.5   *Evaluating covariate effects on* (TPF, FPF) *and on prevalence*

Under some circumstances inference about covariate effects on (DP, FP) do translate into inference about test accuracy. Specifically, when we can assume that prevalence does not depend on the covariate, then covariate effects on DP and/or FP must be due to their effects on classification probabilities. We argued this point earlier when the covariate of interest was 'test type', namely PSA or DRE, in Example 7.4. The following is the more general formal result.

Result 7.8

Under the condition that

$$P[D = 1|Z] = P[D = 1],   \tag{7.18}$$

the parameters β and θ in the detection probability and false referral probability models

$$\log P[D = 1, Y = 1|Z] = \beta_0 + \beta X,$$
$$\log P[D = 0, Y = 1|Z] = \theta_0 + \theta X,$$

respectively, can be interpreted as relating to the parameters of log–linear models for TPF and FPF. That is,

$$\log P[Y = 1|D = 1, Z] = \beta_0^* + \beta X,$$
$$\log P[Y = 1|D = 0, Z] = \theta_0^* + \theta X,$$

where β_0^* and θ_0^* are constants defined below.

Proof The result follows by noting that

$$\log P[Y = 1|D = 1, Z] = \log P[D = 1, Y = 1|Z] - \log P[D = 1|Z]$$
$$= \beta_0 + \beta X - \log P[D = 1]$$
$$= \beta_0^* + \beta X \,,$$

where $\beta_0^* = \beta_0 - \log P[D = 1]$, and

$$\log P[Y = 1|D = 0, Z] = \log P[D = 0, Y = 1|Z] - \log P[D = 0|Z]$$
$$= \theta_0 + \theta X - \log P[D = 0]$$
$$= \theta_0^* + \theta X \,. \qquad \blacksquare$$

A designed experiment is usually required to assure the validity of the condition (7.18). If the covariate is under the control of the investigator and can be assigned to study subjects without influencing risk of disease then the condition can be ensured. For example, the condition holds if X is an indicator of 'test type' and tests are either randomized to subjects or both tests are applied to all subjects. However, if X is a potential risk factor for disease, like race in our example, then the condition cannot be assumed to hold.

Example 7.4 (continued)

Setting the comparison between the PSA test and the DRE test in a regression modeling context, we define the test type covariable X_{Test}, with $X_{\text{Test}} = 1$ for the PSA test. We restrict the analysis to white men only and fit the log–linear models

$$\log P[D = 1, Y = 1|\text{Test}] = \beta_0 + \beta_1 X_{\text{Test}} \,,$$
$$\log P[D = 0, Y = 1|\text{Test}] = \theta_0 + \theta_1 X_{\text{Test}} \,.$$

Each subject contributes two data records to the analysis. Therefore the condition that $P[D = 1|X_{\text{Test}} = 1] = P[D = 1|X_{\text{Test}} = 0]$ holds trivially because the disease prevalence among records relating to the PSA test is exactly the same as that among records relating to the DRE test. The fitted parameter values are $\hat{\beta}_1 = 0.34$, with 90% confidence interval $(0.25, 0.43)$, and $\hat{\theta}_1 = -0.26$, with 90% confidence interval $(-0.33, -0.20)$. By Result 7.8 we can interpret these as estimates and confidence intervals for $\log r\text{TPF}(\text{PSA}, \text{DRE})$ and $\log r\text{FPF}(\text{PSA}, \text{DRE})$. Note that estimated values are the same as the empirical values presented in Section 7.2.3. However, here the estimated standard errors, which are based on the robust sandwich variance from the marginal regression analysis, are larger than those employed earlier. This is a small sample phenomenon. The procedures are asymptotically equivalent. $\blacksquare$

We saw above that if prevalence does not depend on Z then inference about covariate effects on DP can be interpreted as inference for TPF. Conversely, if the TPF of a test does not vary with the covariate, then inference about covariate effects on DP can be interpreted as inference about disease risk. That is, if increasing values of X are associated with increasing detection probabilities but the sensitivity of the test is constant across values of X, then the only explanation is that increasing X corresponds to increasing prevalence of disease.

Similar considerations apply to the FP. The formal statement is provided in the next result.

Result 7.9

(a) Under the condition that TPF does not depend on Z, namely

$$P[Y = 1 | D = 1, Z] = P[Y = 1 | D = 1],$$

the parameter β in the detection probability model

$$\log P[D = 1, Y = 1 | Z] = \beta_0 + \beta X$$

can be interpreted as relating to the risk of disease, i.e.

$$\log P[D = 1 | Z] = \beta_0^{**} + \beta X.$$

(b) Under the condition that FPF does not depend on Z, namely

$$P[Y = 1 | D = 0, Z] = P[Y = 1 | D = 0],$$

the parameter θ in the false referral probability model

$$\log P[D = 0, Y = 1 | Z] = \theta_0 + \theta X$$

can be interpreted as relating to the risk of disease, i.e.

$$\log P[D = 0 | Z] = \theta_0^{**} + \theta X. \qquad \blacksquare$$

The proof is analogous to that of Result 7.8. Observe that the key assumption for this result is that the sensitivity (or specificity) remains constant across co-variate values. We caution about making this assumption lightly and refer back to Chapter 3 for a pertinent discussion.

7.2.6 *Evaluating covariate effects on* $(\text{rTPF}, \text{rFPF})$

We now consider in more detail the problem of comparing the accuracies of two tests. We ask if covariates affect the relative performance of two tests. In our first example we ask if the performance of PSA relative to the DRE test is different in blacks than in whites.

As usual, the notation 'Test' (and X_{Test}) is used to indicate test type. We let Z (and X) denote the other covariates (and covariables). The basic idea is to fit log–linear models to the detection probability and the false referral probability that include interactions between covariates and test type. The interactions quantify covariate effects on relative performance as long as, given the values of other covariates, the prevalence of disease is similar among observations corresponding to the two test types. The proof of this result, stated formally below, is left as an exercise.

Result 7.10

Let us assume that
$$P[D = 1|Z, \text{Test}] = P[D = 1|Z].$$

(a) In the log–linear model for the DP

$$\log P[D = 1, Y = 1|Z, \text{Test}] = \alpha_0 + \alpha_1 X + \beta_0 X_{\text{Test}} + \beta_1 X X_{\text{Test}},$$

the parameter β_1 is interpreted as the effect of the covariate Z on the rTPF:

$$\log \text{rTPF}(Z) \equiv \log \left(\frac{P[Y = 1|D = 1, Z, X_{\text{Test}} = 1]}{P[Y = 1|D = 1, Z, X_{\text{Test}} = 0]} \right) = \beta_0 + \beta_1 X.$$

(b) The parameter θ_1 in the log–linear model for the FP

$$\log P[D = 0, Y = 1|Z, X_{\text{Test}}] = \gamma_0 + \gamma_1 X + \theta_0 X_{\text{Test}} + \theta_1 X X_{\text{Test}}$$

is interpreted as the effect of Z on the rFPF:

$$\log \text{rFPF}(Z) = \log \left(\frac{P[Y = 1|D = 0, Z, X_{\text{Test}} = 1]}{P[Y = 1|D = 0, Z, X_{\text{Test}} = 0]} \right) = \theta_0 + \theta_1 X. \quad \blacksquare$$

Observe that the log detection probability for the baseline test is $\alpha_0 + \alpha_1 X$. Therefore, α_1 quantifies the effect of X on the detection probability for the baseline test. Factors influencing disease prevalence will contribute to this, as will factors influencing the accuracy of the baseline test. The parameter β_0 is the rTPF of the two tests when $X = 0$ and β_1 quantifies the change in this as X changes. Similar considerations apply to the FP model.

Example 7.4 (continued)

To evaluate whether or not the relative accuracy of the PSA to the DRE test is different in blacks than in whites, we fit the following model to the detection probability:

$$\log P[D = 1, Y = 1|\text{Race}, \text{Test}] = \alpha_0 + \alpha_1 X_R + \beta_0 X_{\text{Test}} + \beta_1 X_R X_{\text{Test}},$$

where as before X_R is an indicator of race ($X_R = 1$ for blacks) and X_{Test} is an indicator of test type ($X_{\text{Test}} = 1$ for PSA). We estimate that $\beta_1 = 0.41$ and test the null hypothesis $H_0 : \beta_1 = 0$ (p value $= 0.08$). Thus there is a strong suggestion that the rTPF(PSA, DRE) is higher in blacks than it is in whites. $\quad \blacksquare$

Example 7.5

The next example pertains to a multicenter study to compare two screening tests for cervical cancer. The data shown in Table 7.5 were simulated based on the proposed design of a study submitted for consideration by the United States Food and Drug Administration. For proprietary reasons we do not describe the specific details of the tests or the protocol. Three study sites each enrol 5000 subjects and test them with two screening tests labeled as A and B. Those testing positive on at least one test are given the definitive diagnostic procedure. The data for analysis are displayed.

We let X_{S1} and X_{S2} be dummy variables indicating study site: $X_{S1} = I[\text{Site} = 1]$ and $X_{S2} = I[\text{Site} = 2]$. Again X_{Test} indicates test type, with $X_{\text{Test}} = 1$ for test A.

We fit the log–linear model to the detection probabilities:

$$\log \text{DP} = \alpha_0 + \alpha_1 X_{S1} + \alpha_2 X_{S2} + \beta_0 X_{\text{Test}} + \beta_1 X_{S1} X_{\text{Test}} + \beta_2 X_{S2} X_{\text{Test}}.$$

The results are shown in Table 7.6. We find that the relative true positive fraction does not vary across study sites. A test of the null hypothesis $H_0 : \beta_1 = 0 = \beta_2$ yields a p value of 0.81 using the Wald test. Therefore we fit a reduced model to the data:

$$\log \text{DP} = \alpha_0 + \alpha_1 X_{S1} + \alpha_2 X_{S2} + \beta_0 X_{\text{Test}}.$$

The pooled estimate of the relative true positive fraction is $\exp \hat{\beta}_0 = \text{r}\hat{\text{TPF}}(A, B)$ = 1.05 with 95% confidence interval $(1.02, 1.09)$.

Observe that the baseline detection probabilities do vary across sites, with sites 1 and 2 having detection probabilities that are lower than site 3 ($\alpha_1 = -0.57$ and $\alpha_2 = -0.85$). It may be that prevalence of disease is simply lower at sites 1 and 2 and/or that the screening tests when performed at site 3 detect disease better than at the other two sites. Nevertheless, test A appears to be better than test B at detecting disease at all three sites and the pooled $\text{r}\hat{\text{TPF}}(A, B)$ provides a reasonable overall summary of relative performance. ∎

Table 7.5 *Data from a comparative study of tests A and B conducted at three sites, with $N = 5000$ subjects screened at each site*

		Diseased		Non-diseased	
		$Y_B = 0$	$Y_B = 1$	$Y_B = 0$	$Y_B = 1$
Site 1	$Y_A = 0$	?	14	?	50
	$Y_A = 1$	27	171	50	165
Site 2	$Y_A = 0$	?	9	?	41
	$Y_A = 1$	17	132	54	173
Site 3	$Y_A = 0$	?	29	?	51
	$Y_A = 1$	43	304	50	211

Table 7.6 *Results of the log–linear DP model applied to data from a multicenter study to compare two tests*

	Parameter	Parameter estimate	Exponentiated estimate	95% CI
Full model	α_0	−2.71	0.067	(0.060, 0.074)
	α_1	−0.59	0.560	(0.47, 0.66)
	α_2	−0.86	0.42	(0.35, 0.51)
	β_0	0.04	1.04	(0.99, 1.09)
	β_1	0.03	1.03	(0.95, 1.11)
	β_2	0.01	1.01	(0.93, 1.10)
Reduced model	α_0	−2.71	0.066	(0.060, 0.073)
	α_1	−0.57	0.56	(0.48, 0.67)
	α_2	−0.85	0.43	(0.35, 0.51)
	β_0	0.05	1.05	(1.02, 1.09)
	β_1	–	–	–
	β_2	–	–	–

Example 7.6

An important type of covariate discussed in previous chapters is specific to the diseased (or non-diseased) state. In particular, when comparing two tests, it is often important to delineate if the relative TPF depends on the characteristics of disease. The data in Table 7.7 (DeSutter *et al.*, 1998) concerns $N = 4964$ subjects who were given two screening tests for cervical cancer, namely cytology and cervicography. All 228 subjects that tested positive on one or both tests were biopsied, and if they were found positive for cancer the disease was classified as high or low grade.

In this setting we define four indicator variables for each subject, one for each test type (Test) and disease grade (G) combination. Let X_G be an indicator of grade ($X_G = 1$ for high-grade disease and $X_G = 0$ for low-grade disease) and

Table 7.7 *Data on two screening tests for cervical cancer, namely cytology (Y_A) and cervicography (Y_B). Results for subjects with disease are shown separately for high- and low-grade lesions*

Disease status		Test results $Y_B = 0$	$Y_B = 1$
High grade	$Y_A = 0$	?	4
$(D = 1, X_G = 1)$	$Y_A = 1$	15	14
Low grade	$Y_A = 0$	?	48
$(D = 1, X_G = 0)$	$Y_A = 1$	29	6
No lesions	$Y_A = 0$	?	81
$(D = 0)$	$Y_A = 1$	20	11

define $X_{\text{Test}} = 1$ for the cytology test. For each test type and grade consider the indicators $I[D_G = 1, Y = 1]$, where $D_G = 1$ if the subject has disease and the disease is grade G. Consider the model

$$\log \text{P}[D_G = 1, Y_{\text{Test}} = 1] = \alpha_0 + \alpha_1 X_G + \beta_0 X_{\text{Test}} + \beta_1 X_{\text{Test}} X_G.$$

The parameter β_0 is the $\log \text{rTPF}$(cytology, cervicography) in low-grade lesions, while $\beta_0 + \beta_1$ is the $\log \text{rTPF}$ in high-grade lesions.

The result of fitting this model to the data yields $\hat{\beta}_1 = 0.91$ ($p < 0.001$). Thus the rTPF does differ with grade of lesion. We calculate that it is 1.61 ($p = 0.014$) in high-grade lesions but 0.65 ($p = 0.03$) in low-grade lesions. ∎

7.2.7 *Alternative strategies*

The methods presented so far concern inference about marginal probabilities (DP, FP) with log–linear methods. Much of this material can be found in Pepe and Alonzo (2001*b*). Two other strategies have been proposed for inference with data from studies where only screen positives are verified for disease status.

For paired study designs Cheng and Macaluso (1997) proposed the use of conditional logistic regression models (Breslow and Day, 1980) to evaluate covariate effects on the relative performance of two tests. This methodology considers the pair of test results $(Y_{A,i}, Y_{B,i})$ from the ith subject as a matched pair. Assuming the subject-specific model

$$\text{logit P}[Y_{\text{Test},i} = 1 | D_i = 1, X_{\text{Test}}, X_i] = \alpha_i + \beta_1 X_{\text{Test}} + \beta_2 X_i X_{\text{Test}} \qquad (7.19)$$

for Test $= A$ and B, conditional logistic regression provides estimates of β_1 and β_2. Cheng and Macaluso (1997) note that, since only discordant pairs enter into the analysis, that is, observations for which $(Y_A, Y_B) = (0, 1)$ or $(1, 0)$, this approach accommodates the designs considered in this section, where subjects screening negative on both tests are not verified.

The main concern that we have with this approach has to do with the interpretation of β_1 and β_2 as subject-specific parameters. They quantify the odds of a positive result on test A versus test B when both are performed on the same subject. However, it is the relative test performance in the population that is of primary interest rather than the within-individual relative performance. See Pepe and Alonzo (2001*b*) for further discussion and an application of this approach to the St Louis prostate cancer screening data.

Another strategy is to assume some structure for the probabilistic association between test results conditional on disease status $\text{P}[Y_A, Y_B | D]$. When such structure is assumed it is possible to estimate absolute true and false positive fractions and to evaluate covariate effects on them. This general approach, often called latent class analysis, will be discussed at length in the next section for the setting in which D is missing for all subjects. We refer to Cheng *et al.* (1999), Walter (1999) and Pepe and Alonzo (2001*b*) for discussions of the latent class analysis of studies where only screen positives are verified. Although attractive from a theoretical point of view, Cheng *et al.* (1999) and ourselves feel that inference is highly dependent on the assumed probabilistic structure for associations between tests. Moreover, since the true statistical association between the tests cannot be identified from the data, there are serious concerns about the impact of these unverifiable assumptions on inference.

7.3   Imperfect reference tests

For many diseases it is impossible to determine true disease status. The best available reference tests may themselves be subject to error. When used as a reference against which new tests are compared, error in the reference test can influence the perceived accuracy of new tests. Kraemer (1992) provides an interesting discussion of this, and appears to be of the opinion that true disease status can almost never be ascertained. She suggests that one should distinguish between disease (which is unobservable) and the diagnosis (which is observable). We take a less extreme point of view and define the disease, D, to be the diagnosis when a definitive test exists. In this section, we consider statistical issues when a definitive test does not exist. The focus is again on inference about classification probabilities.

7.3.1   *Examples*

There are numerous examples of diagnostic tests that are imperfect. The following are a few common examples.

(a) *Bacterial infection*   The gold standard assessment is usually a culture from a sample of blood, urine or tissue. However, even when the subject is infected, the culture test may not be positive if the sample of blood, urine or tissue does not contain bacteria or if the sample does contain bacteria but they do not grow in the culture.

(b) *Audiology*   The gold standard for young children is the VRA test. However, it can indicate deafness when the child can hear but does not cooperate or pay attention.

(c) *Cancer*   The gold standard test is the pathologic review of a biopsy specimen. However, similar to (a), if the biopsy is not taken from exactly the right location it can miss the cancer.

(d) *Alcoholism*   This is usually assessed with questionnaires. However, a questionnaire can identify someone who drinks a lot and regularly as being an alcoholic when in fact they are not compulsive about drinking. Questions can also miss identifying alcoholics who lie in response to questions or who fail to recognize their behaviors.

7.3.2   *Effects on accuracy parameters*

We continue to use D to denote true disease status and use R to denote the result of the *observed reference* test which, like D, is assumed to be binary in this chapter. The result of the investigational screening test is, as usual, denoted by Y. To illustrate that error in R can bias estimates of accuracy for Y, consider the following hypothetical data.

Example 7.7

	$D = 0$	$D = 1$		$R = 0$	$R = 1$
$Y = 0$	70	20		74	16
$Y = 1$	30	80		46	64
	100	100		120	80

Suppose that the prevalence of disease is 50% and that the new test is in truth 80% sensitive and 70% specific as shown. Consider a reference test that misses disease when it is there 20% of the time but that never falsely indicates disease. Relative to such a reference test, the new test is still 80% ($= 64/80$) sensitive, but only 62% ($= 74/120$) specific. The new test appears to be worse than it is. Moreover, disease prevalence will appear to be less than it truly is, namely 40% ($= 80/200$) as opposed to the true value of 50%. It makes intuitive sense in this case that observed prevalence is biased too low because the only error in the reference is that it sometimes misses disease.

Suppose now that the same screening test is being evaluated (as shown above) and that, as before, the only error in the reference test is that it misses disease 20% of the time. However, now suppose that the error in R is related to the error in Y. In particular, the reference test always identifies disease when disease is present and Y is positive, but never when disease is present and Y is negative. This might occur if both Y and R are better at detecting severe disease, say, or some particular manifestation of disease. Then, relative to R, the test Y will appear to be 100% ($= 80/80$) sensitive and 75% ($= 90/120$) specific, when in fact it is only 80% sensitive and 70% specific. Thus, in this case the new test appears to be better than it truly is.

As a final illustration consider the case where the new test is perfect, i.e. Y is 100% sensitive and 100% specific. If the reference test is imperfect, its errors are interpreted as errors in the new test and the new test is not seen to be as valuable as it is. For instance, if the reference is 90% sensitive and 90% specific, the new test appears to be only 90% sensitive and only 90% specific even if it is 100% sensitive and specific. It is not unusual for a new test to be better than the best available standard test. ∎

The example illustrates that sensitivity and specificity can be biased in either direction, depending on the error in the reference. We now give some general results about the direction of the bias.

Result 7.11

If, conditional on D, the results of R and Y are statistically independent, then it is likely that observed sensitivity is decreased and observed specificity is decreased. Formally, if *conditional independence* holds:

$$P[Y, R|D] = P[Y|D]P[R|D], \tag{7.20}$$

then assuming that $P[Y = 1|D = 0] < P[Y = 1|D = 1]$ we have

$$P[Y = 1|R = 1] < P[Y = 1|D = 1], \tag{7.21}$$

and assuming that $P[Y = 0|D = 1] < P[Y = 0|D = 0]$ we have

$$P[Y = 0|R = 0] < P[Y = 0|D = 0]. \tag{7.22}$$

∎

The assumption of conditional independence, (7.20), is frequently made. However, in my opinion, it is only likely to be true in unusual cases. If, for example, both R and Y more easily detect disease when it is advanced or severe, then the conditional independence assumption will fail. Similarly, if they both detect only certain manifestations of disease, they will be correlated. As another example, if contamination of a specimen causes both to be positive when no disease is present, then they will be conditionally dependent. These scenarios clearly often occur in practice. Thus, in the more likely event of positive correlation we have the next general result. Let us first define *positive dependence for sensitivity* as

$$P[Y = 1|R = 1, D = 1] > P[Y = 1|D = 1], \tag{7.23}$$

and *positive dependence for specificity* as

$$P[Y = 0|R = 0, D = 0] > P[Y = 0|D = 0]. \tag{7.24}$$

Result 7.12

(a) If the reference test is 100% specific but not 100% sensitive, then the observed sensitivity is inflated under (7.23).

(b) If the reference test is 100% sensitive but not 100% specific, then the observed specificity is inflated under (7.24).   ∎

We need to recognize that bias in the anti-conservative direction, i.e. with classification probabilities appearing to be better than they truly are, is at least as likely in practice as bias in the conservative direction, despite commonly held beliefs about error generally attenuating associations. The example and results above suggest that sources of error in the reference and their relation to those of the new test need to be considered very carefully.

The terms *relative sensitivity* and *relative specificity* are sometimes used for sensitivity and specificity when the reference test is subject to error. These terms are not to be confused with the relative performance parameters, (rTPF, rFPF), that compare the sensitivities and specificities of two tests. For the data in Example 7.7, the new test Y has a relative sensitivity of 80% with respect to the reference test R. However, since the sensitivities of both R and Y relative to D are 80%, their rTPF is 80%/80% = 100%.

7.3.3   *Classic latent class analysis*

We now consider a popular approach to the assessment of diagnostic tests when a gold standard measure of disease is not available.

The unobserved disease status D is a latent, or unobserved, variable. The reference R can be considered as a diagnostic test for D, just as Y is a diagnostic test for D. If one assumes a structure for the probabilistic mechanism from whence R and Y, and possibly other diagnostic tests, are derived from D, then it is sometimes possible to estimate this statistical distribution from observed data on the diagnostic tests. The marginal relationships between D and each of the diagnostic tests can then be calculated. This sort of analysis is referred to as latent class analysis.

Suppose that there are P diagnostic tests $Y_1, \ldots, Y_P$ (one of which may be R) and that each of N individuals yields data $(Y_{1i}, \ldots, Y_{Pi})$, $i = 1, \ldots, N$. We wish to estimate the prevalence of disease, $\rho = \mathrm{P}[D = 1]$, and the true and false positive fractions

$$\phi_k = \mathrm{TPF}_k = \mathrm{P}[Y_k = 1 | D = 1],$$
$$\psi_k = \mathrm{FPF}_k = \mathrm{P}[Y_k = 1 | D = 0],$$

respectively, for each of the tests, where $k = 1, \ldots, P$.

The earliest work on latent class analysis relied on the assumption of conditional independence (Walter and Irwig, 1988). We mentioned conditional independence in Section 7.3.2 in relation to the reference R and Y. Since in this section all observed tests are acknowledged to have error and are denoted similarly (i.e. R is one of the Ys), we state the more general definition.

Definition   Conditional independence

$$\mathrm{P}[Y_{1i}, \ldots, Y_{Pi} | D] = \prod_{k=1}^{P} \mathrm{P}[Y_{ki} | D]. \qquad (7.25)$$

∎

Simply stated, conditional on a subject's true disease status, the results of the P tests are independent. Conditional independence implies that, if a subject's true disease status is known, then knowledge of the result of one test is not informative about the result of any of the other tests. Let us now consider likelihood-based inference when the assumption holds.

For the ith subject, the likelihood of his/her observed data on P test results is

$$
\begin{aligned}
\mathcal{L}_i &= \mathrm{P}[Y_{1i}, \ldots, Y_{Pi}] \\
&= \mathrm{P}[D_i = 1]\mathrm{P}[Y_{1i}, \ldots, Y_{Pi} | D_i = 1] + \mathrm{P}[D_i = 0]\mathrm{P}[Y_{1i}, \ldots, Y_{Pi} | D_i = 0] \\
&= \mathrm{P}[D_i = 1]\prod_{Y_{ki}} \mathrm{P}[Y_{ki} | D_i = 1] + \mathrm{P}[D_i = 0]\prod_{Y_{ki}} \mathrm{P}[Y_{ki} | D_i = 0]
\end{aligned}
$$

$$= \rho \prod_{Y_{ki}} \phi_k^{Y_{ki}} (1 - \phi_k)^{1-Y_{ki}} + (1 - \rho) \prod \psi_k^{Y_{ki}} (1 - \psi_k)^{1-Y_{ki}} .$$

One can estimate ρ and $\{(\phi_k, \psi_k), k = 1, \ldots, P\}$ by maximizing the likelihood function $\mathcal{L}(\rho, \phi, \psi) = \prod_{i=1}^{N} \mathcal{L}_i$ with respect to these parameters. The variance–covariance matrix is calculated using either the Hessian matrix if observations are independent or a robust version if observations are clustered. The likelihood does not yield explicit analytic expressions for parameter estimates.

Result 7.13

Data from at least three diagnostic tests are required for identifiability of true and false positive fractions from latent class analysis under the conditional independence assumption, i.e. $P \geqslant 3$ is required for parameter identifiability.

Proof The informal argument is based on relating the number of parameters to be estimated to the number of degrees of freedom available in the data. We note that formally the identifiability of parameters (ρ, ϕ, ψ) is defined as, the derivative of the log likelihood yielding solutions $(\partial/\partial(\rho, \phi, \psi)) \log \mathcal{L}(\rho, \phi, \psi) = 0$.

When $P = 1$, i.e. only one test, Y_1, is available, then only one frequency can be estimated. We can estimate $P[Y_1 = 1] = \rho\phi_1 + (1 - \rho)\psi_1$ from the data. Therefore, we cannot identify ρ, ϕ_1 and ψ_1, but only the composite $\rho\phi_1 + (1-\rho)\psi_1$. Formally, the likelihood is a function of this composite and we cannot calculate derivatives with respect to its elements.

When 2 tests, (Y_1, Y_2), are available, $P = 2$ and Table 7.8 indicates that again the number of parameters exceeds the degrees of freedom in the data. Three distinct frequencies can be estimated from the tabulated data. That is, we can estimate only three distinct combinations of $(\rho, \phi_1, \phi_2, \psi_1, \psi_2)$. This implies that we cannot solve for the five distinct parameters of interest.

When $P = 3$ tests are available, we see that the degrees of freedom in the data are seven, which is the same as the number of parameters to be estimated. We can therefore estimate the parameters when $P = 3$.   ∎

Example 7.8

Infection with chlamydia bacteria often occurs without the presence of signs and symptoms. However, the bacteria can cause or increase the risk of pelvic inflammatory disease and other ill effects. The standard test for chlamydia is a bacterial culture. Culture is known to be less than 100% sensitive and is considered a bronze (rather than gold) standard for infection. The data in Table 7.9 (Wu *et al.*, 1992) show the results of a new ELISA immune assay (EIA) test compared with culture for $N = 324$ specimens from two clinics in Taiwan and China. With culture as the reference test, we calculate the prevalence of chlamydia infection to be $\rho = 7.1\%$, and the operating characteristics of the EIA test as $\mathrm{TPF}_{\mathrm{EIA}} = 87\%$ and $\mathrm{FPF}_{\mathrm{EIA}} = 2\%$.

Table 7.8 *An informal proof of Result 7.13*

Tests	Data tabulation	Degrees of freedom	Parameters
1	$Y_1 = 0$ $\boxed{n^-}$ $Y_1 = 1$ $\boxed{n^+}$	1	ρ, ϕ_1, ψ_1
2	$Y_2 = 0$ $\quad$ $Y_2 = 1$ $Y_1 = 0$ $\boxed{n^{--}}$ $\boxed{n^{-+}}$ $Y_1 = 1$ $\boxed{n^{+-}}$ $\boxed{n^{++}}$	3	$\rho, \phi_1, \psi_1, \phi_2, \psi_2$
3	$Y_3 = 0$ $Y_2 = 0$ $\quad$ $Y_2 = 1$ $Y_1 = 0$ $\boxed{n^{---}}$ $\boxed{n^{-+-}}$ $Y_1 = 1$ $\boxed{n^{+--}}$ $\boxed{n^{++-}}$ $Y_3 = 1$ $Y_2 = 0$ $\quad$ $Y_2 = 1$ $Y_1 = 0$ $\boxed{n^{--+}}$ $\boxed{n^{-++}}$ $Y_1 = 1$ $\boxed{n^{+-+}}$ $\boxed{n^{+++}}$	7	$\rho, \phi_1, \psi_1, \phi_2, \psi_2, \phi_3, \psi_3$

Table 7.9 *Results of testing for chlamydia bacteria with culture (Y_{CLT}), ELISA immunoassay (Y_{EIA}) and polymerase chain reaction (Y_{PCR})*

		Culture	
		$Y_{\mathrm{CLT}} = 0$	$Y_{\mathrm{CLT}} = 1$
Combined PCR	$Y_{\mathrm{EIA}} = 0$	294	3
	$Y_{\mathrm{EIA}} = 1$	7	20
PCR positive only	$Y_{\mathrm{EIA}} = 0$	2	2
	$Y_{\mathrm{EIA}} = 1$	4	20
PCR negative only	$Y_{\mathrm{EIA}} = 0$	292	1
	$Y_{\mathrm{EIA}} = 1$	3	0

An additional test based on polymerase chain reaction (PCR) was also performed on the specimens. The availability of three tests presents the opportunity to perform a latent class analysis that acknowledges the potential error in the standard reference test, namely culture. The results are shown in Table 7.10.

Interestingly, the results are consistent with popular beliefs about the tests. The PCR test is very sensitive to detecting bacteria (if it is in the clinical specimen), whereas culture is less so. False positive results caused by contamination are rare for both culture and PCR. The results for the EIA test are somewhat different depending on whether culture is used as a reference or if the latent class analysis is performed. The latent class approach suggests a higher prevalence of disease and better performance of the test.

Table 7.10 *Estimated prevalence of chlamydia and test classification probabilities using culture as the reference (bronze standard analysis) and using latent class analysis*

Bronze standard analysis	Latent class analysis
$\hat{\rho} = 7.1\%$	$\hat{\rho} = 8.1\%$
$\hat{\text{TPF}}_{\text{EIA}} = 87\%$	$\hat{\text{TPF}}_{\text{EIA}} = 91\%$
$\hat{\text{FPF}}_{\text{EIA}} = 2\%$	$\hat{\text{FPF}}_{\text{EIA}} = 1\%$
	$\hat{\text{TPF}}_{\text{PCR}} = 100\%$
	$\hat{\text{FPF}}_{\text{PCR}} = 0.5\%$
	$\hat{\text{TPF}}_{\text{CLT}} = 83\%$
	$\hat{\text{FPF}}_{\text{CLT}} = 0.3\%$

The latent class analysis, however, depends on the conditional independence assumption, which is unlikely to hold. In particular, it is probable that some subjects are infected but that the specimens collected from them do not contain bacteria. This would induce false negatives in all three tests. The extent of this bias cannot be assessed from the data at hand. Another issue that this analysis raises concerns the interpretation of the latent variable D. It has no clinical definition in this analysis. This leads to ambiguity in the interpretation of the parameters relating to D, namely all the parameters of interest, prevalence and true and false positive fractions. We will discuss this further later in Section 7.3.5. ∎

7.3.4 *Relaxing the conditional independence assumption*

Recognizing that the conditional independence assumption often fails in practice, various researchers have investigated the robustness of inference to departures from this assumption. There is evidence that results are highly dependent on it. A simple illustration can be found in the next example. Extensive simulation studies are reported in Vacek (1985) and in Torrance-Rynard and Walter (1997).

Example 7.9

Consider the neonatal audiology study dataset described in Section 1.3.7. True hearing status is known, along with the results of three diagnostic tests labeled A, B and C. Here we only include data for ears on which all three tests are performed. Estimates of disease prevalence and test accuracy parameters are shown in Table 7.11.

Suppose now that the gold standard, D, had not been measured. Cross-tabulations of data for (Y_A, Y_B, Y_C) are displayed in Table 7.12. Using latent class analysis (assuming conditional independence), we find that the estimated values for prevalence and accuracy are very different from the true values. We find that the performances of all three tests appear to be better than they really are.

Table 7.11 *Results of a latent class analysis compared with the standard analysis that uses the gold standard assessment of hearing status*

Estimated parameters	Standard analysis (D observed)	Latent class analysis (D unobserved)
Prevalence	42%	54%
TPF$_A$, FPF$_A$	66%, 40%	84%, 13%
TPF$_B$, FPF$_B$	62%, 36%	76%, 13%
TPF$_C$, FPF$_C$	75%, 54%	90%, 31%

Table 7.12 *Results of three tests (A, B and C) for hearing status. Data are only included for ears that have all three tests measured and true hearing status, D, is ignored (hypothetically unobserved)*

	$Y_B = 0$			$Y_D = 1$		
	$Y_C = 0$	$Y_C = 1$		$Y_C = 0$	$Y_C = 1$	
$Y_A = 0$	162	85		29	50	
$Y_A = 1$	31	75		27	207	
			353			313

In this example, the conditional independence assumption clearly does not hold. In fact, there appears to be some positive dependence between test results (data not shown). The effect is to bias the estimated test performance towards higher apparent accuracy with latent class analysis. This agrees with the simulation results of Torrance-Rynard and Walter (1997). ■

One approach to relaxing the conditional independence assumption is to use a study design that yields more degrees of freedom, thereby allowing estimation of more parameters. Some parameters can be used to quantify correlations between test results given disease status. For example, if four tests are performed there are $2^4 - 1 = 15$ degrees of freedom. In addition to the nine parameters quantifying prevalence, TPF and FPF values, there are six degrees of freedom available for conditional dependence parameters. Without any structure imposed on the dependence, there are $2 \times \binom{4}{2} = 12$ dependence parameters that quantify pairwise dependence between tests within the diseased and non-diseased populations. In addition, there are parameters quantifying higher-order dependence. Clearly some considerable structure must be imposed on the dependence in order that parameters can be estimated from the six degrees of freedom available in the data. Whatever these assumptions are, it is possible that they will have a strong influence on the analysis, in much the same way as we saw that the conditional independence assumption had a strong influence on the analysis in the simpler three test scenario.

The availability of covariates can also increase the degrees of freedom in the data. Models that incorporate covariate effects on test results and that require conditional independence to hold, conditional on covariates as well as disease status, are discussed by Kosinski and Flanders (1999). This approach allows one to adjust for sources of correlation that can be observed and documented (i.e. that can be included as covariates in the analysis), but cannot account for unobserved sources of correlation.

Unobserved sources of correlation are modeled with random effects by Qu *et al.* (1996) and by Qu and Hadgu (1998). The structure in this setting is imposed by assuming that subject-specific random effects explain the conditional dependence between tests, assuming a simple subject-specific model for test results and assuming a probability distribution for the random effects in the population. Yang and Becker (1997) also pursue this approach and use a modeling technique that leads to easier, intuitively appealing inference.

Another strategy for relaxing the conditional independence assumption is to incorporate information into the analysis that is external to the study data. In particular, 'prior' information can be incorporated using Bayesian methods (Joseph *et al.*, 1995). Such information might include plausible ranges for disease prevalence in the population, for example. Alternatively, investigators might be willing to specify likely ranges for test accuracy parameters. Dendukuri and Joseph (2001) describe an implementation of such Bayesian methodology when results from two imperfect tests are available for each study subject. Georgiadis *et al.* (2003) discuss a similar approach when testing is performed in two populations. They describe an appealing approach to specifying prior distributions. The Bayesian approach yields a posterior distribution (or belief function) for parameters, including prevalence and test accuracy parameters. In small samples the prior will influence the posterior distribution. In large samples it will not. Note, however, that the asymptotic behavior of the posterior distribution is not necessarily concentrated at the true parameters in large samples. Rather, as Dendukuri and Joseph (2001) point out, it will concentrate in a subregion of the parameter space that is consistent with the data. That is, the non-identifiability problem remains with the Bayesian method unless sufficient structure is imposed on the probabilistic behavior to yield identifiability, as we have discussed before. We refer to the papers cited above for illustrations of the Bayesian approach that allow relaxation of the conditional independence assumption.

An approach which is similar in spirit, but less sophisticated than the Bayesian methodology, is to fix a subset of parameters at certain values and to estimate the remaining parameters from the data. We refer to a seminal article on latent class analysis by Gart and Buck (1966) who provide a solution using this approach. Mantel (1951), Staquet *et al.* (1981) and Thibodeau (1981) also pursue this idea. One might, for example, assume certain values for the prevalence and the (TPF, FPF) of the reference test and then calculate estimates of (TPF, FPF) for an investigational test. Presenting results under a variety of assumptions about the fixed parameters might be wise since there will undoubtedly be differing opinions about likely values for these quantities. The Bayesian approach can be considered as a device to summarize such results across different assumed scenarios. Baker (1991) discusses the problem when estimates of (TPF, FPF) are available for the reference test.

There is clearly a large literature on the latent class analysis approach to evaluating diagnostic tests when the reference test is subject to error. Hui and Zhou (1998) provide a review and a bibliography.

7.3.5 *A critique of latent class analysis*

Although latent class analysis appears to solve a major problem in the evaluation of diagnostic tests, there are some fundamental concerns about the use of latent class analysis in practice that are not widely appreciated. The biggest concern is not so much a statistical issue but a more basic scientific concern. For a latent class analysis, disease is not defined in a clinical sense. Rather, it is an implicit mathematically defined entity, a random variable, which we call 'disease'. However, disease can mean different things to different people. One clinician might define cancer as 'having one or more malignant cells', whereas another clinician could define it as 'a malignant disease which will be fatal if left untreated'. In latent class analysis we make no clinical definition for D. This ambiguity is a major scientific problem. The parameters which we estimate, namely prevalence, test sensitivity and test specificity, are not well defined because they relate to D which is itself not well defined. The interpretations given to TPF and FPF by investigators will vary with their own conceptual definition for disease. Therefore, it is important to discuss the interpretations of results in this regard when reporting a latent class analysis.

The second concern is that latent class analysis requires that a model be specified for the joint distribution of test results conditional on disease status. The validity of components of this model, however, cannot be tested. For example, when $P = 3$ the conditional independence assumption is required for identifiability of parameters, but there is no way to assess if conditional independence is valid. With larger numbers of tests we still need to make assumptions about the underlying model which cannot be confirmed, although, as we have discussed, the assumptions may involve higher-order dependencies.

Example 7.10

Consider the data for the two scenarios displayed in Table 7.13 (Pepe and Alonzo, 2001*a*). They both yield the same observed data for the marginal frequencies, i.e. the same observed data if D is not observed (see Table 7.14). Therefore, results of latent class analysis, which here assumes conditional independence, are the same for both scenarios (see Table 7.15). However, similar to the earlier audiology data, the results are quite different from the truth in both cases. Moreover, there is no way to determine from the observed data whether the assumed latent class model is incorrect, i.e. that the conditional independence assumption fails. ∎

The fact that results are not robust to misspecification of the assumed latent class model and that the validity of the model cannot be assessed directly suggest

Table 7.13 *Two different truths that yield the same observed test result data, i.e. marginal frequencies associated with tests A, B and C*

| | | | $Y_C = 0$ | | $Y_C = 1$ | |
			$Y_B = 0$	$Y_B = 1$	$Y_B = 0$	$Y_B = 1$
Non-diseased	Scenario 1	$Y_A = 0$	520	10	5	0
		$Y_A = 1$	50	10	5	20
	Scenario 2	$Y_A = 0$	530	100	0	0
		$Y_A = 1$	150	110	0	0
Diseased	Scenario 1	$Y_A = 0$	10	90	5	5
		$Y_A = 1$	100	100	20	50
	Scenario 2	$Y_A = 0$	0	0	10	5
		$Y_A = 1$	0	0	25	70

Table 7.14 *Marginal frequencies from Table 7.13*

| | $Y_C = 0$ | | $Y_C = 1$ | |
	$Y_B = 0$	$Y_B = 1$	$Y_B = 0$	$Y_B = 1$
$Y_A = 0$	530	100	10	5
$Y_A = 1$	150	110	25	70

Table 7.15 *Estimated test accuracy under latent class analysis (LCA) compared with true values*

	ρ	TPF_A	TPF_B	TPF_C	$1 - \text{FPF}_A$	$1 - \text{FPF}_B$	$1 - \text{FPF}_C$
Scenario 1					Estimated parameters		
Truth	0.38	0.71	0.65	0.21	0.86	0.94	0.95
LCA estimates	0.22	0.95	0.75	0.44	0.81	0.85	0.98
Scenario 2							
Truth	0.11	0.86	0.68	1.00	0.71	0.76	1.00
LCA estimates	0.22	0.95	0.75	0.44	0.81	0.85	0.98

that considerable caution should be exercised in using the latent class model approach in practice.

Finally, note that estimated parameters from the latent class analysis are not explicit functions of the observed data. This renders it difficult to understand how the data affect parameters, or what factors influence results. The approach yields estimates that are derived from a black box and are not intuitively well connected with the data. This is a drawback to the practitioner. Efforts towards understanding how observed data influence parameter estimates would be worthwhile and might help to clarify the implicit mathematical definition of D. This

Table 7.16 *The discrepant resolution algorithm*

	Unresolved data $R = 0$	$R = 1$			Resolved data $R^* = 0$	$R^* = 1$
$Y = 0$	a	b	$\longrightarrow$		$a + b^1$	$b - b^1$
$Y = 1$	c	d			$c - c^1$	$d + c^1$

seems like a necessary step before latent class analysis should be promoted for widespread use.

7.3.6 *Discrepant resolution*

Discrepant resolution, also known as discrepant analysis, is another commonly used but problematic attempt to rectify problems with an imperfect reference test. When the results of new and reference tests are discrepant the idea is to try to resolve which one is correct using another test, which we call the resolver test.

The procedure is best described with an illustration. Consider the tabulation of Y by R in Table 7.16, where cell frequencies are denoted by a, b, c and d.

Samples where the results are discrepant, $(Y = 0, R = 1)$ and $(Y = 1, R = 0)$, are tested with the resolver. If the result is positive then the resolved reference, denoted by R^*, is defined as positive, and vice versa. We use the notation b^1 and c^1 to denote the numbers of observations whose reference test results are changed by the resolver, as shown in Table 7.16. The parameters TPF and FPF are calculated empirically according to the resolved data table.

Example 7.11

Consider again testing for chlamydia (Wu *et al.*, 1992), where R is the culture test, which is very specific but not 100% sensitive. Test results in cell c are possibly from diseased subjects but are not detected with R. Testing with PCR, the resolver test in this example, yields more subjects detected with disease from cell c, with $c^1 = 4$. One subject from cell b is negative using the PCR test (Table 7.17). As we saw before, TPF is estimated to be $20/23 = 87\%$ with the culture reference. It increases to $24/26 = 92\%$ with the resolved reference. Specificity also increases from $294/301 = 98\%$ with culture to $295/298 = 99\%$ with discrepant resolution. ∎

Table 7.17 *Discrepant resolution applied to chlamydia data. The culture test, R, is resolved with PCR*

	$R = 0$	$R = 1$	$R^* = 0$	$R^* = 1$
$Y_{\text{EIA}} = 0$	294	3	$294 + 1$	$3 - 1$
$Y_{\text{EIA}} = 1$	7	20	$7 - 4$	$20 + 4$

There are some aspects of the discrepant resolution approach that are very attractive and intuitively appealing to researchers. The first stage is performed with an 'imperfect' standard test that is often inexpensive. This picks out the tough cases that need resolving. One then need only apply the more laborious or expensive resolver test to specimens or subjects in discrepant off-diagonal cells which occur with low frequency. Moreover, the algorithm at face value seems like an improvement over using the imperfect reference test R alone because there is an attempt to resolve those tough cases.

However, there are obvious statistical problems with discrepant resolution which are discussed by Hadgu (1996, 1997) and Miller (1998a, 1998b), amongst others. Most importantly, the procedure biases towards improving the apparent accuracy of the new test. Only observations in the off-diagonal cells are potentially reclassified with the procedure and movement is therefore always towards increasing the numbers in the diagonal cells of the table. Note that bias occurs even if the resolver is a perfect gold standard. A second issue is that the reference R^* is not well defined. Therefore definitions for the TPF and FPF parameters calculated are elusive. Even more importantly, R^* depends on the results of the new test under investigation. Clearly this violates first principles for evaluating a test against a reference. Finally, we note that, if errors in the resolver are like those in the new test, then this can further bias the new test towards appearing to be better than it really is. Discrepant resolution as a statistical procedure can rarely, if ever, be justified.

7.3.7 *Composite reference standards*

Although discrepant resolution itself is problematic, it introduces the idea of defining a reference test based on the results of multiple imperfect reference tests. Alonzo and Pepe (1999) call a reference test that is defined on the basis of multiple references (excluding of course the new investigational tests) a composite reference standard test. The hope is that the new composite reference is better than a single reference test and hence a better reflection of true disease status. In the chlamydia example, a sensible composite reference is defined as positive if either culture or PCR indicate the presence of bacteria and negative if both do not indicate infection.

Example 7.11 (continued)

In the case presented in Table 7.18, relative to the composite reference the estimated TPF = 83% and FPF = 1%.   ∎

An important feature of the composite reference approach is that the reference is explicitly defined. Thus a working clinical definition of 'disease' is available which is essential for interpretation and appropriate communication of accuracy parameters. This contrasts with latent class analysis where disease is not defined clinically. In contrast with discrepant resolution, the definition of disease is not dependent on the results of the diagnostic test under investigation, Y.

Table 7.18 *Classification for the EIA test compared with culture as the reference, and with the composite reference standard denoted by D*

	Culture		Composite reference	
	$R = 0$	$R = 1$	$D = 0$	$D = 1$
$Y_{\mathrm{EIA}} = 0$	294	3	292	5
$Y_{\mathrm{EIA}} = 1$	7	20	3	24

In adopting the composite reference approach, we acknowledge that a reference needs an explicit clinical definition and that it needs to be observable. This is a good thing. Definitions of disease are often difficult to arrive at. However, by using an approach that avoids making a definition, one simply buries one's head in the sand. It is better to have a working definition than to have none at all. That the definition be based on observable quantities seems to be a rather minimal requirement too. If the disease as defined is not observable, then one cannot gauge how close the new test reflects disease. Common sense indicates that one can only compare the new test with observable quantities.

One attraction of discrepant resolution is that most subjects are tested only with the imperfect reference. Only a small subset require testing with the resolver test. Sometimes a composite reference is defined so that, with sequential application of the reference tests that comprise the composite, not all subjects will need to be tested with all of the references. For instance, consider if the composite is defined on the basis of references A and B, with the rule for positivity of the composite being 'A or B positive'. One could apply test A first and avoid testing with B those subjects who test positive with A. If the rule for positivity is that 'A and B are positive', then subjects who test negative with A do not need to be tested with B. Alonzo and Pepe (1999) provide further discussion of sequential testing in this context.

7.4 Concluding remarks

In this chapter issues surrounding incomplete ascertainment of true disease status have been discussed. Sections 7.1, 7.2 and 7.3 dealt with progressively more difficult problems: verification biased sampling (VBS), verification of only positive testers (VOPT) and missing gold standards (MGS), respectively. Inference about a single test was considered in Section 7.1, while the focus in Section 7.2 was on the comparison of two tests. This is because VOPT only allows for inference about relative performance, $(\mathrm{rFPF}, \mathrm{rTPF})$, while estimation of the performance parameters themselves, $(\mathrm{FPF}, \mathrm{TPF})$, is feasible in principle with VBS. Interestingly, if the purpose of a study is to compare tests, then there is no gain from a VBS study in which some screen negatives are verified for disease status compared with a VOPT study that ignores them (see Sections 8.4.1 and 8.4.4).

In theory, latent class analysis allows one to both estimate and compare the performance parameters of tests. However, I am rather doubtful about the ability to do either in a valid way when one is not willing to define a gold standard explicitly from observable quantities. Others are more hopeful than I, as is evident from the many statistical methodology articles on latent class analysis. For some practical substantive applications of these methods, see papers by Walter *et al.* (1991), Ferraz *et al.* (1995), Szatmari *et al.* (1995) and Mahoney *et al.* (1998).

The discussion throughout has focused on inference about the classification probabilities, (FPF, TPF). With VBS the predictive values, (PPV, NPV), can be directly estimated, while for VOPT studies the PPV but not the NPV can be estimated. When the gold standard is missing, latent class analysis provides estimates of both predictive values because they can be calculated from the estimates of ρ, TPF and FPF.

Inference about ROC curves from verification biased studies was discussed in Section 7.1.8. Little work has been done concerning ROC analysis for the VOPT and MGS problems. Baker and Pinsky (2001) show that the ratio of partial areas under two ROC curves can be estimated with a VOPT design, thus providing a generalization of Result 7.6 to continuous tests. Henkelman *et al.* (1990) propose using latent class models to estimate an ROC curve when no gold standard reference test is available. The model assumes that test results are normally distributed conditional on true disease status. Begg and Metz (1990) voice some of the same concerns about this approach that I have voiced about latent class analysis in general.

The key assumption necessary for inference with verification biased studies is the MAR assumption (7.2). This is relaxed to (7.5) when auxiliary variables exist that also affect efforts to assess disease status. Baker (1995) shows that MAR can be relaxed further if one is willing to model the missing data mechanism and make some assumptions about interactions between D and (Y, A) on the verification probabilities. Such assumptions cannot be tested with the data at hand, and so this methodology must be viewed with caution. It has been suggested that two-stage VBS study designs might be more cost efficient than simple cohort studies because only a fraction of screen negatives undergo costly procedures for assessing disease status. Unfortunately, work by Irwig *et al.* (1994a) and Obuchowski and Zhou (2002) suggests that two-stage designs can rarely be used to reduce costs. The reduced sampling of screen negatives implies that the overall size of the cohort study must be increased to the extent that little reduction in total study cost is achieved. This will be discussed again in Chapter 8 (see Section 8.4.4).

In conclusion, statistical inference about diagnostic accuracy is possible to varying extents with incomplete and imperfect data on the reference test. Several major questions remain for the practitioner, however. We have highlighted difficulties with inference in VBS studies, lack of methodology for ROC analysis in VOPT studies, and so forth. For the MGS problem the key question is 'does latent class analysis provide a useful solution to the problem of imperfections in the reference test?' At this point I believe that much more empirical evidence in favor of latent class analysis is needed before it can be recommended for practice.

7.5 Exercises

1. A cohort study is proposed to compare the classification probabilities of two tests, A and B. The prevalence of disease is low, 0.5%, and ascertainment of the gold standard is expensive. The study can enrol 10 000 subjects for screening with both tests, and definitive diagnostic testing for all subjects that screen positive on either A or B will be paid for by health insurance. Investigators are willing to pay for definitive diagnostic testing for a random sample of 500 subjects that screen negative on both tests if it will provide useful information. It is anticipated that the tests will have classification probabilities $(\text{FPF}_A, \text{TPF}_A) = (0.1, 0.7)$ and $(\text{FPF}_B, \text{TPF}_B) = (0.1, 0.9)$. Do you, as the study statistician, recommend that the validation of 500 screen negatives should proceed? How about if 5000 screen negatives can be validated?

2. Suppose that we seek to estimate the (FPF, TPF) of a screening test for a disease with prevalence 5% in the population. The cost of the screening test is $10, while definitive diagnostic testing costs $1000. It is anticipated that the test will have $(\text{FPF}, \text{TPF}) = (0.1, 0.8)$ and the study must estimate both parameters with standard errors of no more than 2.5%. Calculate the required sample size for the simple cohort study and the anticipated cost of the study. Two-stage study designs have been proposed to possibly lead to cost-efficient study designs. Assuming that all screen positives will be referred for definitive testing, calculate the cohort sample size and validation fraction, $P[V = 1|Y = 0]$, that lead to the study with minimum cost among one- or two-stage studies having standard errors of up to 2.5% for $\hat{\text{FPF}}$ and $\hat{\text{TPF}}$. Discuss the reductions in cost. See Irwig *et al.* (1994a) and Obuchowski and Zhou (2002) for related discussions. See Reilly and Pepe (1995) for related work on optimizing cost for two-stage studies in more standard (non-diagnostic testing) applications.

3. In studies with extreme verification biased sampling we have discussed the comparison of tests based on their detection and false referral probabilities on multiplicative scales. Consider instead using $\text{DP}_A - \text{DP}_B$ and $\text{FP}_A - \text{FP}_B$ to compare tests. Are there advantages to the interpretations of absolute differences? Can these parameters be estimated from a paired study without assessing disease status for subjects who test positive on both tests A and B? Provide an interpretation for the ratio $(\text{DP}_A - \text{DP}_B)/(\text{FP}_A - \text{FP}_B)$ that can be understood easily by a clinical audience.

4. There has been a great deal of debate in the literature about bias induced by the discrepant resolution procedure. See, for instance, a recent series of letters (Green *et al.*, 2001; Hadgu, 2001; Schachter, 2001). Proponents of the approach suggest that there is little bias when the reference and investigational tests are highly specific. Do you agree? Can one bound the bias induced by discrepant analysis in this case? See also simulation studies presented in Green *et al.* (1998).

5. Consider diagnostic testing when a gold standard is not available. Suppose that two binary tests, (Y_A, Y_B), are performed on subjects in two different populations. Write the data as $\{(k_i, Y_{Ai}, Y_{Bi}),\ i = 1, \ldots, N_1 + N_2\}$, where k_i denotes the population to which the ith subject belongs and N_k subjects are tested in the kth population, where $k = 1, 2$. Assume that the classification probabilities for the tests are the same in the two populations but that disease prevalence differs. Write down the likelihood for the unknown parameters $\{(\mathrm{FPF}, \mathrm{TPF}), \rho_1, \rho_2\}$. Are there sufficient degrees of freedom to estimate the parameters?

6. Consider latent class analysis when three tests are performed on each of N subjects. Write down expressions for the likelihood score equations assuming that the conditional independence assumption holds. From these expressions, is it obvious that estimates of sensitivity and specificity will be biased towards higher values if test results are positively correlated?

7.6   Proofs of theoretical results

Proof of Result 7.1   We prove the first result and the second is proven similarly. We have

$$
\begin{aligned}
\mathrm{P}[Y = 1 | D = 1, V = 1] &= \frac{\mathrm{P}[Y = 1, D = 1, V = 1]}{\mathrm{P}[V = 1, D = 1]} \\
&= \frac{\mathrm{P}[Y = 1, D = 1]\mathrm{P}[V = 1 | Y = 1, D = 1]}{\mathrm{P}[D = 1]\mathrm{P}[V = 1 | D = 1]} \\
&= \mathrm{TPF}\frac{\mathrm{P}[V = 1 | Y = 1, D = 1]}{\mathrm{P}[V = 1 | D = 1]} \\
&\geqslant \mathrm{TPF},
\end{aligned}
$$

the last inequality following from (7.1) and the fact that

$$
\begin{aligned}
\mathrm{P}[V = 1 | D = 1] = {} &\mathrm{P}[V = 1 | Y = 1, D = 1]\mathrm{P}[Y = 1 | D = 1] \\
&+ \mathrm{P}[V = 1 | Y = 0, D = 1]\mathrm{P}[Y = 0 | D = 1]. \qquad \blacksquare
\end{aligned}
$$

Proof of Result 7.2   First suppose that (7.2) holds. We then have

$$
\begin{aligned}
\mathrm{P}[D = 1 | V = 1, Y] \\
&= \frac{\mathrm{P}[D = 1, V = 1, Y]}{\mathrm{P}[V = 1, Y]} \\
&= \frac{\mathrm{P}[D = 1, V = 1, Y]}{\mathrm{P}[D = 1, V = 1, Y] + \mathrm{P}[D = 0, V = 1, Y]} \\
&= \frac{\mathrm{P}[V = 1 | D = 1, Y]\mathrm{P}[D = 1, Y]}{\mathrm{P}[V = 1 | D = 1, Y]\mathrm{P}[D = 1, Y] + \mathrm{P}[V = 1 | D = 0, Y]\mathrm{P}[D = 0, Y]} \\
&= \frac{\mathrm{P}[D = 1, Y]}{\mathrm{P}[D = 1, Y] + \mathrm{P}[D = 0, Y]}
\end{aligned}
$$

$$= \frac{P[D = 1, Y]}{P[Y]}$$

$$= P[D = 1|Y],$$

since, by MAR, $P[V = 1|D = 1, Y] = P[V = 1|D = 0, Y]$. Hence MAR implies (7.3). Let us now suppose that (7.3) holds. Then

$$P[V = 1|D, Y] = \frac{P[V = 1, D, Y]}{P[D, Y]}$$

$$= \frac{P[D|V = 1, Y]P[V = 1, Y]}{P[D|V = 1, Y]P[V = 1, Y] + P[D|V = 0, Y]P[V = 0, Y]}$$

$$= \frac{P[V = 1, Y]}{P[V = 1, Y] + P[V = 0, Y]}$$

$$= P[V = 1|Y],$$

since (7.3) implies that $P[D|V = 1, Y] = P[D|V = 0, Y]$.   ∎

Proof of Result 7.3   Observe that

$$P[D, Y] = P[D|Y]P[Y] = P[D|Y, V = 1]P[Y]$$

$$= \frac{P[D, Y, V = 1]P[Y]}{P[Y, V = 1]}$$

$$= \frac{P[D, Y, V = 1]}{P[V = 1|Y]}. \qquad (7.26)$$

Thus, at the population level, by replacing each observed data cell $P[D, Y, V = 1]$ by its inverse probability weighted version $P[D, Y, V = 1]/P[V = 1|Y]$, we correct for bias since the resultant probability frequency, $P[D, Y]$, reflects the population frequency.

Now let $\hat{P}$ denote observed empirical probability frequencies and let $\hat{P}_{\mathrm{IPW}}$ be the empirical inverse probability weighted frequencies. The inverse probability weighted estimates of $\mathrm{TPF} = P[Y = 1|D = 1]$ can then be written as

$$\hat{\mathrm{TPF}}_{\mathrm{IPW}} = \frac{\hat{P}_{\mathrm{IPW}}[D = 1, Y = 1]}{\hat{P}_{\mathrm{IPW}}[D = 1, Y = 1] + \hat{P}_{\mathrm{IPW}}[D = 1, Y = 0]}.$$

According to our definition of inverse probability weighting, this is

$$\frac{\hat{P}[D = 1, Y = 1, V = 1]}{\hat{P}[V = 1|Y = 1]} \bigg/ \left(\frac{\hat{P}[D = 1, Y = 1, V = 1]}{\hat{P}[V = 1|Y = 1]} + \frac{\hat{P}[D = 1, Y = 0, V = 1]}{\hat{P}[V = 1|Y = 0]} \right)$$

$$= \frac{\hat{P}[D = 1|Y = 1, V = 1]\hat{P}[Y = 1]}{\hat{P}[D = 1|Y = 1, V = 1]\hat{P}[Y = 1] + \hat{P}[D = 1|Y = 0, V = 1]\hat{P}[Y = 0]},$$

where the last equality follows by the same algebraic argument as (7.26) applied to the sampled data. Observe that this latter quantity is the Begg and Greenes estimator, $\hat{\mathrm{TPF}}_{\mathrm{BG}}$. Similar arguments verify the identity for FPF.   ∎

Proof of Result 7.4 Let $\hat{\tau}$, $\hat{\phi}$ and $\hat{\psi}$ denote the empirical estimates of τ, $\phi = \mathrm{PPV}$ and $\psi = 1 - \mathrm{NPV}$, respectively. We have

$$\hat{\mathrm{TPF}}_{\mathrm{BG}} = \frac{\hat{\phi}\hat{\tau}}{\hat{\phi}\hat{\tau} + \hat{\psi}(1 - \hat{\tau})}.$$

Therefore

$$\frac{\hat{\mathrm{TPF}}_{\mathrm{BG}}}{1 - \hat{\mathrm{TPF}}_{\mathrm{BG}}} = \left(\frac{\hat{\tau}}{1 - \hat{\tau}}\right) \frac{\hat{\phi}}{\hat{\psi}}.$$

We write

$$\log\left(\frac{\hat{\mathrm{TPF}}_{\mathrm{BG}}}{1 - \hat{\mathrm{TPF}}_{\mathrm{BG}}}\right) = \log\left(\frac{\hat{\tau}}{1 - \hat{\tau}}\right) + \log\hat{\phi} - \log\hat{\psi}$$

and note that $\hat{\tau}$, $\hat{\phi}$ and $\hat{\psi}$ are uncorrelated. Thus the variance of the left-hand side is the sum of the variances of the components on the right-hand side. Using the delta method we have

$$\mathrm{var}\left\{\log\left(\frac{\hat{\mathrm{TPF}}_{\mathrm{BG}}}{1 - \hat{\mathrm{TPF}}_{\mathrm{BG}}}\right)\right\} = \frac{\mathrm{var}(\hat{\tau})}{\tau^2(1 - \tau^2)} + \frac{\mathrm{var}(\hat{\phi})}{\phi^2} + \frac{\mathrm{var}(\hat{\psi})}{\psi^2}$$

$$= \frac{1}{N}\left\{\frac{\tau(1-\tau)}{\tau^2(1-\tau)^2} + \frac{\phi(1-\phi)}{\phi^2\tau P_1^V} + \frac{\psi(1-\psi)}{\psi^2(1-\tau)P_0^V}\right\}$$

$$= \frac{1}{N}\left\{\frac{1}{\tau(1-\tau)} + \frac{1-\phi}{\phi\tau P_1^V} + \frac{1-\psi}{\psi(1-\tau)P_0^V}\right\},$$

since each of $\hat{\tau}$, $\hat{\phi}$ and $\hat{\psi}$ is a binomial proportion with approximate sample sizes N, $N\tau P_1^V$ and $N(1-\tau)P_0^V$, respectively. ∎

Proof of Result 7.5 The expectation can be written as

$$\mathrm{E}\left\{\mathrm{E}\left\{\frac{I[V=1]}{\mathrm{P}[V=1|Y,A,X]}S_\beta(D,Y,X)\bigg| D,Y,A,X\right\}\right\}$$

$$= \mathrm{E}\left\{\frac{S_\beta(D,Y,X)}{\mathrm{P}[V=1|Y,A,X]}\mathrm{E}\left\{I[V=1]|D,Y,A,X\right\}\right\}$$

$$= \mathrm{E}\left\{S_\beta(D,Y,X)\right\} = 0,$$

since under MAR, i.e. (7.8), $\mathrm{E}\{I[V=1]|D,Y,A,X\} = \mathrm{P}[V=1|Y,A,X]$.

Observe that without the inverse probability weighting the expectation is not necessarily 0 because

$$\mathrm{E}\{I[V_i=1]S_\beta(D_i,Y_i,X_i)\} = \mathrm{P}[V_i=1]\mathrm{E}\{S_\beta(D_i,Y_i,X_i)|V_i=1\} \neq 0$$

in general. ∎

Proof of Result 7.11   We prove the result for attenuated sensitivity. We have

$$P[Y = 1|R = 1] = P[Y = 1, D = 1|R = 1] + P[Y = 1, D = 0|R = 1]$$
$$= P[Y = 1|D = 1, R = 1]P[D = 1|R = 1]$$
$$+ P[Y = 1|D = 0, R = 1]P[D = 0|R = 1].$$

Since the conditional independence assumption implies that $P[Y = 1|D = 1, R = 1] = P[Y = 1|D = 1]$, we have

$$P[Y = 1|R = 1]$$
$$= P[Y = 1|D = 1]P[D = 1|R = 1] + P[Y = 1|D = 0]P[D = 0|R = 1]$$
$$< P[Y = 1|D = 1]P[D = 1|R = 1] + P[Y = 1|D = 1]P[D = 0|R = 1]$$
$$= P[Y = 1|D = 1] \{P[D = 1|R = 1] + P[D = 0|R = 1]\}$$
$$= P[Y = 1|D = 1].$$ ∎

Proof of Result 7.12

(a) The observed sensitivity is $P[Y = 1|R = 1]$ and, since R is 100% specific,

$$P[Y = 1|R = 1] = P[Y = 1|R = 1, D = 1]$$
$$> P[Y = 1|D = 1] = \text{TPF}.$$

(b) The observed specificity is $P[Y = 0|R = 0]$ and, since R is 100% sensitive,

$$P[Y = 0|R = 0] = P[Y = 0|D = 0, R = 0]$$
$$> P[Y = 0|D = 0] = 1 - \text{FPF}.$$ ∎

8

STUDY DESIGN AND HYPOTHESIS TESTING

8.1 The phases of medical test development

8.1.1 *Research as a process*

The development of a medical test is a process. At the beginning of the process there are small exploratory studies that seek to identify how best to apply the test and whether or not it has potential for use in practice. At the end of the process there are studies that seek to determine the value of the test when applied in particular populations. In this chapter we first outline the series of research steps involved in developing a test.

It is important to have this 'big picture' in mind when designing a particular study. Where the study fits into the development process is critical for defining appropriate scientific objectives for a study, and consequently its design and evaluation. We categorize here the development process for a medical test into five distinct phases. Later in this chapter we will discuss sample size calculations. It facilitates our discussion of sample size calculations to consider them separately for studies in each phase.

Those familiar with therapeutic research will recognize that there is already an analogous well-established paradigm for the development of a new therapeutic agent. The research process for therapeutic drugs is categorized into five phases: a preclinical testing phase, three clinical phases prior to regulatory approval, known as phases 1, 2 and 3, and a post-marketing surveillance phase, sometimes called phase 4. The process is so well established that regulatory agencies in Europe, the United States and Japan have outlined a joint document with guidelines for study design and evaluation at each phase (ICH, 1999). Preclinical testing involves *in vitro* and animal studies of toxicity and biologic efficacy. Phase 1 studies typically involve establishing pharmacokinetic profiles, toxicity parameters and preliminary measures of biologic efficacy in humans. Appropriate doses, routes and regimens for administering the drug are also determined in phase 1. Phase 2 studies evaluate biologic efficacy. That is, the effects of the treatment on biologic measures of disease, which are supposedly targeted by the drug, are determined. If the treatment is successful in phase 2 then a comprehensive and usually large phase 3 study is undertaken to determine if the treatment is better than existing therapies in ways that tangibly benefit the patient. Clinical efficacy in phase 3 is often defined by mortality or quality of life parameters. A treatment approved in phase 3 for marketing will need to be monitored for low-frequency adverse effects that occur when the treatment is made available on a large scale. Such effects observed in this so-called post-marketing phase 4 may not be apparent in the studies at earlier phases conducted with limited sample sizes.

Categorizing the research development process for therapeutic agents has lead to widely accepted standards for study design and evaluation, and a development process that is regarded as reasonably rigorous and efficient. In a similar vein, categorizing the phases of development for a medical test can help clarify study objectives and streamline the development process, potentially making the process more rigorous and efficient.

8.1.2 Five phases for the development of a medical test

The phases shown in Table 8.1 were proposed for cancer biomarker research (Pepe et al., 2001). We adapt this structure here for more general tests. Although this paradigm will not apply exactly to all tests, the basic structure is useful to consider for many tests.

Phase 1 is the initial phase. Its purpose is basically exploratory, to see if the test might be worth developing and evaluating rigorously. It is therefore appropriate to study the test in a wide range of circumstances (Guyatt et al., 1986). Subjects with a variety of characteristics should be tested. In particular, subjects with diverse manifestations and severities of disease are tested. Non-diseased subjects with conditions that might be confused with disease should be tested in order to gain some insight into the limitations of the test for distinguishing disease from non-disease. The test should be implemented in a variety

Table 8.1 *Phases of research for the development of a medical test*

Phase	Description	Typical objectives	Typical design
1	Exploratory investigations	Identify promising tests and settings for application	Case-control study with convenience sampling
2	Retrospective validation	Determine if minimally acceptable (FPF_0, TPF_0) are achieved	Population-based case-control sampling
3	Retrospective refinement	Define criteria for screen positivity. Determine covariates affecting $S_{\bar{D}}$ and ROC. Compare promising tests. Develop algorithms for combining tests	Large-scale comprehensive population-based case-control study
4	Prospective application	Determine positive predictive values, detection and false referral probabilities when the test is applied in practice	Cohort study
5	Disease impact	Determine effects of testing on cost and mortality associated with disease	Randomized prospective trial comparing new test with standard of practice

of settings and by a variety of test operators. The operating parameters for the test can be varied. For example, the frequency and/or intensity of the auditory stimulus might be varied for a hearing test. The protocol for collecting and storing the clinical specimen might be varied for a laboratory test. In summary, one should determine at this early phase if the test is reasonably robust to the circumstances under which it is performed or if it only operates well in particular settings. The reproducibility of results is an important factor to address in phase 1, and the test should be improved in this regard if necessary. Often, at the exploratory phase, subjects and samples that are conveniently available (e.g. from a clinic or blood bank) are studied. Rigorous evaluation of a test in a well-defined sense begins in the next phase.

Phase 2 is called the validation phase to contrast it with the exploratory (hypothesis generating) phase 1. Selection criteria for cases and controls, the tester (if applicable) and the protocol for performing the test are specified in rigorous detail in phase 2. This allows the results to be interpreted without ambiguity and as pertaining to a relevant well-defined population. Sampling of cases and controls was discussed in the early chapters of this book. The choice of tester (e.g. technician and radiologist in an imaging study) is also an important factor to consider. In phase 2, expert testers might be employed in contrast to later phases where testers might be population based. We discussed common sources of bias of which investigators should be aware in Chapter 1. Care must be taken to avoid these in phase 2, as in all phases of development. A key objective of phase 2 is to ascertain true and false positive fractions of the test in a particular setting. Thus, in order to design a phase 2 study, some minimally acceptable true and false positive fractions should be specified in advance. The study can then be designed with adequate sample sizes, so that conclusions can be drawn from it with regard to the test meeting these minimal operating characteristics or not.

A test that meets these criteria in phase 2 and appears promising for further development should undergo thorough evaluation in more comprehensive case-control studies before it proceeds to be applied as a practical testing tool in prospective studies at phase 4. We call phase 3 this intermediate phase. Often a primary objective of phase 3 is to determine criteria that should be used for defining screen positivity in phase 4. ROC curves can be employed to determine an operating point with desirable trade-offs between the TPF and the FPF, and the corresponding threshold can then be used as the positivity criterion in phase 4. Factors affecting test results from non-diseased subjects should be determined at this stage. If necessary, covariate-specific thresholds can then be defined. In addition, covariates that affect the TPFs or the ROC curve should be identified so that the populations or circumstances in which the test is performed can be optimized in phase 4. Tests are often compared in case-control studies. We consider such studies to be part of phase 3 also, because the purpose is usually to select tests that should undergo prospective phase 4 evaluation. In addition, algorithms for combining tests to define a useful composite for application in phase 4 may be developed in phase 3.

Phases 1, 2 and 3 are typically retrospective case-control studies. Testing is therefore done only for research purposes (the disease status of the patient is already determined by other means). In contrast, the prospective cohort studies of phase 4 apply the test to subjects whose disease status is generally unknown at the time of testing. The results of the test frequently determine if further diagnostic work-up is even undertaken for a patient. Due to their prospective nature, the care of the patient enters into consideration when designing phase 4 studies. For example, definitive diagnostic testing may not be undertaken for subjects that screen negative in phase 4, or may only be undertaken for a subset of such patients, as discussed in Chapter 7. The objective of phase 4 is to determine the operating characteristics of the test when used as a diagnostic tool in a designated patient population. The extent and characteristics of disease detected with the test are determined. The false referral probability and characteristics of subjects that falsely screen positive must be determined. Promising tests are often compared in phase 4, because this is the phase where their practical performances as diagnostic tools are measured, and hence where the most relevant comparisons can be made.

Although a test accurately diagnoses disease, this does not necessarily mean that there is benefit to the patient. As delineated in Chapter 1 (see Table 1.1), effective treatment must be available for the disease detected with the test. Testing, work-up and treatment must be affordable and acceptable to patients, and so on. Ideally, the test is evaluated for its impact on the patient population before becoming part of routine healthcare. Its impact can be measured in terms of disease outcomes (mortality and quality of life) and cost. Such can be done through a randomized clinical trial, for example. Studies that evaluate the overall impact of the test on the population are called phase 5 studies.

Some general principles of study design were discussed in Chapter 1. These apply to studies at all phases of test development, but particularly starting at phase 2. Rigorous definitions of disease, clear protocols for applying the test, criteria for enrolling subjects and so forth must be undertaken with the same sort of care that is typically required for therapeutic studies. Sources of bias (see Section 1.2.5) must be minimized. Efforts should include blinding, for example. Comparative studies of test accuracy should be undertaken following the principles discussed in Section 3.1. Finally, in phase 5, randomized trials with mortality and cost as outcome measures are ideal and the reader is referred to the large body of literature on the design of randomized trials for study design principles (see Pocock, 1982, for example).

We focus in this chapter on the sample size calculations needed to ensure that conclusions can be drawn from a study. Sample size calculations for phases 2, 3 and 4 are considered in detail in Sections 8.2, 8.3 and 8.4, respectively. The following section describes matching and stratification as two additional issues that can be considered in study design.

8.2   Sample sizes for phase 2 studies

A phase 1 study is exploratory by definition. Its design is not based on a specific well-defined hypothesis. Rather, its purpose is to generate such a hypothesis for testing in phase 2. Thus formal sample size calculations are not considered here for phase 1, and we begin with phase 2. Multiple strategies are possible for sample size calculations. There are at least as many possibilities as there are for data analysis! We first describe a strategy that we find particularly straightforward and conceptually appealing for binary tests. It is extended to continuous tests in Section 8.2.2. Another strategy that has been proposed is described in Section 8.2.3.

8.2.1   *Retrospective validation of a binary test*

A phase 2 study is designed when a well-defined test and its target population are already identified. Assume that random samples of cases and controls will be drawn from the population and estimates of test accuracy will be made. In this section we assume that Y is binary, and therefore estimates of (FPF, TPF) will be made.

One needs to identify values for (FPF, TPF) that are minimally acceptable in order to design the study. Let $(\text{FPF}_0, \text{TPF}_0)$ denote such values. These are specified by the investigators and depend on the trade-off between false positives and true positives that are acceptable within the context of the test, disease, available resources and the population in which it is to be applied (Baker, 2000). Suppose that the goal of the phase 2 study is to determine if the test meets these minimal criteria.

Formally, the study will test the null hypothesis depicted in Fig. 8.1, namely

$$H_0 : \{\text{TPF} \leqslant \text{TPF}_0 \quad \text{or} \quad \text{FPF} \geqslant \text{FPF}_0\}. \tag{8.1}$$

From a study that rejects H_0 it will be concluded that $\text{TPF} > \text{TPF}_0$ and $\text{FPF} < \text{FPF}_0$, i.e. that the test meets minimal criteria.

The hypothesis can be tested by calculating a joint $1 - \alpha$ confidence region for (FPF, TPF), as described in Section 2.2.2. When the null hypothesis is one-sided, a rectangular confidence region made up of the cross-product of two one-sided, $1 - \alpha^* = \sqrt{1 - \alpha}$ confidence intervals is appropriate, as shown in Fig. 8.2. If the $1 - \alpha$ confidence region for (FPF, TPF) lies entirely within the region of acceptable values (unshaded region in Fig. 8.1), one can reject H_0 and make a positive conclusion about the test. We refer the reader back to Chapter 2 for a discussion of confidence interval construction.

The sample sizes for the phase 2 study, n_D and $n_{\bar{D}}$, should be chosen sufficiently large to ensure that a positive conclusion will be drawn with power $1 - \beta$ if the accuracy of the test is in fact at some specified, desirable levels. We denote these desirable classification probabilities by $(\text{FPF}_1, \text{TPF}_1)$. These reflect a test with levels of performance sufficiently good that the research community would want it to undergo further development. In summary, we require that

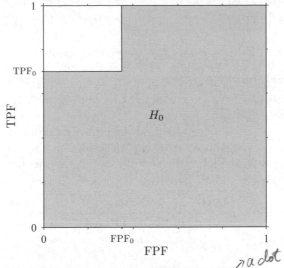

↗ a dot

FIG. 8.1. Regions in the (FPF, TPF) space for a binary test that correspond to unacceptable tests (H_0, shaded region) and acceptable tests (unshaded region)

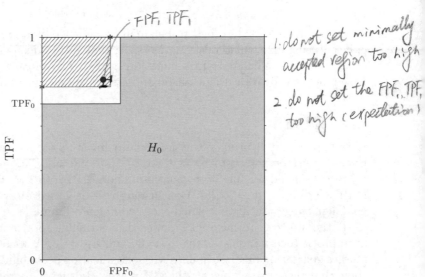

: FPF, TPF,

1. do not set minimally accepted region too high

2. do not set the FPF, TPF, too high (expectation)

FIG. 8.2. A one-sided rectangular confidence region for (FPF, TPF) of the exercise stress test calculated from the CASS data. The classification probabilities meet the minimal criteria: FPF $\leqslant$ 0.35 and TPF $\geqslant$ 0.70. The points indicated with asterisks represent $\left(\mathrm{FPF}_U^{\alpha^*} \text{ and } \mathrm{TPF}_L^{\alpha^*}\right)$, the upper and lower $\alpha^* = 1 - \sqrt{1 - \alpha}$ confidence limits for FPF and TPF, respectively

CI: $1 - \alpha^* = \sqrt{1 - \alpha}$ 95% CI

$$1 - \beta = P[\text{TPF}_L^{\alpha^*} > \text{TPF}_0 \quad \text{and} \quad \text{FPF}_U^{\alpha^*} < \text{FPF}_0 | \text{FPF}_1, \text{TPF}_1]$$
$$= P[\text{TPF}_L^{\alpha^*} > \text{TPF}_0 | \text{TPF}_1] P[\text{FPF}_U^{\alpha^*} < \text{FPF}_0 | \text{FPF}_1],$$

where $\text{TPF}_L^{\alpha^*}$ and $\text{FPF}_U^{\alpha^*}$ denote the lower and upper one-sided limits of the confidence intervals for TPF and FPF, respectively. If n_D is chosen so that $P[\text{TPF}_L^{\alpha^*} > \text{TPF}_0 | \text{TPF}_1] = \sqrt{1 - \beta}$ and $n_{\bar{D}}$ so that $P[\text{FPF}_U^{\alpha^*} < \text{FPF}_0 | \text{FPF}_1] = \sqrt{1 - \beta}$, then this ensures adequate study power $1 - \beta$ since the product is $1 - \beta$. We define $\beta^* = 1 - \sqrt{1 - \beta}$.

If the confidence limits are based on asymptotic normal distribution theory for the estimates, then sample sizes can be based on the asymptotic variance formulae. These yield the following sample size requirements:

one sample z test for proportion

$$n_D = \frac{\left(Z^{1-\alpha^*}\sqrt{\text{TPF}_0(1 - \text{TPF}_0)} + Z^{1-\beta^*}\sqrt{\text{TPF}_1(1 - \text{TPF}_1)}\right)^2}{(\text{TPF}_1 - \text{TPF}_0)^2} \quad (8.2)$$

and *independent*

$$n_{\bar{D}} = \frac{\left(Z^{1-\alpha^*}\sqrt{\text{FPF}_0(1 - \text{FPF}_0)} + Z^{1-\beta^*}\sqrt{\text{FPF}_1(1 - \text{FPF}_1)}\right)^2}{(\text{FPF}_1 - \text{FPF}_0)^2}, \quad (8.3)$$

normal distribution

where $Z^{1-\alpha^*} = \Phi^{-1}(1 - \alpha^*)$ and $Z^{1-\beta^*} = \Phi^{-1}(1 - \beta^*)$.

Since phase 2 studies tend to be small, confidence limits may be better calculated using exact methods. Sample sizes that yield adequate power for such analysis can be calculated with simulation studies. The above asymptotic theory-based formulae provide useful starting points for simulation studies, as illustrated next.

Example 8.1

It is hoped that a urinary test for chlamydia is 95% specific and 90% sensitive. It must be shown to be at least 80% specific and 75% sensitive in order to be considered for further evaluation. Thus $(\text{FPF}_1, \text{TPF}_1) = (0.05, 0.90)$ and $(\text{FPF}_0, \text{TPF}_0) = (0.20, 0.75)$. Conclusions will be based on a 90% rectangular confidence region using one-sided exact confidence limits.

If the study is to have 90% power, the formulae (8.2) and (8.3) based on asymptotic theory indicate that $n_D = 64$ and $n_{\bar{D}} = 46$. A set of 5000 simulation studies generating binary test data with classification probabilities $(\text{FPF}_1, \text{TPF}_1)$ show that these sample sizes yield 88% power. Raising the sample sizes to $n_D = 70$ and $n_{\bar{D}} = 50$ increases the power to 91%. Therefore, about 70 cases and 50 controls should be enrolled in the phase 2 validation study. ∎

8.2.2 *Retrospective validation of a continuous test*

When Y, the result of the test, is on a continuous scale, the question to answer is whether or not, for some threshold c, the dichotomized test, $I[Y > c]$, has

$P(T > c | D)$

$P(T > c | \bar{D})$

acceptable performance. That is, can the test operate at TPF and FPF values
that reach or exceed the minimal criteria? In Fig. 8.3 the shaded region again
corresponds to unacceptable test performance while performance parameters in
the unshaded region are acceptable. If the ROC curve for Y passes through this
unshaded region, then it is an acceptable test, because for some threshold it has
acceptable (FPF, TPF) values. On the other hand, if the ROC curve lies entirely
in the shaded region, then the test is unacceptable. For the ROC curves in Fig.
8.3, we see that test A meets the minimal criteria but test B does not.

Observe that the ROC curve for a test crosses the unshaded region if and
only if $\mathrm{ROC}(\mathrm{FPF}_0) \geqslant \mathrm{TPF}_0$. An equivalent formulation is that $\mathrm{ROC}^{-1}(\mathrm{TPF}_0) \leqslant$
FPF_0. We write the null hypothesis as

$$H_0 : \mathrm{ROC}(\mathrm{FPF}_0) \leqslant \mathrm{TPF}_0. \tag{8.4}$$

$H_1 : ROC (FPF_0) > TPF_0$

Under the null hypothesis, the ROC curve for Y lies fully in the unacceptable
region of the (FPF, TPF) space. A hypothesis test can be based on the lower
$(1 - \alpha)$-level confidence limit for $\mathrm{ROC}(\mathrm{FPF}_0)$. If this lower limit exceeds TPF_0,
then (8.4) is rejected and we conclude that the test meets the minimal criterion
for further development. In Fig. 8.4 we show the 95% lower confidence limit for
the ROC(0.2) of the CA-19-9 marker for pancreatic cancer based on data from
Wieand *et al.* (1989). If the minimally acceptable levels for the (FPF, TPF) of a
pancreatic cancer biomarker were (0.2, 0.6), say, we would conclude that CA-19-9
meets these criteria. That is, we reject $H_0 : \mathrm{ROC}(0.2) \leqslant 0.6$.

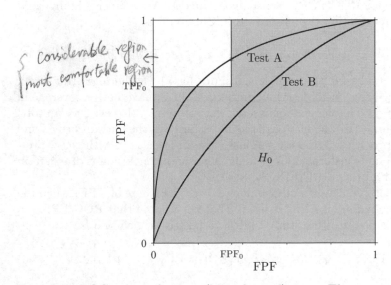

considerable region
most comfortable region

FIG. 8.3. ROC curves for two (hypothetical) tests. The upper one meets the
    minimally acceptable criterion that it can attain operating points which ex-
    ceed (FPF$_0$, TPF$_0$), whereas the lower one does not

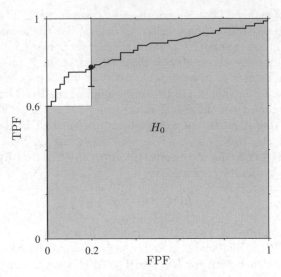

FIG. 8.4. A test of the null hypothesis that, at the threshold corresponding to $\text{FPF}_0 = 0.2$, the TPF does not exceed 0.6 for the CA-19-9 marker of pancreatic cancer. Shown is the lower 95% confidence limit for $\text{ROC}(0.2)$ using data from Wieand *et al.* (1989)

Turning now to sample size calculations, we need to consider how the lower confidence limit for $\text{ROC}(\text{FPF}_0)$ will be constructed. A confidence limit based on asymptotic distribution theory derived in Chapter 5 is

$$\text{ROC}(\text{FPF}_0)^{\alpha}_L = \hat{\text{ROC}}(\text{FPF}_0) - \Phi^{-1}(1-\alpha)\sqrt{\text{var}\{\hat{\text{ROC}}(\text{FPF}_0)\}}.\qquad(8.5)$$

In practice, we find that the confidence limits based on the logit transform, $\text{logit}\,\hat{\text{ROC}}(\text{FPF}_0)$, that were described in Section 5.2.3, have better coverage in small samples and we implement analyses with these limits. However, asymptotic theory-based sample size calculations are similar for both the untransformed and transformed approaches. Thus, for simplicity, we proceed here with the expression (8.5) for the untransformed lower limit. A positive conclusion is drawn from the study if we find that $\text{ROC}(\text{FPF}_0)^{\alpha}_L > \text{TPF}_0$.

Suppose that the diagnostic test, in fact, has a TPF value of TPF_1 when the threshold corresponding to FPF_0 is used. That is, suppose that $\text{ROC}(\text{FPF}_0) = \text{TPF}_1$. Then, the power of the study to draw a positive conclusion is

$$P\left[\hat{\text{ROC}}(\text{FPF}_0) - \Phi^{-1}(1-\alpha)\sqrt{\text{var}\{\hat{\text{ROC}}(\text{FPF}_0)\}} > \text{TPF}_0\right]\qquad(8.6)$$

where the probability is calculated assuming that $\text{TPF}_1 = \text{ROC}(\text{FPF}_0)$.

With the power (8.6) specified at some desired level $1 - \beta$, this implies that the sample sizes n_D and $n_{\bar{D}}$ should be chosen to satisfy

$$\frac{V_1}{n_D} \left(\Phi^{-1}(1-\alpha) + \Phi^{-1}(1-\beta) \right)^2 = (\text{TPF}_0 - \text{TPF}_1)^2 ,$$

where V_1/n_D is the asymptotic theory-based expression for $\text{var}\{\hat{\text{ROC}}(\text{FPF}_0)\}$ calculated under the alternative hypothesis $\text{ROC}(\text{FPF}_0) = \text{TPF}_1$. Using the empirical ROC curve estimator, $\hat{\text{ROC}}_e(\text{FPF}_0)$, and the analytic form for its asymptotic variance derived in Result 5.1, we write *only sensitivity was included*

$$V_1 = \text{TPF}_1(1 - \text{TPF}_1) + \kappa r_1^2 \text{FPF}_0(1 - \text{FPF}_0) , \qquad (8.7)$$

Can be data driven and based on previous data

where r_1 denotes the slope of the ROC curve at FPF_0 and κ denotes the ratio of cases to controls, $n_D/n_{\bar{D}}$. The next result summarizes the discussion.

Result 8.1

If study conclusions are based on $\text{ROC}(\text{FPF}_0)_L^\alpha$ exceeding TPF_0, where $\text{ROC}(\text{FPF}_0)_L^\alpha$ is the lower $1 - \alpha$ confidence interval calculated with the empirical ROC curve, then in order to achieve power $1 - \beta$ when $\text{TPF}_1 = \text{ROC}(\text{FPF}_0)$ we require that

$$n_D = \frac{\{\Phi^{-1}(1-\alpha) + \Phi^{-1}(1-\beta)\}^2}{(\text{TPF}_0 - \text{TPF}_1)^2} V_1 , \qquad (8.8)$$

where V_1 is defined in (8.7).   ∎

Example 8.2

The largest acceptable false positive fraction for a test based on a new biomarker is $\text{FPF}_0 = 0.10$. It is anticipated that it will be 95% sensitive ($\text{TPF}_1 = 0.95$) at the threshold corresponding to $\text{FPF} = 0.10$, but it must be shown to be at least 75% sensitive there ($\text{TPF}_0 = 0.75$) in order to proceed with further development. The study will enrol equal numbers of cases and controls ($\kappa = 1$) and we choose $\alpha = 0.05$ and $\beta = 0.10$. All components of the sample size formula (8.8) are now defined except for r_1, the slope of the ROC curve at FPF_0. We have

$$n_D = \frac{(1.64 + 1.28)^2 \{(0.95)(0.05) + (r_1)^2(0.10)(0.90)\}}{(0.95 - 0.75)^2} .$$

Suppose that the biomarker is anticipated to have a binormal ROC curve, $\text{ROC}(t) = \Phi(a + b\Phi^{-1}(t))$. Then by the chain rule we have

density

$$r_1 = \frac{\delta}{\delta t} \text{ROC}(t) = b \frac{\phi(a + b\Phi^{-1}(t))}{\phi(\Phi^{-1}(t))} .$$

Suppose further that we anticipate the slope parameter $b = 1$ under both the null and alternative hypotheses. Under these assumptions we can determine the values of a that correspond to each of the hypotheses. We do this by noting that $\text{ROC}(\text{FPF}_0) = \Phi(a + \Phi^{-1}(\text{FPF}_0)) = 0.75$ under the null, which implies that

pnorm   qnorm

$a = 1.96$. Similarly, under the alternative $\text{ROC}(\text{FPF}_0) = 0.95$, which implies that $a = 2.93$. Substituting $b = 1$ and these values for a into the expression for r_1 yields corresponding values of 1.81 and 0.58 for r_1. To be conservative, we use the larger value, having found from experience that this generally provides a better sample size calculation. Substituting $r_1 = 1.81$ into the expression for n_D we find $n_D = 73$. The choice $\kappa = 1$ implies that $n_{\bar{D}} = 73$ also.

This sample size calculation is based on asymptotic distribution theory. Simulation studies are used to assess the adequacy of the calculations. In particular, we generate data under H_1 and calculate the empirical power as the proportion of simulated studies in which a positive conclusion is drawn. Data for $n_D = 73$ cases and $n_{\bar{D}} = 73$ controls are generated from the binormal model with ROC intercept $a = 2.93$ and slope $b = 1$, as we assumed in the sample size calculations above. Normal distributions are used, with $Y_{\bar{D}} \sim \text{N}(0, 1)$ and $Y_D \sim \text{N}(a/b, 1/b^2)$. Recall that, since the analysis uses only the ranks of the data, the Gaussian distributional forms used in the simulations are irrelevant. The study power, calculated as 89%, appears to be adequate.

Additional simulations are performed under the null hypothesis, simply to check if inference using the confidence limits is valid with sample sizes of 73. That is, we wish to confirm that the size of the test procedure using the 95% lower confidence limit is the nominal 5%. Data are generated from the binormal model under the null. Hence we choose $a = 1.96$ and $b = 1.0$ so that $\text{ROC}(\text{FPF}_0) = \text{TPF}_0$. The null hypothesis is rejected in 6% of simulations, close enough to the nominal level. We reiterate that these confidence limits, based on the logit transform, are better behaved in small samples than are those based on the untransformed estimate of $\text{ROC}(\text{FPF}_0)$. The null is rejected in 10% of simulations that used the latter confidence limits, which is unacceptably large compared with the nominal 5% level.   ∎

8.2.3 *Sample size based on the AUC*

A non-binary diagnostic test can also be evaluated by comparing its AUC or other ROC summary index with a value that is considered to be minimally acceptable. Specifying a minimally acceptable AUC may be more difficult, in my opinion, than specifying a minimally acceptable (FPF, TPF) combination. However, the strategy does have the advantage of incorporating information across multiple operating points of the test, rather than being limited to only one point, as in the previous subsection.

Suppose that we estimate the AUC either with nonparametric or other methods and compare the estimate with the minimally acceptable value, which we denote by AUC_0. To test

$$H_0 : \text{AUC} \leqslant \text{AUC}_0$$

the $1 - \alpha$ lower confidence limit is calculated and H_0 is rejected if it exceeds AUC_0. In practice, we use confidence limits based on logit $\widehat{\text{AUC}}$, but again, to simplify the sample size calculations, we suppose that the lower limit of the confidence interval is based on asymptotic normality of the untransformed estimate, $\widehat{\text{AUC}}$. That is, we reject H_0 if

$$\widehat{\text{AUC}} - \Phi^{-1}(1 - \alpha)\sqrt{\hat{\text{var}}(\widehat{\text{AUC}})} > \text{AUC}_0\,,$$

where $\hat{\text{var}}(\widehat{\text{AUC}})$ denotes the estimated variance.

To calculate sample sizes using standard calculations so that a power of $1-\beta$ is achieved when the AUC is at some desirable value, AUC_1, the following equation must be satisfied:

$$\frac{\text{var}(\widehat{\text{AUC}})\left(\Phi^{-1}(1 - \alpha) + \Phi^{-1}(1 - \beta)\right)^2}{(\text{AUC}_1 - \text{AUC}_0)^2} = 1\,. \tag{8.9}$$

Once α, β, AUC_0 and AUC_1 are specified, the remaining task is to postulate a value for the variance. This is not a simple task because the variance depends, not only on the sample sizes and postulated AUCs, but on the underlying probability distributions. The next result shows that for the empirical AUC estimate, $\widehat{\text{AUC}}_e$, the asymptotic variance expression can be written in terms of the ROC curve. Therefore, if one postulates an ROC curve under the null and alternative, the asymptotic variance can be calculated and so approximate sample sizes can be derived.

Result 8.2

In large samples,

$$\text{var}(\widehat{\text{AUC}}_e) = \text{var}_D / n_{\bar{D}} + \text{var}_{\bar{D}} / n_D\,,$$

where

$$\text{var}_D = \int_0^1 (\text{ROC}(t))^2 \, dt - \text{AUC}^2\,,$$

$$\text{var}_{\bar{D}} = \int_0^1 (\text{ROC}^{-1}(t))^2 \, dt - (1 - \text{AUC})^2\,.$$

Proof   Consider the expression for $\text{var}(\widehat{\text{AUC}}_e)$ given in Result 5.5:

$$\text{var}(\widehat{\text{AUC}}_e) = \frac{\text{var}\left(S_{\bar{D}}(Y_D)\right)}{n_D} + \frac{\text{var}\left(S_D(Y_{\bar{D}})\right)}{n_{\bar{D}}}\,.$$

Observe that

$$\begin{aligned}
\text{var}\left(S_D(Y_{\bar{D}})\right) &= \text{E}\left\{S_D(Y_{\bar{D}})\right\}^2 - \left[\text{E}\left\{S_D(Y_{\bar{D}})\right\}\right]^2 \\
&= -\int_{-\infty}^{\infty} S_D^2(y) \, dS_{\bar{D}}(y) - \text{AUC}^2 \\
&= \int_0^1 S_D^2\left(S_{\bar{D}}^{-1}(t)\right) dt - \text{AUC}^2 \\
&= \int_0^1 (\text{ROC}(t))^2 \, dt - \text{AUC}^2\,.
\end{aligned}$$

Similarly

$$\text{var}\left(S_{\bar{D}}(Y_D)\right) = \text{E}\left\{S_{\bar{D}}(Y_D)\right\}^2 - \left[\text{E}\left\{S_{\bar{D}}(Y_D)\right\}\right]^2$$
$$= \int_0^1 \left\{\text{ROC}^{-1}(t)\right\}^2 \, \mathrm{d}t - \left\{\int_0^1 \text{ROC}^{-1}(t) \, \mathrm{d}t\right\}^2$$

and the second term is $(1 - \text{AUC})^2$.   ∎

As a consequence of (8.9) and Result 8.2, we have the following expression for sample sizes:

$$n_D = (\kappa \, \text{var}_D + \text{var}_{\bar{D}}) \left\{\frac{\Phi^{-1}(1 - \alpha) + \Phi^{-1}(1 - \beta)}{\text{AUC}_1 - \text{AUC}_0}\right\}^2, \qquad (8.10)$$

where $\kappa = n_D/n_{\bar{D}}$. Approximations to $\text{var}(\hat{\text{AUC}}_e)$ have been reported previously. Hanley and McNeil (1982) assume exponential probability distributions for Y_D and $Y_{\bar{D}}$ to derive an expression. Obuchowski (1994) found that the Hanley and McNeil approximation performed poorly for binormal ROC curves and proposed an alternative expression suitable for the binormal setting. Our Result 8.2 is much more general than either of theirs.

Given an assumed ROC curve, one can calculate $\text{var}(\hat{\text{AUC}}_e)$ in at least two ways. One can use the expressions in Result 8.2 directly and numerically integrate the squared terms. Another tactic is to simulate large amounts of data from the ROC model, transform the raw data to placement values and calculate the variance terms $\text{var}(S_{\bar{D}}(Y_D))$ and $\text{var}(S_D(Y_{\bar{D}}))$ empirically. We take the latter approach in the next example.

Example 8.3

Suppose that the standard biomarker has a binormal ROC curve with $a = 0.545$ and $b = 1.0$. That is, its AUC is $\Phi\left(a/\sqrt{1 + b^2}\right) = 0.65$. A new biomarker will be considered for further development if its AUC is shown to be greater than this value. Thus, the minimally acceptable AUC is $\text{AUC}_0 = 0.65$. The new biomarker is anticipated to have a binormal ROC curve with $a = 1.19$ and $b = 1.0$. Thus, we identify AUC_1 as 0.80.

Let us calculate the variance components in Result 8.2, assuming that the ROC curve for the biomarker is what we anticipate it will be: $\text{ROC}(t) = \Phi(1.19 + \Phi^{-1}(t))$. We generated $10\,000$ disease and non-disease observations from the binormal ROC curve, with $Y_{\bar{D}} \sim N(0, 1)$ and $Y_D \sim N(1.19, 1)$. Recall again that, because the ROC curve is a function of only the ranks of the data, the actual distributional forms chosen are irrelevant. All that matters is that the ROC curve is of the stipulated form. The placement values calculated have variances

$$\text{var}(S_{\bar{D}}(Y_D)) = 0.048 \quad \text{and} \quad \text{var}(S_D(Y_{\bar{D}})) = 0.045 \, .$$

Therefore, if the biomarker is as good as we hope, we will have

$$\text{var}(\text{A}\hat{\text{U}}\text{C}_e) = \frac{0.048}{n_D} + \frac{0.046}{n_{\bar{D}}}.$$

Suppose that equal numbers of cases and controls will be enrolled to the study. Substituting into eqn (8.8), with $\alpha = 0.05$ and $\beta = 0.10$, yields

$$n_D = \frac{(1.64 + 1.28)^2}{(0.80 - 0.65)^2}(0.048 + 0.046) = 36.$$

Asymptotic theory therefore suggests that 36 cases and 36 controls be enrolled, in order to be 90% sure that the lower 95% confidence limit for the AUC based on the empirical estimator will exceed AUC_0.

The calculations are based on asymptotic theory that may not hold exactly in small samples. They provide starting points for simulation studies that fine tune the sample size calculations. Data are generated from the binormal model as before, but now using sample sizes $n_D = n_{\bar{D}} = 36$ and repeated 500 times. The lower 95% confidence limit for the AUC exceeds 0.65 with a rate of only 81%. This power is not as large as desired. We therefore increase the sample sizes to $n_D = n_{\bar{D}} = 50$, repeat the simulation study and find that the power is 90%. Thus sample sizes of $n_D = n_{\bar{D}} = 50$ are recommended. Finally, data are generated under the null hypothesis and confirm that the rejection rate is adequate for the study. It is 5.4%, a value that is close enough to the nominal level. ∎

Our development of sample size calculations is based on the nonparametric estimate of the AUC. If a parametric estimator of the AUC is to be used for inference, then sample size calculations could acknowledge the smaller variance that such an estimator is likely to have relative to that of $\text{A}\hat{\text{U}}\text{C}_e$. Obuchowski (1994) provides a variance formula for the fully parametric AUC estimator that assumes normal distributions for test results, namely $Y_D \sim \text{N}(\mu_D, \sigma_D^2)$ and $Y_{\bar{D}} \sim \text{N}(\mu_{\bar{D}}, \sigma_{\bar{D}}^2)$. As described in Example 5.3, this AUC estimator has the form

$$\text{A}\hat{\text{U}}\text{C}_N = \Phi\left(\frac{\hat{\mu}_D - \hat{\mu}_{\bar{D}}}{\sqrt{\hat{\sigma}_D^2 + \hat{\sigma}_{\bar{D}}^2}}\right),$$

where parameters are estimated with sample means and variances. Obuchowski's expression for $\text{var}(\text{A}\hat{\text{U}}\text{C}_N)$ relies on the asymptotic joint normal distribution for $\{\hat{\mu}_D, \hat{\sigma}_D^2, \hat{\mu}_{\bar{D}}, \hat{\sigma}_{\bar{D}}^2\}$ and the delta method. Variance formulae for parametric distribution-free estimates of the AUC (see Section 5.5) have not been derived and may be complicated. We suggest that $\text{A}\hat{\text{U}}\text{C}_e$ be used for sample size calculations, even if a fully parametric or a parametric distribution-free estimator will be used for analysis. The rationale is based on the observation that $\text{A}\hat{\text{U}}\text{C}_e$ is very efficient, at least under the normal theory model (Dodd, 2001). Therefore, calculated sample sizes will not be that much larger than required for those AUC estimators that make parametric assumptions.

Summary measures other than the AUC can be used to quantify the accuracy of a test and may also provide the basis for power calculations. The principles for power calculations are the same. However, since we often do not have explicit analytic expressions for variances, the calculations must be done entirely using simulation studies. For instance, when using nonparametric estimates of the partial AUC, a simulation-based sample size calculation seems to be the only currently available option. Obuchowski and McClish (1997) and Obuchowski (1998) present analytic expressions for variances of fully parametric estimates of the partial AUC from which sample sizes can then be calculated. These might provide useful starting points for simulation-based calculations of sample sizes needed for studies that will use semiparametric or nonparametric inference about the partial AUC.

Use of an ROC summary index such as the AUC or pAUC is likely to be more efficient than the use of a single ROC point for inference. Therefore the strategy of the previous section is likely to require larger sample sizes than the calculations in the current section. To illustrate, consider the assumed binormal curves of Example 8.3. The ROC point at $FPF_0 = 0.1$ corresponds to TPFs of $TPF_0 = 0.23$ under H_0 and $TPF_1 = 0.46$ under the alternative. The asymptotic theory-based calculations for testing $ROC(FPF_0) = TPF_0$ with 90% power at $\alpha = 0.05$ yield $n_D = n_{\bar{D}} = 115$. These are substantially larger than the AUC-based sample sizes calculated in Example 8.3.

The main disadvantage of basing inference on the AUC or pAUC is that these measures are less clinically relevant than the measure considered in the previous section, namely the TPF corresponding to the minimally acceptable FPF. In my opinion, specification of a practically meaningful improvement in the AUC (i.e. AUC_1) is likely to be more difficult than specification of an improvement in the TPF (i.e. TPF_1) corresponding to the minimally acceptable false positive fraction, $ROC(FPF_0)$. However, others may disagree with me on this point. Perhaps experience with the AUC index in a specific context may lead one to an intuition for the magnitudes of improvement that correspond to clinically meaningful improvements in test performance in that context.

8.2.4 *Ordinal tests*

Sample size calculations geared specifically towards ordinal tests have not received sufficient attention in the literature. Obuchowski has been the main contributor to this area. She employs ROC summary indices as the basis for inference. Her calculations, however, use variances that apply to continuous data and are based on the assumption that test results have normal distributions. She implicitly assumes that these apply to ROC summary indices estimated from ordinal data with the Dorfman and Alf (1968) binormal distribution-free method. Simulation studies (Obuchowski and McClish, 1997) suggest that these variances for continuous data underestimate the actual variances of summary indices calculated from ordinal study data. Nevertheless, the continuous data sample size formulae may provide reasonable starting points for simulation-based calculations of sample size for ordinal tests. Obuchowski and McClish refer to the simulation program ROCPWR, which is part of the ROC software developed primarily for ordinal data by Metz and colleagues at the University of Chicago.

Another approach is to dichotomize the ordinal test for the purposes of sample size calculations. The methods described in Section 8.2.1 can then be employed. This requires one to specify an appropriate category as the threshold for defining the binary test. Further work to allow some flexibility in this regard would be worthwhile.

8.3   Sample sizes for phase 3 studies

The types of objectives for a phase 3 study are more varied than they are for phase 2. We consider here sample size calculations for studies that address three different types of objectives. First, there are studies that seek to compare two different tests. We assume that a paired case-control study design is employed. The two different tests may actually be the same test, but done at different time points or under different circumstances on the same subject. The key is that within-subject comparisons are to be made. Next, case-control studies that seek to compare tests in different subpopulations will be considered in order to determine if subject characteristics affect test performance. The key statistical aspect here is that comparisons are made between subjects, not within subjects. The sample size calculations would also apply to the comparison of two tests in an unpaired design. Lastly, we consider estimation of the threshold value corresponding to a pre-specified false positive fraction, one important component of the effort in phase 3 to define a screen positive criterion that can be employed in phase 4.

8.3.1   *Comparing two binary tests—paired data*

In this book we have emphasized the multiplicative scale for quantifying the relative performance of two tests. Thus, for the two tests under consideration, test A and test B, we base inference on $\text{rTPF}(A, B) = \text{TPF}_A/\text{TPF}_B$ and $\text{rFPF}(A, B) = \text{FPF}_A/\text{FPF}_B$. Other scales can be used. In particular, absolute differences, $(\text{FPF}(A) - \text{FPF}(B), \text{TPF}(A) - \text{TPF}(B))$, have been used (Obuchowski, 1998; Obuchowski and Zhou, 2002). Their large sample theory calculations yield sample sizes that are similar to ours because the test procedures are asymptotically equivalent under the null hypothesis.

Some comparative studies seek to determine if one test is superior to the other. However, in some instances a test might be preferable to another even if its accuracy parameters are not superior. For example, if an existing test is costly or invasive, then a new inexpensive noninvasive test may be preferable to the existing test as long as its accuracy is not substantially less. In this case the scientific objective is to determine if the accuracy of the new test is substantially inferior to the standard or not.

Therapeutic clinical trials are often classified as superiority studies or as non-inferiority (equivalence) studies (ICH, 1999). The same idea is pertinent to comparative studies of diagnostic tests, as has been described by Obuchowski (1997b) and by Alonzo et $al.$ (2002b). If the null hypothesis relating to the TPFs is

$$H_0 : \mathrm{rTPF}(A, B) \leqslant 1 \,,$$

then the study is considered a superiority study on the TPF dimension, because rejecting H_0 allows one to conclude that TPF_A is larger than TPF_B. A non-inferiority study on the TPF dimension would use as the null hypothesis

$$H_0 : \mathrm{rTPF}(A, B) \leqslant \delta_0^T \,, \tag{8.11}$$

where δ_0^T is some value close to but less than one. The magnitude of δ_0^T is such that, if $\mathrm{rTPF}(A, B) = \delta_0^T$, then one can conclude that test A is, in a practical sense, no worse than test B. That is, investigators consider a true positive fraction of $\delta_0^T \mathrm{TPF}_B$ to be adequately close to TPF_B. If H_0 is rejected, one can conclude that $\mathrm{rTPF}(A, B) > \delta_0^T$ and hence that test A is not inferior to test B.

In general, we set up the null hypothesis comparing the TPFs of two tests to be of the form (8.11), where $\delta_0^T = 1$ indicates that a superiority study is under consideration, while $\delta_0^T < 1$ indicates a non-inferiority study. To keep the exposition simple we only consider one-sided hypotheses, and note that the extra steps for two-sided hypotheses are straightforward.

One must simultaneously compare tests with regards to their FPFs and TPFs. Because smaller FPFs are more desirable, the null hypotheses for superiority and non-inferiority of FPFs are

$$H_0 : \mathrm{rFPF}(A, B) \geqslant 1$$

and

$$H_0 : \mathrm{rFPF}(A, B) \geqslant \delta_0^F \,, \tag{8.12}$$

respectively, where δ_0^F is some value close to but greater than one.

A study may be designed as a superiority study in one dimension and as a non-inferiority study in the other. For instance, suppose it is hoped that a new test, test A, will decrease the false positive fraction relative to the standard test B. It must also be shown that its true positive fraction is not substantially less than that of the standard. In this case, the null hypotheses are

$$H_0^T : \mathrm{rTPF}(A, B) \leqslant \delta_0^T \quad \text{and} \quad H_0^F : \mathrm{rFPF}(A, B) \geqslant 1 \,,$$

where $\delta_0^T < 1$. By rejecting both H_0^T and H_0^F we can conclude that test A has a lower false positive fraction than test B and that its true positive fraction is at least δ_0^T times that of test B. On the other hand, if a new test is substantially cheaper or less invasive than the standard, then the study might seek to determine non-inferiority on both dimensions.

We define the general composite null hypothesis to be

$$H_0 : \left\{ \mathrm{rTPF}(A, B) \leqslant \delta_0^T \quad \text{or} \quad \mathrm{rFPF}(A, B) \geqslant \delta_0^F \right\} . \tag{8.13}$$

The hypothesis is tested using joint confidence limits for $\mathrm{rTPF}(A, B)$ and rFPF(A, B). In particular, if the $1 - \alpha^*$ lower limit for $\log \mathrm{rTPF}(A, B)$ is denoted by $(\log \mathrm{rTPF})_L^{\alpha^*}$, and the upper limit for $\log \mathrm{rFPF}(A, B)$ is denoted by $(\log \mathrm{rFPF})_U^{\alpha^*}$, then we reject H_0 if

$$(\log \mathrm{rTPF})_L^{\alpha^*} > \log \delta_0^T \quad \text{and} \quad (\log \mathrm{rFPF})_U^{\alpha^*} < \log \delta_0^F . \tag{8.14}$$

The study must be designed so that the probability is high, $1 - \beta$ say, that both the criteria of (8.14) will be satisfied for a test A with desirable operating characteristics.

Let $\delta_1^T = \mathrm{rTPF}(A, B)$ and $\delta_1^F = \mathrm{rFPF}(A, B)$ be the anticipated or desired relative performance parameters. We require that

$$\sqrt{1 - \beta} = \mathrm{P}\left[(\log \mathrm{rTPF})_L^{\alpha^*} > \log \delta_0^T | \mathrm{rTPF}(A, B) = \delta_1^T\right]$$

and

$$\sqrt{1 - \beta} = \mathrm{P}\left[(\log \mathrm{rFPF})_U^{\alpha^*} < \log \delta_0^F | \mathrm{rFPF}(A, B) = \delta_1^F\right],$$

so that $1 - \beta$ is the power of the study to yield an overall positive conclusion if test A meets the desired performance levels. Suppose that the confidence limits are based on asymptotic normality of the empirical estimates of $\log \mathrm{rTPF}(A, B)$ and $\log \mathrm{rFPF}(A, B)$ and their variance estimators, given in Chapter 3, as follows:

$$(\log \mathrm{rTPF})_L^{\alpha^*} = \log \mathrm{r\hat{T}PF}(A, B) - \Phi^{-1}(1 - \alpha^*)\sqrt{\mathrm{v\hat{a}r}(\log \mathrm{r\hat{T}PF}(A, B))},$$

$$(\log \mathrm{rFPF})_U^{\alpha^*} = \log \mathrm{r\hat{F}PF}(A, B) + \Phi^{-1}(1 - \alpha^*)\sqrt{\mathrm{v\hat{a}r}(\log \mathrm{r\hat{F}PF}(A, B))} .$$

Then sample size requirements are given in the next result.

Result 8.3

In a paired comparative study to test the null hypothesis (8.13), the numbers of diseased and non-diseased subjects required are

$$n_D = \left\{\frac{\Phi^{-1}(1 - \beta^*) + \Phi^{-1}(1 - \alpha^*)}{\log\left(\delta_1^T / \delta_0^T\right)}\right\}^2 \frac{\left(\delta_1^T + 1\right)\mathrm{TPF}_B - 2\mathrm{TPPF}}{\delta_1^T \mathrm{TPF}_B^2} , \tag{8.15}$$

where $\mathrm{TPPF} = \mathrm{P}[Y_A = 1, Y_B = 1 | D = 1]$, and

$$n_{\bar{D}} = \left\{\frac{\Phi^{-1}(1 - \beta^*) + \Phi^{-1}(1 - \alpha^*)}{\log\left(\delta_1^F / \delta_0^F\right)}\right\}^2 \frac{\left(\delta_1^F + 1\right)\mathrm{FPF}_B - 2\mathrm{FPPF}}{\delta_1^F \mathrm{FPF}_B^2} , \tag{8.16}$$

where $\mathrm{FPPF} = \mathrm{P}[Y_A = 1, Y_B = 1 | D = 0]$, respectively. Here $1 - \alpha^* = \sqrt{1 - \alpha}$ and $1 - \beta^* = \sqrt{1 - \beta}$. ∎

In practice, the correlation between test results within an individual is often unknown. Lower bounds for TPPF and FPPF can be used in practice. One lower bound for both TPPF and FPPF is, of course, 0. Another derives from the fact that $\text{TPPF} \geqslant \text{TPF}_A + \text{TPF}_B - 1 = (1 + \delta_1^T)\text{TPF}_B - 1$ and similarly $\text{FPPF} \geqslant (1 + \delta_1^F)\text{FPF}_B - 1$ (Alonzo *et al.*, 2002*b*). We use these in the next example. If it can be assumed that there is a positive dependence between tests conditional on disease status, with $\mathcal{A}_D(A, B) \geqslant 1$ and $\mathcal{A}_{\bar{D}}(A, B) \geqslant 1$ in the notation of Section 3.3.5, then lower bounds are given by $\text{TPPF} \geqslant \text{TPF}_A\text{TPF}_B = \delta_1^T(\text{TPF}_B)^2$ and $\text{FPPF} \geqslant \text{FPF}_A\text{FPF}_B = \delta_1^F(\text{FPF}_B)^2$. A positive association may be reasonable to assume if the two tests measure similar aspects or manifestations of disease. However, if they measure different aspects then a negative association conditional on disease status can occur.

Example 8.4

The standard test for vision impairment in children is 70% sensitive and 90% specific. We write $\text{TPF}_B = 0.70$ and $\text{FPF}_B = 0.10$. It is anticipated that a new, more sophisticated test will be more sensitive, $\text{TPF}_A = 0.90$, but that its false positive fraction will be similar, $\text{FPF}_A = 0.10$. In order to proceed with further development of the test, the study investigators have decided that they would need to draw the following conclusions from a study:

(i) the new test, test A, is more sensitive than test B; and

(ii) the FPF is not increased by more than 50%.

Translating these criteria into a formal null hypothesis, we have

$$H_0 : \{\text{rTPF}(A, B) \leqslant 1.0 \ \text{ or } \ \text{rFPF}(A, B) \geqslant 1.5\}.$$

That is, $\delta_0^F = 1.5$ and $\delta_0^T = 1.0$. Both components of H_0 must be rejected to draw a positive conclusion.

The study should have 90% power to draw a positive conclusion if the new test is as good as it is expected to be, namely $\text{TPF}_A = 0.90$ and $\text{FPF}_A = 0.10$. Thus $\delta_1^T = (0.90/0.70) = 1.30$ and $\delta_1^F = (0.10/0.10) = 1.00$.

All components of formulae (8.15) and (8.16) are now specified except for the components that relate to the correlation between the two tests. To be conservative we do not make assumptions about the association between the tests and use the lower limit $\text{TPPF} = (1 + \delta_1^T)\text{TPF}_B - 1 = 0.61$. For FPPF we use the value 0 because the lower limit $\text{FPPF} = (1 + \delta_1^F)\text{FPF}_B - 1$ is negative.

With significance level $\alpha = 0.05$ and power $1 - \beta = 0.90$, we calculate

$$n_D = \left(\frac{1.95 + 1.63}{\log 1.3}\right)^2 \frac{(1.3 + 1)(0.7) - 2(0.61)}{1.3(0.70)^2} = 114,$$

$$n_{\bar{D}} = \left(\frac{1.95 + 1.63}{-\log 1.5}\right)^2 \frac{(1.0 + 1)(0.10)}{1.0(0.10)^2} = 1565.$$
∎

8.3.2 *Comparing two binary tests—unpaired data*

The discussion in the previous section about setting up the null and alternative hypotheses pertains equally well to unpaired study designs as it does to paired study designs. The only difference is in the analytic expressions for the variances, $\mathrm{var}(\log r\hat{\mathrm{TPF}}(A, B))$ and $\mathrm{var}(\log r\hat{\mathrm{FPF}}(A, B))$. By substituting the expressions from Result 3.1 for unpaired data we arrive at the following sample size formulae (Alonzo *et al.*, 2002*b*).

Result 8.4

When comparing two binary tests using an unpaired study design, the sample sizes necessary for testing with each test are

$$n_D = \left\{ \frac{\Phi^{-1}(1 - \alpha^*) + \Phi^{-1}(1 - \beta^*)}{\log\left(\delta_1^T / \delta_0^T\right)} \right\}^2 \frac{1 + \delta_1^T - 2\delta_1^T \mathrm{TPF}_B}{\delta_1^T \mathrm{TPF}_B}, \qquad (8.17)$$

$$n_{\bar{D}} = \left\{ \frac{\Phi^{-1}(1 - \alpha^*) + \Phi^{-1}(1 - \beta^*)}{\log\left(\delta_1^F / \delta_0^F\right)} \right\}^2 \frac{1 + \delta_1^F - 2\delta_1^F \mathrm{FPF}_B}{\delta_1^F \mathrm{FPF}_B}, \qquad (8.18)$$

yielding a required total of $2n_D + 2n_{\bar{D}}$ subjects for the study. ∎

Example 8.4 (continued)

Suppose that the tests for the vision impairment study interfere with each other, in the sense that a subject's experience with one test influences his responses to the second. Then an unpaired study is required. The sample sizes for an unpaired study are

$$n_D = 99 \quad \text{and} \quad n_{\bar{D}} = 1409$$

subjects per test for a total of 198 cases and 2818 controls. These correspond to increases of 38% in the number of impaired subjects and 80% in the number of non-impaired control subjects relative to a paired study. However, note that the total numbers of tests required with the unpaired design are less, $198 + 2818 = 3016$ versus $2(114 + 1565) = 3358$ with the paired design.

In making the sample size calculations for the paired design, if we could assume that the tests are conditionally independent or positively associated then we could use larger lower bounds for TPPF and FPPF, namely $\mathrm{TPPF} \geqslant \delta_1^T (\mathrm{TPF}_B)^2$ and $\mathrm{FPPF} \geqslant \delta_1^F (\mathrm{FPF}_B)^2$. This strategy yields a paired design with the same number of tests as the unpaired design. See Section 3.3.5 for discussion of the efficiency of paired versus unpaired designs. ∎

8.3.3 *Evaluating population effects on test performance*

Suppose that we want to compare the operating characteristics of a test in two populations. For example, we want to determine if $\mathrm{TPF}_A = \mathrm{TPF}_B$ and $\mathrm{FPF}_A = \mathrm{FPF}_B$, where, in this subsection, the subscripts A and B denote the population.

More generally, we might want to quantify the relative performance of the test when performed in the two populations. That is, we wish to estimate $\text{rTPF}(A, B)$ and $\text{rFPF}(A, B)$.

From a statistical point of view, the problem is essentially the same as the comparison of two tests with an unpaired study design. Two independent groups of subjects are compared with regards to test TPFs and with regards to test FPFs. Thus the sample size formulae of Result 8.4 also apply to this setting. We illustrate with an example.

Example 8.5

A new simple serum test for type II diabetes has been developed in adults, and it is thought to be 80% sensitive and 95% specific. Type II diabetes has recently been recognized as a problem in adolescent children and it is hoped that the serum test will perform as well in this population as it does in adults. Even if sensitivity and specificity are reduced to 70% and 85%, respectively, the test would still be considered worthwhile relative to current standard tests in children. With subscripts A and B denoting children and adults, respectively, the null hypothesis which we hope to reject is

$$H_0 : \{\text{rTPF}(A, B) \leqslant 0.70/0.80 = 0.875 \quad \text{or} \quad \text{rFPF}(A, B) \geqslant 0.15/0.05 = 3.0\}.$$

The null hypothesis δ values are $\delta_0^T = 0.875$ and $\delta_0^F = 3.0$. The values for δ_1^T and δ_1^F are both 1.0 because it is anticipated that the new test will perform equally well in children as it does in adults. Thus the expressions of Result 8.4 yield

$$n_D = \left(\frac{1.95 + 1.63}{\log 0.875}\right)^2 \frac{1 + 1 - 2(0.80)}{0.80} = 360$$

and

$$n_{\bar{D}} = \left(\frac{1.95 + 1.63}{\log 3.0}\right)^2 \frac{1 + 1 - 2(0.05)}{3(0.05)} = 405.$$

In all, the study will require the enrolment of 720 diseased and 810 non-diseased subjects, with half of each group enrolled from the adolescent population. ∎

8.3.4 *Comparisons with continuous test results*

We now turn to phase 3 studies of tests with *continuous* outcomes. Sample size calculations for studies to compare two tests are a relatively straightforward extension of those developed for single test phase 2 studies. Rather than considering a single ROC index, as we considered in phase 2, we now consider two such estimated indices, one for each test. To keep the discussion general, we use $\hat{X}$ to denote the indices, so that $\hat{X}_A$ and $\hat{X}_B$ are used for tests A and B, respectively. We might take $\hat{X}$ to be $\hat{\text{ROC}}_e(\text{FPF}_0)$, $\hat{\text{AUC}}_e$ or $\hat{\text{pAUC}}_e$, for example.

Traditionally, simple differences between ROC indices for each test are taken as the basis for inference (Obuchowski, 1998). To allow for more generality we consider $g(X_A, X_B)$, where g denotes a specified function. For example, if $X = \text{ROC}(\text{FPF}_0)$ and $g(X_A, X_B) = \log X_A - \log X_B$, then the comparison between tests is based on the logarithm of $\text{rTPF}(A, B)$ when the thresholds for both tests are set to yield a common false positive fraction of FPF_0. On the other hand, if $X = \text{AUC}$ and $g(X_A, X_B) = X_A - X_B$, then the comparison is based on the more traditional difference in AUC indices.

Result 8.5

Suppose that

$$H_0 : g(X_A, X_B) = g_0$$

and that H_0 will be rejected if

$$g(\hat{X}_A, \hat{X}_B) - \Phi^{-1}(1 - \alpha)\sqrt{\hat{\text{var}}(g(\hat{X}_A, \hat{X}_B))} > g_0\,.$$

The numbers of diseased and non-diseased subjects required to reject H_0 with power $1 - \beta$ under assumptions denoted by H_1 are such that the following equation is satisfied:

$$\text{var}(g(\hat{X}_A, \hat{X}_B))\frac{\left(\Phi^{-1}(1 - \alpha) + \Phi^{-1}(1 - \beta)\right)^2}{(g_1 - g_0)^2} = 1\,. \qquad (8.19)$$

Here g_1 denotes the assumed value for $g(X_A, X_B)$ under H_1 and $\text{var}(g(\hat{X}_A, \hat{X}_B))$ is calculated under H_1 as follows:

$$\text{var}(g(\hat{X}_A, \hat{X}_B)) = (g_A^1)^2\,\text{var}(\hat{X}_A) + (g_B^1)^2\,\text{var}(\hat{X}_B) + 2(g_A^1)(g_B^1)\,\text{cov}(\hat{X}_A, \hat{X}_B)\,,$$

where g_A^1 and g_B^1 are the partial derivatives of $g(X_A, X_B)$ with respect to X_A and X_B, respectively. ∎

If an unpaired study design is employed, then $\hat{X}_A$ and $\hat{X}_B$ are statistically independent and the covariance term involving $\text{cov}(\hat{X}_A, \hat{X}_B)$ is zero. For paired designs the covariance term is typically very difficult to anticipate prior to performing the study. The amount of correlation between test results, Y_A and Y_B, is rarely known in advance, and analytic forms for the covariance of summary indices, $\text{cov}(\hat{X}_A, \hat{X}_B)$, are typically complicated. Pilot studies that can adequately quantify the covariance may need to be quite large. One strategy is to assume that $\text{cov}(\hat{X}_A, \hat{X}_B) = 0$ when calculating sample sizes. If it can be assumed that the actual correlation is positive and that the signs of g_A^1 and g_B^1 are opposite, as is typically the case when comparing tests, then this results in a conservative sample size calculation.

Example 8.6

A new screening test (A) for coronary artery disease is anticipated to have AUC = 0.90 for detecting disease in post-menopausal women. A standard test (B) is anticipated to have AUC = 0.80 and will be compared with the new test using an unpaired randomized trial. We will use the empirical AUCs for estimation (we drop the 'e' subscript in favor of that which now indexes the test) and compare them on the multiplicative scale using $\log(\hat{\text{AUC}}_A/\hat{\text{AUC}}_B)$. In the notation of Result 8.5, $\hat{X} = \hat{\text{AUC}}$ and $g(X_A, X_B) = \log X_A - \log X_B$. Also $g_0 = 0$, while $g_1 = \log 0.9 - \log 0.8 = 0.118$.

Assume that the ROC curves are binormal, $\text{ROC}(t) = \Phi(a + b\Phi^{-1}(t))$, with slope parameter $b = 1$. Writing $\text{AUC} = \Phi(a/\sqrt{1+b^2})$, which is assumed to be equal to 0.8 for test B, we can solve the resulting equation $0.8 = \Phi(a/\sqrt{2})$ to yield $a = 1.188$. Thus, under the null hypothesis, the ROC curve for both tests is $\text{ROC}(t) = \Phi(1.188 + \Phi^{-1}(t))$. Under the alternative, the standard test, B, has the same ROC curve and the new test, A, has $\text{ROC}(t) = \Phi(1.810 + \Phi^{-1}(t))$, since AUC = 0.9 yields $a = 1.810$. Equal numbers of cases and controls will be enrolled and they will be equally distributed to the two testing modalities. Write the number of cases per study arm as m. Under the alternative hypothesis and using Result 8.2, we calculate

$$\text{var}(\hat{\text{AUC}}_A) = \frac{0.04}{m} \quad \text{and} \quad \text{var}(\hat{\text{AUC}}_B) = \frac{0.10}{m}.$$

Observe that, since $g(\text{AUC}_A, \text{AUC}_B) = \log(\text{AUC}_A/\text{AUC}_B)$, we have $g_A^1 = 1/\text{AUC}_A$ and $g_B^1 = -1/\text{AUC}_B$. Thus $g_A^1 = 1/0.9 = 1.11$ and $g_B^1 = -1/0.8 = -1.25$. Hence

$$\text{var}(g(\hat{X}_A, \hat{X}_B)) = \frac{(1.11)^2(0.04)}{m} + \frac{(1.25)^2(0.10)}{m},$$

where the covariance term is zero because of the unpaired design employed.

Substituting into eqn (8.19) we find that the required number of cases per arm is

$$m = \frac{\left\{\Phi^{-1}(1-\alpha) + \Phi^{-1}(1-\beta)\right\}^2 (0.21)}{(\log(0.9/0.8))^2}.$$

Asymptotic theory therefore indicates that, for a power of 90% with a one-sided 0.05 level test, the study requires the enrolment of $m = 123$ cases and controls to each study arm for a total of 492 study subjects. If a paired study can be performed, then half of this number of subjects would be needed.

We ran a small simulation study to verify the adequacy of these calculations. When unpaired data were simulated under the null configurations and the lower 5th percentile of the bootstrap distribution of the relative area $\hat{\text{AUC}}_A/\hat{\text{AUC}}_B$ was used for testing the null hypothesis (rejecting if it exceeds 1), the observed significance level was 0.05. The power calculated using a similar simulation study was 0.92. The large sample theory approximations provided reasonable values for sample sizes in this case.   ∎

For further discussion of comparative studies with continuous tests we refer the reader to a series of papers by Obuchowski and colleagues (Obuchowski and McClish, 1997; Obuchowski, 1998). As noted earlier, Obuchowski only gives formulae for comparisons based on fully parametric estimates of summary indices. Methods for ordinal test results are not well developed at this time, and we refer back to the discussion in Section 8.2.4 because the same points apply to phase 3 studies as to phase 2 studies.

8.3.5 *Estimating the threshold for screen positivity*

One frequent important goal of phase 3 is to determine the criterion that will be used in phase 4 for classifying subjects as positive or negative for disease on the basis of the new test. A reasonable strategy in some settings (particularly in disease screening) is to set the false positive fraction at some tolerable value, FPF_0 say, and to choose the criterion accordingly. In particular, the screen positivity rule

$$\text{screen positive if } \quad Y > S_{\bar{D}}^{-1}(FPF_0)$$

may be a reasonable criterion. An objective of a phase 3 study might therefore be to estimate $q = S_{\bar{D}}^{-1}(FPF_0)$.

Suppose that the following empirical quantile estimator will be used, where $\hat{S}_{\bar{D}}$ is the empirical survivor function for Y in the non-disease sample:

$$\hat{q} = \hat{S}_{\bar{D}}^{-1}(FPF_0).$$

The study must be designed so that q is estimated with adequate precision. The desired precision is more naturally expressed in terms of the actual false positive fraction of the recommended rule $Y > \hat{q}$, rather than in terms of the variability of the estimate $\hat{q}$. This latter quantity is measured on the scale for the test result itself, whereas the former is the practically relevant quantity. We choose $n_{\bar{D}}$ large enough so that

$$P[Y_{\bar{D}} > \hat{q}] \leqslant FPF_0 + \varepsilon,$$

where ε is some specified allowable error in the false positive fraction for the binary test recommended for phase 4.

Observe that we can write $P[Y_{\bar{D}} > \hat{q}] = S_{\bar{D}}(\hat{S}_{\bar{D}}^{-1}(FPF_0))$. Asymptotic distribution theory for empirical quantiles indicates that

$$\sqrt{n_{\bar{D}}}(\hat{S}_{\bar{D}}^{-1}(FPF_0) - q) \sim N\left(0, FPF_0 \frac{1 - FPF_0}{\{f_{\bar{D}}(q)\}^2}\right),$$

where $f_{\bar{D}}$ is the probability density for $Y_{\bar{D}}$. Hence

$$\sqrt{n_{\bar{D}}}\left[S_{\bar{D}}(\hat{S}_{\bar{D}}^{-1}(FPF_0)) - FPF_0\right] \sim N(0, FPF_0(1 - FPF_0)).$$

The sample size formula in the following result can then be derived.

Result 8.6

In order to guarantee with probability $1 - \beta$ that the false positive fraction associated with the threshold $\hat{q} = \hat{S}_{\bar{D}}^{-1}(\text{FPF}_0)$ is no more than $\text{FPF}_0 + \varepsilon$, the study should enrol

$$n_{\bar{D}} = \left(\frac{\Phi^{-1}(1 - \beta)}{\varepsilon} \right)^2 \text{FPF}_0 (1 - \text{FPF}_0) \qquad (8.20)$$

subjects.   ∎

Example 8.7

Suppose that a false positive fraction of no more than 5% can be tolerated in a phase 4 study, but that a rate of 3% is thought to be necessary in order for the sensitivity of the test to be adequate. Then the target false positive fraction is $\text{FPF}_0 = 3\%$ and the maximum error in the false positive fraction is $\varepsilon = 2\%$. For an assurance level of $1 - \beta = 95\%$, Result 8.6 yields

$$n_{\bar{D}} = \left(\frac{1.64}{0.02} \right)^2 (0.03)(0.97) = 196 \,.$$ ∎

8.3.6   *Remarks on phase 3 analyses*

The purpose of phase 3 is to make preparations for phase 4. Since phase 3 studies have case-control designs, they tend to be smaller and less expensive than phase 4 studies. Moreover, they usually do not interfere with the medical care of the patient. In contrast, phase 4 cohort studies are often massive undertakings. The importance of having prepared adequately before undertaking a phase 4 study cannot be emphasized enough. The implication is that one should learn as much as possible from phase 3 retrospective studies before proceeding further.

In this section we have discussed case-control study designs that allow paired or unpaired comparisons. Such designs can be used to compare different tests, to compare the same test operating under different conditions, and to assess if patient or other characteristics affect the operating characteristics. This knowledge can be used to pick optimal conditions for phase 4. Although we emphasize simple comparative inference for the purposes of sample size calculations, more generally, the regression analytic methods described in Chapters 3 and 6 will be employed for the analysis of data from phase 3 studies. We also discuss the identification of a criterion for defining screen positivity in phase 4. Our focus on the false positive fraction, for this purpose, is probably over-simplified because the trade-off with the true positive fraction will also be a factor in choosing the threshold. Nevertheless, it provides an approach for calculating sample sizes which is adequate to address one aspect, i.e. the FPF aspect, of the screen positivity criterion. Again, in practice, regression methods may be used for data analysis in order to evaluate factors affecting the false positive fractions and/or for defining covariate-specific screen positive criteria (Chapter 6).

8.4 Sample sizes for phase 4 studies

In phase 4, subjects are enrolled into a cohort study and evaluated for disease with both the gold standard procedures and with the investigational diagnostic test or tests. Since we assume that the test positivity criterion has been defined in phase 3, only binary tests are considered here. Recall that the key objectives in this phase are to determine test operating characteristics when the test is applied prospectively in a defined population. Since cohort studies allow the flexibility to estimate predictive values, in this section we consider designs based on these parameters. First, however, we consider studies that seek to make inferences about the test classification probabilities.

8.4.1 *Designs for inference about* (FPF, TPF)

The diseased subjects, identified from the study cohort, serve to estimate and compare TPFs, while the remaining subjects provide data for estimation and comparison of FPFs. Sample size formulae for n_D and $n_{\bar{D}}$ from Section 8.2.1 can be used when estimation of classification probabilities is of primary interest, while those in Sections 8.3.1 to 8.3.3 can be used when comparisons between tests or between populations are to be made. Note that these entities are non-random and under the control of investigators in the case-control studies of phases 2 and 3. In contrast, n_D and $n_{\bar{D}}$ are random variables in a cohort study.

In a phase 4 cohort study, only the total sample size, $N = n_D + n_{\bar{D}}$, can be specified as part of the design. Let n_D^* and $n_{\bar{D}}^*$ denote, respectively, the calculated case and control sample sizes required for adequate power to make inferences about (FPF, TPF). Assuming that disease prevalence, ρ, is known, one could choose N so that the random variables n_D and $n_{\bar{D}}$ will have appropriate expectations. That is, if we choose

$$N = \max\left(n_D^*/\rho,\; n_{\bar{D}}^*/(1-\rho)\right), \tag{8.21}$$

then

$$\mathrm{E}(n_D) = N\rho \geqslant n_D^* \quad \text{and} \quad \mathrm{E}(n_{\bar{D}}) = N(1-\rho) \geqslant n_{\bar{D}}^*,$$

with equality holding for at least one.

Schatzkin *et al.* (1987) note, however, that sampling variability can lead to observed values of n_D or $n_{\bar{D}}$ that are less than those required. If $n_D < n_D^*$ or $n_{\bar{D}} < n_{\bar{D}}^*$, then the study is underpowered. They suggest choosing a value for N which is slightly larger than (8.21) in order to guarantee, with some probability $1 - \gamma$, that the realized values of n_D and $n_{\bar{D}}$ are *at least* as large as required. We state the adjustment formally in the next result.

Result 8.7

If N is chosen to satisfy the inequalities

$$N \geqslant \frac{n_D^*}{\rho} + \Phi^{-1}(1-\gamma)\sqrt{\frac{1-\rho}{\rho}N}, \qquad (8.22)$$

$$N \geqslant \frac{n_{\bar{D}}^*}{1-\rho} + \Phi^{-1}(1-\gamma)\sqrt{\frac{\rho}{1-\rho}N}, \qquad (8.23)$$

then

$$P\left[n_D > n_D^*\right] \geqslant 1 - \gamma \quad \text{and} \quad P\left[n_{\bar{D}} > n_{\bar{D}}^*\right] \geqslant 1 - \gamma.$$

Proof Consider the first inequality relating to n_D. The normal approximation to the binomial distribution of n_D implies that

$$\frac{n_D - N\rho}{\sqrt{N\rho(1-\rho)}} \sim N(0,1).$$

Thus, if N is chosen to satisfy (8.22), then

$$\frac{n_D^* - N\rho}{\sqrt{N\rho(1-\rho)}} \leqslant \Phi^{-1}(\gamma) = -\Phi^{-1}(1-\gamma)$$

and $P[n_D > n_D^*] \geqslant 1 - \gamma$. A similar argument proves the result for $n_{\bar{D}}$. ∎

Example 8.8

Consider the standard Pap screening test for cervical cancer, which is thought to have sensitivity of about 60% and a false positive fraction of 5%. From phase 3 studies, a new test appears to have sensitivity of 85% and a false positive fraction of 2%. Setting up the null hypothesis as

$$H_0 : \{\mathrm{rTPF} < \delta_0^T = 1 \quad \text{or} \quad \mathrm{rFPF} > \delta_0^F = 1\}$$

and specifying the δ values as

$$\delta_1^T = \frac{0.85}{0.60} = 1.42, \qquad \delta_1^F = \frac{0.02}{0.05} = 0.4,$$

with $\alpha = 0.05$ and $1 - \beta = 0.90$, we calculate

$$n_D^* = 115 \quad \text{and} \quad n_{\bar{D}}^* = 1080$$

on the basis of Result 8.3 and assuming minimum values for TPPF and FPPF. Thus, 115 cases and 1080 controls are required.

Suppose that the study is to be conducted in a cohort where the prevalence of cervical cancer is 2%. Then, the required number of cases will drive the size of the cohort study. A cohort of size $n_D^*/\rho = 5750$ will yield an expected number of cases equal to 115, but the numbers that arise in the actual cohort may be less. Solving eqn (8.22) for N with $\gamma = 0.10$, we find that a cohort of size $N = 6471$ will be required so that at least 115 cases will be enrolled with probability $1 - \gamma = 90\%$. Substituting this value of N into (8.23), we see that, even for very small γ, the inequality is satisfied and therefore the required number of non-disease subjects

will also almost certainly be enrolled with the proposed cohort of 6471 subjects.
∎

In the proposed study of the above example, note that it is not necessary to ascertain disease status for subjects that screen negative on both tests. As discussed earlier in Section 7.2, those data do not enter into inference about $\mathrm{rFPF}(A, B)$ and $\mathrm{rTPF}(A, B)$. They are ignored even if they are ascertained. This is the case not just when inference is based on the relative classification probabilities. If the comparison between tests is based on absolute differences, $\mathrm{FPF}_A - \mathrm{FPF}_B$ and $\mathrm{TPF}_A - \mathrm{TPF}_B$, then subjects testing negative on both tests are also ignored. If the primary purpose of a cohort study is to *compare* tests, a valid comparison can be made and huge cost savings are to be gained by selecting only those that screen positive for ascertainment of the gold standard, D. However, if an objective of the study is the *estimation* of the classification probabilities, then ascertainment of D for subjects that test negative is required. Identifiability of $(\mathrm{FPF}, \mathrm{TPF})$ depends on the availability of such data.

8.4.2 *Designs for predictive values*

Methods for making inferences about predictive values are, for the most part, analogous to those for classification probabilities, with the roles of Y and D interchanged. Consider, for instance, a cohort study that seeks to determine if the positive and negative predictive values, PPV and NPV, are above some minimally acceptable values, PPV_0 and NPV_0, respectively. By analogy with Section 8.2.1, we set up the null hypothesis as

$$H_0 : \{\mathrm{PPV} \leqslant \mathrm{PPV}_0 \ \ \mathrm{or} \ \ \mathrm{NPV} \leqslant \mathrm{NPV}_0\}$$

and reject it on the basis of a joint $1 - \alpha$ rectangular confidence region for $(\mathrm{PPV}, \mathrm{NPV})$, with $1 - \alpha^*$ confidence limits for each component. Suppose that we wish to have power $1 - \beta$ when the predictive values are at some desirable levels $(\mathrm{PPV}_1, \mathrm{NPV}_1)$. With n^+ and n^- denoting the numbers of positive and negative test results, respectively, this power is guaranteed if

$$n^+ = \frac{\left(Z^{1-\alpha^*}\sqrt{\mathrm{PPV}_0(1 - \mathrm{PPV}_0)} + Z^{1-\beta^*}\sqrt{\mathrm{PPV}_1(1 - \mathrm{PPV}_1)}\right)^2}{(\mathrm{PPV}_1 - \mathrm{PPV}_0)^2}, \qquad (8.24)$$

$$n^- = \frac{\left(Z^{1-\alpha^*}\sqrt{\mathrm{NPV}_0(1 - \mathrm{NPV}_0)} + Z^{1-\beta^*}\sqrt{\mathrm{NPV}_1(1 - \mathrm{NPV}_1)}\right)^2}{(\mathrm{NPV}_1 - \mathrm{NPV}_0)^2}, \qquad (8.25)$$

where $1 - \alpha^* = \sqrt{1 - \alpha}$ and $1 - \beta^* = \sqrt{1 - \beta}$.

These formulae are the predictive value analogues of (8.2) and (8.3). The discussion in Section 8.4.1, about choosing a big enough cohort sample size N to guarantee that n_D and $n_{\bar{D}}$ are sufficiently large, also applies here to n^+ and n^-. That is, n^+ and n^- are random in a cohort study. If $\tau = \mathrm{P}[Y = 1]$ is known, then, rather than choosing $N = n^+/\tau$ or $N = n^-/(1 - \tau)$, an adjustment analogous to that of Result 8.7 is made to ensure that observed (n^+, n^-) will reach, or exceed, their required values. We illustrate this with an example.

Example 8.9

Suppose that a new clinical criterion is proposed for triaging injury patients for bone X-ray in a critical care clinic unit. The outcome variable, D, indicates whether or not a bone fracture is observed on the X-ray. The diagnostic test being evaluated is the clinical criterion, with the result $Y = 1$ if the criterion is met for going forward with the X-ray procedure. A review of patient charts in the clinic indicates that 20% of patients meet the criterion. That is $\tau = 20\%$. This criterion will be employed if its PPV is shown to be at least 60%, while its NPV must be shown to be at least 80%. Therefore $PPV_0 = 0.60$ and $NPV_0 = 0.80$. It is anticipated that the criterion has much higher predictive values, namely $PPV_1 = 0.80$ and $NPV_1 = 0.90$. For a study with statistical power of 90% and $\alpha = 5\%$ we calculate

$$n^+ = 66 \quad \text{and} \quad n^- = 164 \,.$$

In a study of $N = n^+/\tau = 330$ we therefore expect to see $n^+ = 66$ patients that meet the criterion and $N(1 - \tau) = 264$ that do not. The Schatzkin adjustment with $\gamma = 0.10$ yields that N satisfies the predictive value analogue of (8.22):

$$\frac{n^+}{\tau} \leqslant N - \Phi^{-1}(1 - \gamma)\sqrt{\frac{1 - \tau}{\tau}N} \,. \tag{8.26}$$

The smallest value of N that satisfies this is $N = 380$. A study with this sample size is 90% sure to yield $n^+ \geqslant 66$, the required number of patients meeting the clinical criterion. Such a cohort will also yield the required number of criterion-negative patients for inference about NPV, since it satisfies the second Schatzkin inequality

$$\frac{n^-}{1 - \tau} \leqslant N - \Phi^{-1}(1 - \gamma)\sqrt{\frac{\tau}{1 - \tau}N} \,. \tag{8.27}$$

∎

Sample size calculations for studies that seek to compare predictive values can proceed by analogy with those described in Section 8.3.2 for classification probabilities, when *unpaired* study designs are employed. The predictive value analogues of Result 8.4 yield the number of subjects to be tested in each arm with positive and negative test results. The Schatzkin-adjusted values for the total numbers of subjects to be tested in each arm, N_A and N_B, are then calculated.

The analogy between classification probability calculations and predictive value calculations breaks down for *paired* comparative study designs. Analytic expressions for the variance of estimated relative predictive values are not available (see Section 3.6.2). Consequently, we cannot provide simple formulae for sample sizes. One strategy would be to use the formulae for an unpaired study design and to refine the sample size calculations with simulation studies.

A cohort study that does not measure D on subjects testing negative with Y cannot be used for inference about NPV. We noted this in Chapter 7. Inference about PPV is, however, still possible. In addition, inference about τ would be of interest. One might consider a study design to estimate τ and to determine if PPV exceeds a minimally acceptable value. The principles used for cohort studies of (FPF, TPF) and (PPV, NPV) would also apply to the sample size calculation for such a study. We leave this as an exercise.

8.4.3   Designs for (FP, DP)

The detection and false referral probabilities can also be estimated from a cohort study when D is not ascertained for those with negative test results, $Y = 0$. We discussed this previously in Chapter 7 and noted that these are key parameters which can be estimated in such studies. Even when ascertainment of D is feasible for all study subjects, DP and FP may be regarded as primary parameters of interest. We now consider sample size calculations for making inferences about (FP, DP).

The (FP, DP) parameters are multinomial probabilities. Joint inference for them is therefore complicated by the correlation between their estimators, $(\hat{\text{FP}}, \hat{\text{DP}})$. This contrasts with the (FPF, TPF) parameters, whose estimators are independent given n_D and $n_{\bar{D}}$. Therefore, testing of a joint null hypothesis and the associated sample size calculations are not as straightforward for (FP, DP) as they are for the classification probabilities.

If one considers only a single parameter, then sample size calculations are simple. Standard methods for a binomial probability apply. For example, suppose that $H_0^D : \text{DP} \leqslant \text{DP}_0$, where DP_0 is a minimally acceptable value, and DP_1 is the anticipated desired value. With inference based on the $1 - \alpha$ lower confidence limit for DP, a cohort study requires

$$N = \frac{\left(\Phi^{-1}(1-\alpha)\sqrt{\text{DP}_0(1 - \text{DP}_0)} + \Phi^{-1}(1-\beta)\sqrt{\text{DP}_1(1 - \text{DP}_1)}\right)^2}{(\text{DP}_1 - \text{DP}_0)^2} \qquad (8.28)$$

for $1 - \beta$ statistical power. Similarly,

$$N = \frac{\left(\Phi^{-1}(1-\alpha)\sqrt{\text{FP}_0(1 - \text{FP}_0)} + \Phi^{-1}(1-\beta)\sqrt{\text{FP}_1(1 - \text{FP}_1)}\right)^2}{(\text{FP}_1 - \text{FP}_0)^2} \qquad (8.29)$$

yields power $1 - \beta$ for the null hypothesis $H_0^F : \text{FP} > \text{FP}_0$ when in fact $\text{FP} = \text{FP}_1$, where FP_1 is some acceptably low rate of false referrals. These formulae do not acknowledge the joint inference that will be made in practice. One could, nevertheless, use the formulae as starting points for a series of simulation studies to calculate sample sizes. That is, one can use the larger value of N and modify it until it yields appropriate power for a test of the joint null hypothesis

$$H_0 : \{\text{DP} < \text{DP}_0 \ \text{ or } \ \text{FP} > \text{FP}_0\},$$

based on a joint $1 - \alpha$ elliptical confidence region for (DP, FP), say.

Studies can also be designed to compare detection or false referral probabilities. Assuming the relative performance parameters will be the basis for inference, recall that $rDP = rTPF$ and $rFP = rFPF$. One can therefore use the strategy described in Section 8.4.1 for sample size calculations. We also refer the reader to Alonzo *et al.* (2002*b*), who provide sample size formulae directly in terms of the (FP, DP) parameters.

8.4.4 *Selected verification of screen negatives*

We now return to cohort studies where inference about (FPF, TPF) is of interest and ascertainment of D is feasible for study subjects that screen negative. Studies that purposefully select a subset of screen negatives for disease verification have been proposed as possibly yielding a more ethical or cost efficient strategy than studies that require ascertainment of D on all subjects (Obuchowski and Zhou, 2002). As mentioned earlier, for the purposes of comparing the classification probabilities of two tests, there is no statistical value in ascertaining D for any subject who screens negative on both tests. Therefore, we limit our discussion here to studies that seek to estimate classification probabilities.

Obuchowski and Zhou (2002) present analytic sample size formulae for prospective screening studies. Assuming that all subjects who screen positive, as well as a fraction f of screen negatives, have disease ascertained, they apply the variance formula for the adjusted estimators $\widehat{TPF}_{BG}$ and $\widehat{FPF}_{BG}$ (Result 7.4) to calculate the required cohort sample size. They investigate the cost savings for studies that employ a selected verification design compared with those that simply ascertain D for all study subjects. They conclude that the savings are usually small because the reductions in the numbers of subjects that require ascertainment of D is usually offset by the increased size of the total cohort that is required to maintain the variances of the estimates at required levels. Their results indicate that the following conditions are needed in order for nonnegligible benefits to result from selected verification:

  (i) TPF < 70%;

 (ii) FPF > 20%; and

(iii) the cost of verification relative to the cost of screening should exceed 5.

Even then, the savings are modest, rarely exceeding 15%. Irwig *et al.* (1994*a*) arrive at similar conclusions. They find that negligible savings occurred in the total number of subjects verified for disease status when TPF > 80%. Indeed, savings of 20% or more occur for TPF > 50% only if the specificity is very high, FPF < 0.01, or the prevalence of disease is very low, namely less than 0.1%.

The recommendation then seems to be that there is little benefit to be gained from deliberately incorporating a selected verification scheme into the design of a cohort study. For studies that seek to characterize classification probabilities with a certain degree of precision, there is no reduction in cost relative to a study that requires verification of all subjects. Such studies should simply verify all subjects. For studies that seek to compare tests, only those subjects that screen positive need to be verified, because only they contribute useful data for evaluating the relative performance parameters of tests.

8.5   Phase 5

The objective in phase 5 is to evaluate the overall impact of using the new test on the health of a population. Ideally, a randomized trial is performed, with one study arm receiving the diagnostic test and consequent health procedures, while the other study arm receives standard health care in the absence of the test. Clinically important outcomes are the basis for comparing the study arms.

As an example, consider the use of a chest X-ray to detect pneumonia in patients that go to an urgent care clinic because of a cough. Standard care is that patients without the additional symptoms of fever and lethargy are not referred for X-ray, but may be referred later if symptoms develop. To determine if the use of X-rays early in patients with a cough is beneficial, such patients could be randomized to immediate diagnostic work-up with X-ray or not. Clinically meaningful outcomes such as IV-antibiotic treatment for chest infection and/or hospitalization could be used as primary endpoints. If the chest X-ray identifies subjects that are cured with less intense treatment (e.g. oral antibiotics) but who would otherwise progress to infection and require IV antibiotics, then its impact relative to standard care would be positive.

Screening healthy populations for disease is controversial, particularly in light of the enormous costs involved. Randomized trials to determine the value of mammography as a breast cancer screening test have been undertaken (Fletcher et al., 1993). Breast cancer mortality is the outcome measure of choice for evaluating such screening programs. In addition to clinical outcomes, cost and compliance outcomes are often measures of extreme public health importance that must be evaluated in phase 5.

The design of a randomized phase 5 trial of a diagnostic test is essentially no different from any other randomized trial. We refer to Pocock (1982) and Friedman et al. (1996) for in-depth coverage of the design of clinical trials. Sample size calculations depend on the primary clinical outcomes of interest (not test accuracy), and proceed in the standard fashion.

Although ideal in a scientific sense, randomized trials of diagnostic tests are not always deemed to be necessary or ethical. If diagnosis is accurate, treatment is convenient and successful, and consequences of disease in the absence of treatment are severe, then it is probably appropriate to adopt the diagnostic test without a randomized experiment. Recall from Chapter 1 that the PKU test satisfies these criteria and was never subjected to a randomized trial. Tests and treatments for many other diseases are not quite so clear-cut and the decision as to whether or not a randomized trial should be performed can be extremely difficult.

A few other strategies for evaluating the impact of adopting a diagnostic test in medical practice are used. If the test is made available to the medical care community, observational studies can compare clinical outcomes in subjects offered the test to those not offered the test. Such comparisons can be made between concurrent groups, or by comparing with historical data accumulated when the test was not available. The potential biases in these observational studies do, however, limit their usefulness. Nevertheless, careful designs can provide convincing evidence. We refer to Weiss (1997), who points to a clever case-control design by Selby *et al.* (1992) for evaluating colon cancer screening sigmoidoscopy.

The decision to proceed with approval of the test for use in medical practice versus subjecting the test to a randomized trial can be very difficult. An informative exercise, undertaken in such circumstances, is to synthesize what is known about the test, the disease, the treatment, compliance and the clinical outcome in order to estimate the overall impact of the test on the outcome. Effects on costs, both monetary and utilitarian, can be evaluated similarly. Such a synthesis involves making certain assumptions, but, if done carefully and with up-to-date information, the process can lead to rational decision making. Calculations can be undertaken via simulation studies if they seem to be complex. See Etzioni *et al.* (1999*a*) and Ross *et al.* (2000) for some examples in the context of prostate cancer.

8.6   Matching and stratification

We now discuss two additional strategies that can be employed in study design: matching and stratification. These strategies are commonly employed in therapeutic and epidemiologic research and have similar roles to play in the context of diagnostic test evaluation. Matching and stratification are relevant when factors other than disease can affect test results and/or when factors other than test results are associated with disease. Moreover, they can be applied in data analysis as well as in study design.

8.6.1   *Stratification*

Suppose that we are interested in quantifying some measure of test performance, such as the TPF, or a measure of comparative performance, such as rTPF. A *stratified analysis* seeks to determine this measure at fixed covariate-specific levels, i.e. within strata. Moreover, if there is some commonality among the strata in the performance measure, then data can be accumulated across strata to estimate the common measure.

As an example, consider a multi-center paired data cohort study to compare the TPFs of two tests. Such a study was considered in Example 7.5. Study site is a covariate that can affect the test result and/or disease prevalence. We wish to estimate rTPF(A, B) within study sites. Study site is therefore a stratification factor. If the rTPF(A, B) is assumed to be constant across study sites, it can be estimated within each center and averaged across strata to yield an estimate of the common rTPF(A, B). Analysis that ignores the stratification is inappropriate.

As another example, suppose that two study radiologists read images but interpret the rating scales differently. Then a stratified analysis is appropriate, an ROC curve being estimated for each separately. If their ROC curves can be assumed to be equal, then an average of their individual curves yields an estimate of the common curve.

We define a *stratified study design* to be one in which pre-specified numbers of subjects satisfying criteria for each stratum are deliberately enrolled. Because the proportions of study subjects in the different strata may not equal the corresponding population proportions, the study group as a whole will not be representative of the population. Consider a case-control study of mammography with equal numbers of women with cancer enrolled from two age strata, under fifty years and fifty years or above. Since breast cancer is much more prevalent in older women, the study case group will have an age distribution that is different from the population age distribution. Analyses stratified on design factors will be valid, while analyses of pooled data may not (see Fig. 6.2).

What are some reasons for using a stratified study design?

(i) If there is interest in test performance within particular strata and these strata occur with low frequency in the population, one might stratify to oversample these strata for the study. This could allow one to examine test performance in particular strata, which would not be possible if an unstratified design is used.

(ii) Study power can be enhanced by stratification. For example, if disease prevalence varies across strata, a cohort study might oversample the higher-prevalence strata in order to enrol more subjects with disease. Obuchowski and Zhou (2002) showed that this strategy can be beneficial for increasing study power and hence for substantially decreasing sample sizes.

Sample size calculations need to account for the stratification strategies used in both the design and the analysis. Asymptotic formulae can be derived by extending those derived for unstratified settings. The notation becomes cumbersome, however, and we do not pursue this further here. The paper by Obuchowski and Zhou (2002) provides some formulae.

8.6.2 *Matching*

Although stratification may be feasible in phases 3 and beyond, it is usually not feasible in earlier phases because sample sizes are too small. Moreover, quantification of covariate-specific performance measures is not addressed in phases 1 and 2. Nevertheless, one needs to ensure that confounding factors are controlled for adequately in these studies. This is accomplished by matched designs.

In particular, consider a phase 1 or 2 case-control study. Suppose that a covariate, Z, is statistically correlated with both disease status, D, and with the test result, Y. This can lead to an association between Y and D that is due in part to the confounding effect of Z. As an example, suppose that a new potential biomarker for lung cancer is over-expressed in smokers, and subjects with lung cancer are more likely to have smoked than the controls. Smoking can therefore cause a spurious statistical association between the biomarker and lung cancer.

A *matched case-control design* ensures that there is no association between D and Z in the study sample. This is done by selecting a set of controls so that they have the same distribution of Z as the cases. Frequency matching of cases and controls with regards to Z accomplishes this. In the previous example, if half of the cases were smokers, then one would select a set of controls of whom 50% smoked for a frequency matched study design. Any associations between Y and D in a matched study cannot then be caused by statistical associations between Z and D.

The analysis of matched data is well developed in the context of epidemiologic case-control studies of risk factors for disease (Breslow and Day, 1980). In the context of diagnostic test studies, however, there has been little discussion to date. The topic certainly deserves further consideration. One approach is to ignore the matching and to proceed with the analysis of $\{Y_{Di}, i = 1, \ldots, n_D\}$ and $\{Y_{\bar{D}j}, j = 1, \ldots, n_{\bar{D}}\}$ in the usual fashion. Variability of estimates should account for the matching, of course, but the entities estimated ignore Z. The classification probabilities or ROC curve, say, for the test are simply calculated from the study sample. We call this the marginal analysis of the matched study.

The interpretations given to the entities estimated must be carefully considered. They pertain to disease and non-disease populations that have the same distribution of Z. If cases are selected randomly from the disease population and matched controls are selected, then the estimated TPF represents the population TPF but the FPF does not. The estimated FPF pertains to a hypothetical non-disease population whose distribution of Z is the same as that of the disease population. Such a non-disease population does not exist in reality. Similar considerations apply to the interpretation of the marginal ROC curve. At the early stages of test development these marginal entities may be of interest. However, in later phases the classification probabilities and ROC curves that apply to the real non-disease and disease populations should be estimated, possibly with stratification on covariates.

8.7 Concluding remarks

Much of this chapter dealt with sample size calculations. This is clearly an important aspect of study design but certainly there are many other aspects that are dealt with elsewhere in the book. Section 1.2 emphasized biases that should be avoided by design. Section 2.2.5 discussed the choice of sampling scheme, case-control or cohort, and Section 8.6 extended the sampling discussion to considerations of stratified and matched designs. Comparative studies may be paired or unpaired, and the analogies with cross-over versus parallel-arm clinical trial designs were drawn in Section 3.1.

The first key step in deciding upon a design, however, is to define the study objectives. These depend on the phase of development at which the study is being performed. Therefore, recognizing the phase of the research is vital. Broad objectives for each phase were outlined in Section 8.1.2 (Table 8.1). More detailed

Table 8.2 *Summary of sample size formulae*

Phase	Design	Test type	Key parameter	Sample sizes
2	Case-control	Binary	(FPF, TPF)	$n_D = (8.2), \quad n_{\bar{D}} = (8.3)$
2	Case-control	Continuous	$\text{ROC}(\text{FPF}_0)$	$n_D = (8.8)$ with $(8.7), \quad n_{\bar{D}} = n_D/\kappa$
2	Case-control	Continuous	AUC	$n_D = (8.10)$ with Result 8.2 $n_{\bar{D}} = n_D/\kappa$
3	Case-control, paired	Binary	$(\text{rFPF}, \text{rTPF})$	$n_D = (8.15), \quad n_{\bar{D}} = (8.16)$
3	Case-control, unpaired	Binary	$(\text{rFPF}, \text{rTPF})$	$n_D = (8.17), \quad n_{\bar{D}} = (8.18)$
3	Case-control	Continuous	ROC summary	$(n_D, n_{\bar{D}})$ satisfy (8.19)
3	Controls only	Continuous	$S_{\bar{D}}^{-1}(\text{FPF}_0)$	$n_{\bar{D}} = (8.20)$
4	Cohort	Binary	Classification probabilities	$(n_{\bar{D}}, n_D)$ as for phase 2 or phase 3 case-control studies. N satisfies (8.22) and (8.23)
4	Cohort, single arm	Binary	Predictive values	$n^+ = (8.24), \quad n^- = (8.25)$ N satisfies (8.26) and (8.27)
4	Cohort, unpaired	Binary	$(\text{rNPV}, \text{rPPV})$	$N =$ analogue of that for classification probabilities
4	Cohort, paired	Binary	$(\text{rNPV}, \text{rPPV})$	Simulation studies, with unpaired design for initial N
4	Cohort, single arm	Binary	(FP, DP)	(8.28) and (8.29) as starting points for simulation studies
4	Cohort, two arms	Binary	(rFP, rDP)	N same as for $(\text{rFPF}, \text{rTPF})$

objectives must be defined before a study can be designed, and these of course will depend on the medical context. See Pepe *et al.* (2001), where primary and secondary specific aims are detailed for each phase of cancer biomarker development. I think that there are many areas of medicine where tests and biomarkers need development and that reaching a consensus about specific aims for each phase of development would be worthwhile.

The material in this chapter is technical and pertains to a long list of study designs. For ease of reference Table 8.2 is provided. In addition, sample size calculations carried out for a variety of configurations for phase 2 studies are shown in Tables 8.3, 8.4 and 8.5. They relate to the text in Sections 8.2.1, 8.2.2 and 8.2.3, respectively. These sample sizes are based on simulation studies (code available at http://www.fhcrc.org/labs/pepe/book). Formulae based on asymptotic theory will probably be adequate for phases 3 and 4, though

Table 8.3 *Sample sizes, $(n_{\bar{D}}, n_D)$, for a phase 2 study of a binary test, performed with $\alpha = 0.05$ and $\beta = 0.10$. Calculations used simulation studies. Initial values were derived from asymptotic theory*

$(\mathrm{FPF_0}, \mathrm{TPF_0})$	$(\mathrm{FPF_1}, \mathrm{TPF_1})$					
	$(0.05, 0.70)$	$(0.05, 0.80)$	$(0.05, 0.90)$	$(0.10, 0.70)$	$(0.10, 0.80)$	$(0.10, 0.90)$
$(0.10, 0.60)$	$(350, 290)$	$(370, 70)$	$(395, 27)$	–	–	–
$(0.10, 0.70)$	–	$(365, 245)$	$(365, 50)$	–	–	–
$(0.10, 0.80)$	–	–	$(365, 165)$	–	–	–
$(0.20, 0.60)$	$(60, 300)$	$(65, 75)$	$(70, 28)$	$(165, 300)$	$(170, 70)$	$(185, 28)$
$(0.20, 0.70)$	–	$(65, 250)$	$(62, 50)$	–	$(165, 245)$	$(170, 55)$
$(0.20, 0.80)$	–	–	$(60, 180)$	–	–	$(172, 172)$
$(0.30, 0.60)$	$(28, 315)$	$(28, 70)$	$(30, 28)$	$(55, 320)$	$(55, 70)$	$(55, 28)$
$(0.30, 0.70)$	–	$(30, 255)$	$(30, 55)$	–	$(50, 255)$	$(50, 50)$
$(0.30, 0.80)$	–	–	$(28, 175)$	–	–	$(52, 175)$

Table 8.4 *Sample sizes for a phase 2 study of a continuous test using ROC(FPF$_0$) as the basis for inference, with $\alpha = 0.05$ and $\beta = 0.10$. Simulation studies were based on the binormal ROC curve with slope parameter $b = 1$. Initial values were calculated from asymptotic theory. We set $n_D = n_{\bar{D}}$*

$(\mathrm{FPF_0}, \mathrm{TPF_0})$	$\mathrm{TPF_1}$		
	0.70	0.80	0.90
$(0.10, 0.60)$	549	120	51
$(0.10, 0.70)$	–	428	87
$(0.10, 0.80)$	–	–	258
$(0.20, 0.60)$	449	100	43
$(0.20, 0.70)$	–	344	70
$(0.20, 0.80)$	–	–	205

Table 8.5 *Sample sizes for a phase 2 study of a continuous test using the* $\hat{\mathrm{AUC}}_e$ *as the basis for inference, with* $\alpha = 0.05$ *and* $\beta = 0.10$. *Simulation studies were used with the ROC curves assumed to be binormal with intercept and slope parameters* (a, b). *We set* $b = 1$ *and* $n_{\bar{D}} = n_D$. *Initial values were calculated from asymptotic theory*

	AUC_1		
AUC_0	0.70	0.80	0.85
0.5	35	15	10
0.6	125	25	15
0.7	–	90	40
0.8	–	–	270

confirmation with simulation studies is always recommended.

8.8   Exercises

1. When evaluating a binary test or tests, inference must be made about two parameters. These are (FPF, TPF) in Section 8.2.1 and (rFPF, rTPF) in Section 8.3.1. Show that, for any particular values of the parameters that satisfy H_0, the type 1 error associated with the statistical test based on the rectangular joint confidence region is at most $1 - \sqrt{1 - \alpha}$, even for values that lie on the border of the H_0 region of the (FPF, TPF) space. In this sense the procedure is conservative.

2. Consider a phase 2 study of a continuous test where the null hypothesis is $H_0 : \mathrm{ROC}(\mathrm{FPF}_0) = \mathrm{TPF}_0$. We consider rejecting H_0 on the basis of the lower confidence bound for $\mathrm{ROC}(\mathrm{FPF}_0)$. Show that, under the null hypothesis, this is asymptotically equivalent to a procedure based on FPF_0 exceeding the upper confidence bound for $\mathrm{ROC}^{-1}(\mathrm{TPF}_0)$.

3. The comparison of the detection probabilities of two tests with data from a phase 4 cohort study does not require ascertainment of D for subjects that test positive on both tests. We show this when comparisons are based on relative detection probabilities $\mathrm{rDP}(A, B)$. Show that this is also true when comparisons are based on the absolute difference, $\mathrm{DP}_A - \mathrm{DP}_B$. Indeed, show that disease status is only required for those with discordant test results, $(Y_A = 1, Y_B = 0)$ or $(Y_A = 0, Y_B = 1)$, when the absolute differences, $\mathrm{DP}_A - \mathrm{DP}_B$ and $\mathrm{FP}_A - \mathrm{FP}_B$, are of interest.

4. Consider an unpaired comparative phase 3 case-control study to compare the diagnostic likelihood ratios of two binary tests. Suppose that the null hypothesis $H_0 : \{\mathrm{rDLR}^+(A, B) \leqslant 1 \text{ or } \mathrm{rDLR}^-(A, B) \geqslant 1\}$ is to be evaluated. Describe how conclusions will be drawn from data collected in the study and calculate sample sizes which ensure that a positive conclu-

sion will be drawn with power 80% if the classification probabilities are $FPF_A = 0.1$, $FPF_B = 0.2$, $TPF_A = 0.9$ and $TPF_B = 0.7$.

5. Consider a cohort study that is designed to estimate the probability of a positive test, $\tau = P[Y = 1]$, with a 95% confidence interval width of no more than 2%. In addition, it must be determined if the PPV of the test exceeds 70%. A 95% lower confidence limit will be used for this purpose. The study should have 90% power if the PPV is in fact 80%. Assuming that $\tau = 10\%$, calculate n^+ and N that will be sufficient for inference about PPV. Will this value of N be sufficient for the precision with which τ is to be estimated, and, if not, how large should N be?

6. Suppose that a diagnostic test is 80% sensitive and 95% specific at detecting a preclinical condition D. If treated at the preclinical phase, 60% of patients will be cured, while the remaining 40% will proceed to develop clinical disease that requires extensive medical procedures. The prevalence of D in this population is 10%. The cost of the diagnostic test is $10, treatment of preclinical disease costs $200, while treatment of the clinical condition costs $20 000 per patient. Quantify the impact of the test on disease in this population, both in terms of reductions in subjects developing the clinical condition and in terms of health care costs allocated to dealing with this disease. Calculate the sample sizes required to study the impact of the test on the population.

9

MORE TOPICS AND CONCLUSIONS

The evaluation of medical tests has many and varied aspects. We have tried to cover the basic concepts and statistical approaches available in the previous chapters. Some additional topics will be discussed, albeit briefly, in this chapter. We then conclude the chapter, and the book, with thoughts about broader applications for the statistical methodology described.

9.1 Meta-analysis

9.1.1 *Goals of meta-analysis*

The purpose of a meta-analysis is to synthesize the results of many (or all) studies pertaining to the performance of a diagnostic test. A typical study is small and performed at a single center. Inference is limited, not only because of small sample size, but because the population tested may be different from other populations and because the manner in which the test is performed may be different. By gathering together the results of many studies, a meta-analysis can allow stronger, more general conclusions to be drawn about the performance of a test. Some additional benefits of meta-analysis are:

(i) It can make the research community aware of all completed investigations of the test.

(ii) It can help explain discrepancies between study results, often by pointing to differences in design.

(iii) It can help identify common mistakes made in designing studies, thereby providing principles for the better design of future studies.

There are many published examples of meta-analysis for diagnostic tests. Two straightforward meta-analyses that investigated exercise stress tests for diagnosis of coronary artery disease are reports from Fleischmann *et al.* (1998) and Kwok *et al.* (1999). An example that is more ambitious in its objectives is the AHCPR report on cervical cancer screening in the United States (AHCPR, 1999). This synthesized not only results on test accuracy, but also on the cost and cost-effectiveness of tests for cervical cancer. We focus here on accuracy only.

9.1.2 *Design of a meta-analysis study*

The synthesis of results from multiple studies by meta-analysis is not unique to diagnostic tests, but is also well established in therapeutic research and in epidemiologic research. The design of a meta-analysis study should follow similar principles in all applications. The six basic steps are given in Table 9.1.

253

Table 9.1 *Steps in the design of a meta-analysis*

Step	Description
(1)	Define objectives and scope
(2)	Sources of articles identified
(3)	Inclusion criteria defined
(4)	Study characteristics of interest are identified and coded for data collection
(5)	Assemble information
(6)	Analyze data

Some detailed discussion of the steps involved is provided by the Cochrane Methods Group on the Systematic Review of Screening and Diagnostic Tests (Irwig *et al.*, 1994*b*). See the material from this group posted at the website http://www.cochrane.de/cochrane/crgs.htm#MGLIST which includes an excellent bibliography. Vamvakas (1998) also provides a thorough and insightful discussion.

As with any scientific endeavor, the first step is to define the objectives and scope of the study. This entails detailed definitions for disease, for the diagnostic test, for the setting in which the test is used and for what purpose, for the patient populations, for the control populations, and for the time period during which the studies were conducted. Next, the sources for retrieving articles must be identified. Clearly, these should be as inclusive as possible and any efforts to reduce publication bias by, for example, locating funded research proposals, not just publications, should be employed. The criteria for including studies in the meta-analysis will be driven largely by the definitions formulated in step (1). In addition, one might exclude articles on the basis of flaws in study design, such as uncorrected verification biased sampling, or if insufficient data are presented.

The next step is to identify study-specific characteristics that might affect test performance across the studies. Variations in populations, testing techniques and so forth, might account for some heterogeneity across studies and should be incorporated as covariates in the meta-analysis. Such study characteristics, therefore, should be recorded in the meta-dataset. Factors relating to the quality of the study design should also be recorded. These would include the potential for verification bias, the quality of the reference test and the independence of the reference and investigational tests. Finally, the data are assembled. Most studies report the results of a dichotomized test yielding $n_D, n_{\bar{D}}$ and associated estimates $(\mathrm{T\hat{P}F}, \mathrm{F\hat{P}F})$ for each constituent study. We next consider the analysis of a simple meta-dataset $\{(\mathrm{T\hat{P}F}_k, \mathrm{F\hat{P}F}_k, n_{Dk}, n_{\bar{D}k}), \ k = 1, \ldots, K\}$ of K studies. Analytic approaches for more complex datasets that include non-binary tests and covariates have received little attention in the literature.

9.1.3 *The summary ROC curve*

Meta-analyses of therapeutic studies often summarize results by the average treatment effect observed across studies. The average relative risk is a typical summary statistic for epidemiologic meta-analyses. In contrast, for diagnostic tests simple averaging is not used. Instead, a curve is typically used to summarize results. The main reason for this is that there are two dimensions to consider for summarizing diagnostic tests, the FPF and the TPF. Moreover, the false and true positive fractions tend to be positively correlated. One important source of the correlation is that studies vary in their criteria (implicit or explicit) for defining test positivity. Studies that have more stringent positivity criteria will have lower TPF *and* lower FPF values. Studies with more lenient criteria will have higher values for both. Moses *et al.* (1993) therefore proposed that an ROC-like curve be used to summarize study results in meta-analyses of diagnostic tests. Since this so-called summary ROC (sROC) curve, which goes through the scatter plot of points $\{(\text{FPF}_k, \text{TPF}_k),\ k = 1, \ldots, K\}$, is typically concave in shape, it is not well characterized by the average point $(\overline{\text{FPF}}, \overline{\text{TPF}}) = (\sum \text{FPF}_k / K, \sum \text{TPF}_k / K)$.

The following procedure is the current standard of practice for calculating the sROC curve that summarizes the meta-dataset.

Result 9.1

The Moses algorithm for the sROC is to fit a linear model

$$\text{E}\big(\hat{D} | \hat{S}\big) = \alpha + \beta \hat{S}, \tag{9.1}$$

where

$$\hat{D}_k = \text{logit}\,\hat{\text{TPF}}_k - \text{logit}\,\hat{\text{FPF}}_k\,,$$
$$\hat{S}_k = \text{logit}\,\hat{\text{TPF}}_k + \text{logit}\,\hat{\text{FPF}}_k\,,$$

and to plot the induced sROC curve $(\text{FPF}, \text{TPF}) = (t, \text{sROC}(t))$, where

$$\text{logit}\,\text{sROC}(t) = \frac{\alpha}{1 - \beta} + \frac{\beta + 1}{1 - \beta}\,\text{logit}(t)\,. \qquad\blacksquare$$

The logit transforms of $\hat{\text{TPF}}$ and $\hat{\text{FPF}}$ in the Moses procedure could be replaced with alternatives, such as the probit transform. The logit is most popular in meta-analysis. Irwig *et al.* (1995) note that $D_k = \text{logit}\,\text{TPF}_k - \text{logit}\,\text{FPF}_k$ is interpretable as the log odds ratio in the kth study for the association between disease and test result, and consider it to be a valuable measure of the discrimination power of the test in the kth study. The component $S_k = \text{logit}\,\text{TPF}_k + \text{logit}\,\text{FPF}_k$ is interpreted as a measure related to the threshold for classifying a test as positive. Therefore, the regression model fitted in (9.1),

$$D = \alpha + \beta S\,,$$

is an attempt to characterize the discrimination of the test among studies while allowing it to depend on the threshold. Observe that α is the log odds ratio at the point where $S = 0$, i.e. where the specificity is equal to the sensitivity. It is therefore related to the ROC summary index Sym that was defined in Chapter 4. In fact, $\alpha = 2\log(\text{Sym}/(1-\text{Sym}))$. The interpretation for β is less straightforward than that for α. It describes the shape of the curve. In practice, it is not unusual for the regression coefficient β to be near 0 (Irwig et al., 1995; AHCPR, 1999), in which case the common odds ratio, $\exp\alpha$, provides a reasonable overall summary of the results. It characterizes the sROC completely.

Moses et al. (1993) suggest adding 1/2 to the frequencies in the numerators of $\hat{\text{FPF}}$ and $\hat{\text{TPF}}$, and restricting the analysis to only the subset of points $(\hat{\text{FPF}}_k, \hat{\text{TPF}}_k)$ that lie in a range of interest. The former is a modification to stabilize calculations in small samples. The latter suggestion, however, to select only points where the test performs reasonably well, can bias results towards improved performance of the test and it is not endorsed widely (Irwig et al., 1995).

There has been some debate about whether a weighted or unweighted least-squares algorithm should be used for fitting the linear model (9.1). The unweighted approach gives small studies the same weight as larger ones and ignores differences in the precisions with which D_k is estimated, potentially yielding statistically inefficient procedures. The weighted approach acknowledges differences amongst studies in sample sizes $(n_{Dk}, n_{\bar{D}k})$ by weighting according to $\{\text{vâr}(\hat{D}_k)\}^{-1}$, where

$$\text{vâr}(\hat{D}_k) = \left(n_{Dk}\hat{\text{TPF}}_k(1 - \hat{\text{TPF}}_k)\right)^{-1} + \left(n_{\bar{D}k}\hat{\text{FPF}}_k(1 - \hat{\text{FPF}}_k)\right)^{-1}.$$

However, it has been noted that such weighting can bias results because a study with poorer accuracy will be weighted more heavily than one with better accuracy when sample sizes are similar. For example, if $n_{Dk} = n_{\bar{D}k} = 100$, then the weight given a study with $(\hat{\text{FPF}}_k, \hat{\text{TPF}}_k) = (0.01, 0.95)$ is 0.8, while that for a study with $(\hat{\text{FPF}}_k, \hat{\text{TPF}}_k) = (0.3, 0.6)$ is 11.4. The Cochrane group recommend implementing both weighted and unweighted fitting procedures.

Example 9.1

Data from 59 studies of the Papanicolaou (Pap) test for cervical cancer are displayed in Fig. 9.1 (Fahey et al., 1995). The unweighted approach yielded $(\hat{\alpha}, \hat{\beta}) = (1.58, 0.004)$, while for the weighted analysis $(\hat{\alpha}, \hat{\beta}) = (1.73, -0.04)$. Both ROC curves in Fig. 9.1 appear to provide a reasonable summary of the data. As an overall summary, we conclude that the Pap test has an odds ratio of about $\exp 1.65 = 5.2$ for discriminating cancer cases from controls when TPF $= 1-\text{FPF}$. This level of discrimination does not change much by varying the criteria used to classify the cervical cytology smear. ∎

There are a number of unorthodox and technically dissatisfying aspects of the Moses procedure that have been noted (Rutter and Gatsonis, 2001). First, both the dependent variable, $\hat{D}_k$, and the independent variable, $\hat{S}_k$, that enter into the linear regression model are derived from the same random variables

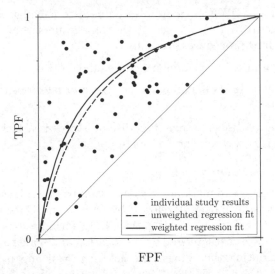

FIG. 9.1. Summary ROC curves for the cervical cancer Pap test. Shown are
curves calculated using weighted and unweighted regression

$(\hat{\mathrm{FPF}}_k, \hat{\mathrm{TPF}}_k)$. Sampling variability induces dependence between $\hat{D}_k$ and $\hat{S}_k$,
even if the true values, D_k and S_k, are unrelated. Second, since $\hat{S}_k$, which is the
covariate in (9.1), is only an estimate of S_k, it is essentially a variable measured
with error. It is well known that covariate measurement error induces bias into
estimates of regression coefficients (Carroll *et al.*, 1995). Third, we have already
mentioned the controversy concerning weighted versus unweighted least-squares
fitting procedures. The extent to which these technical aspects affect the fitted
sROC curves remains to be explored.

   Perhaps of greater concern is the premise upon which the sROC is based. The
rationale provided by Moses *et al.* (1993) and other proponents of the method
is that if the true values $(\mathrm{FPF}_k, \mathrm{TPF}_k)$ were known they would lie *on* the ROC
curve defined by $D_k = \alpha + \beta S_k$. If the only differences amongst studies were
in the threshold criteria for defining test positivity, then the assumption that
the points $(\mathrm{FPF}_k, \mathrm{TPF}_k)$ lie on a single curve would hold. However, in most
settings it is likely that factors other than the threshold criterion also contribute
to variability between studies and that the points $(\mathrm{FPF}_k, \mathrm{TPF}_k)$ are scattered
about a curve. Formal approaches that accommodate between-study variability
in $\{(\mathrm{FPF}_k, \mathrm{TPF}_k), k = 1, \ldots, K\}$, in addition to the within-study sampling variability in $\{(\hat{\mathrm{FPF}}_k, \hat{\mathrm{TPF}}_k), k = 1, \ldots, K\}$, will be discussed in the next section.

   As an informal approach, the sROC can be thought of as simply providing
a curve that goes through the scatter of observed points $(\hat{\mathrm{FPF}}_k, \hat{\mathrm{TPF}}_k)$. Taken
in that sense, it does not really rely on the aforementioned assumption of a
single curve explaining between-study variability. Other statistical smoothing

procedures, such as LOWESS, could also be used to calculate such a summary curve. Some noteworthy advantages of the Moses algorithm relative to these other more standard procedures are that

(i) it provides a monotone summary curve, and

(ii) it is symmetric in its handling of the true and false positive fractions (see Exercise 1).

Since the labeling of disease versus non-disease states is arbitrary, a procedure that is unaffected by the labeling has some appeal.

9.1.4   Binomial regression models

More formal approaches to meta-analysis that employ binomial regression models with random effects have been developed by Rutter and Gatsonis (1995, 2001). Their models are based on the location-scale ROC formulations (see Result 6.4), where ROC curves are characterized by the location and scale parameters $\mu = \mu_D$ and $\sigma = \sigma_D$, adopting the convention that $\mu_{\bar{D}} = 0$ and $\sigma_{\bar{D}} = 1$. That is, $\mathrm{ROC}(t) = S_0(-\mu/\sigma + \sigma^{-1} S_0^{-1}(t))$. They employ the logistic function for $1 - S_0$ and in general allow μ and σ to vary across studies. Thus they write

$$\mathrm{logit\,TPF}_k = (\mathrm{logit\,FPF}_k + \mu_k)\,\sigma_k^{-1}, \tag{9.2}$$

$$= (\theta_k + \mu_k)\,\mathrm{e}^{-b_k}, \tag{9.3}$$

where (θ_k, μ_k, b_k) can be random variables. Observe that, when (μ_k, b_k) are constant, the model asserts that the points $(\mathrm{FPF}_k, \mathrm{TPF}_k)$ fall on an ROC curve, while variability in (μ_k, b_k) allows points to vary around a curve.

Conditional on $(\mathrm{FPF}_k, \mathrm{TPF}_k)$, the data from the kth study are assumed to have binomial distributions. To completely specify the model, distributional forms are assumed for $\{\theta_k, \mu_k, b_k\}$. Rutter and Gatsonis (2001) assume that θ_k and μ_k are independent, with $\mu_k \sim \mathrm{N}(M, \sigma_M^2)$ and $\theta_k \sim \mathrm{N}(\Theta, \sigma_\theta^2)$, and that b_k is a constant, b, across studies. The parameters M, Θ, σ_θ^2, σ_M^2 and b can be estimated from the data with maximum likelihood methods. Alternatively, Bayesian methods can be employed after specification of prior distributions for the unknown parameters. The computational steps are fairly involved and are described in detail by Rutter and Gatsonis (2001).

The study-specific parameters (θ_k, μ_k, b_k) can also be modeled as functions of covariates. In addition to modeling effects of study-specific characteristics (e.g. populations, test operating parameters, etc.), tests can be compared by including test type as a covariate in these models. Rutter and Gatsonis (2001) illustrate this with an application to diagnosing metastasis of cervical cancer with three different imaging modalities.

The binomial regression modeling approach to meta-analysis has several important attributes. First, it accommodates between-study variability that can be modeled with covariates and/or that can be considered random due to unknown sources of variability. The fitting procedures have a sound theoretical basis in maximum likelihood or Bayesian methodology. The drawbacks of the approach appear to be in the computational demands it requires given the limitations of commonly available software, and the complexities involved in assessing the adequacy of the models assumed. The BUGS software package (Spiegelhalter *et al.*, 1996; www.mrc-bsu.cam.ac.uk/bugs/) provides specialized programs that are available for free.

9.2 Incorporating the time dimension

9.2.1 *The context*

Diagnostic tests are often developed to detect or predict the occurrence of an event, such as myocardial infarction, the onset of cancer, infection and so forth. In this context D is a time-dependent variable. Methods that acknowledge the time-dependent nature of the disease state in such settings will be discussed briefly here. Amongst the issues that arise in this context is the following. The time at which the diagnostic test is performed relative to the incidence of the event outcome in general has a big influence on its operating characteristics. To fix ideas, let us consider some examples.

Examples 9.2

1. Cancer, when it is diagnosed clinically, because of its signs or symptoms, is usually quite advanced. Biomarkers, such as serum concentrations of PSA and CA-125, are used to detect cancer before clinical onset, which is the event of interest. Treatment is more successful the longer the lead time gained prior to clinical onset. Unfortunately, biomarker values may not become elevated until the cancer is relatively advanced.

2. Risk factors for myocardial infarction (MI) include high blood pressure and cholesterol levels. These can be regarded as diagnostic tests for a future MI event. Again, measurements close to the time of MI may be more indicative of risk than measurements taken years prior to the MI.

3. The sensitivity of a diagnostic test for infection might increase for a time after the infection event occurs, as the extent of infection worsens, and/or as the body undergoes biological response.   ■

Various proposals for extending notions of accuracy to time-dependent outcomes have been made. We consider two approaches to defining time-dependent classification probabilities in the next two sections. The key differences between the two approaches that we describe is in how the cases and controls are defined over time. In the following section we discuss the concept of time-dependent predictive values.

To fix notation, let the event time variable be denoted by $\mathcal{L}$ and, for the n_D subjects that have events, let $\{\mathcal{L}_i, i = 1, \ldots, n_D\}$ denote their observed event times. We use l to denote the time axis. Suppose that the test, Y, and possibly other covariates, Z, are measured at a baseline time, $l = 0$. These restrictions simplify our initial discussion, although extensions to recurrent events, repeated screening tests and time-dependent covariates are straightforward.

9.2.2 *Incident cases and long-term controls*

Suppose that we define a subject who has an event at time l to be a case at l. Mathematically we write

$$D(l) = 1 \quad \text{if } \mathcal{L} = l.$$

We seek to characterize how well Y, measured at time 0, can detect cases that arise at l. The sensitivity often depends on l, the time-lag between measurement of Y and the onset of disease, i.e. the event. For a binary test, we write the true positive fraction function as

$$\text{TPF}(l) = P[Y = 1|\mathcal{L} = l]. \tag{9.4}$$

Leisenring *et al.* (1997) and Balasubramanian and Lagakos (2001) define time-dependent sensitivity in this fashion. To define the false positive fraction we need to consider what constitutes an appropriate set of controls. Possibilities include: those who do not have disease at l; those who have not developed disease by time l; those who never develop disease during their lifetimes; or those who have not had an event by some large time denoted by $\mathcal{L}^\infty$. Although those who never develop disease may be an ideal group, we use the latter group to define controls:

$$D = 0 \quad \text{if and only if} \quad \mathcal{L} > \mathcal{L}^\infty,$$

because complete lifetime follow-up is rare. We contend that, in applications where subclinical disease may exist, the false positive fraction is probably best characterized by this non-time-dependent control group. Subjects with preclinical disease are eliminated from the control group as far as possible, assuming that $\mathcal{L}^\infty$ is large enough. This is important because positive test results from subjects with preclinical disease should not be counted as false positives. On the contrary, they should count in favor rather than against the test. We define the false positive fraction, FPF, as pertaining to these *long-term controls*:

$$\text{FPF} = P[Y = 1|\mathcal{L} > \mathcal{L}^\infty]. \tag{9.5}$$

Example 9.3

Infection with cytomegalovirus (CMV) is a major concern after patients receive a bone marrow transplant. Using the results of a PCR blood leukocyte test for CMV, Leisenring *et al.* (1997) sought to characterize its diagnostic accuracy. Figure 9.2 shows the incidence of clinical disease in 113 patients. By 100 days after transplant, 90 (80%) had developed an infection, while 23 relatively healthy subjects with functioning immune systems had not developed a CMV infection. These constitute the control group. Only 1 of these subjects had a positive initial PCR test, yielding an estimated FPF = 4% and 90% upper confidence limit equal to 16%.

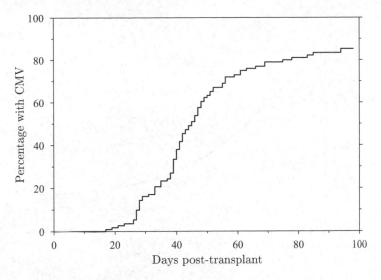

FIG. 9.2. Incidence of cytomegalovirus infection (CMV) for bone marrow transplant patients

The TPF of the PCR test depends on the time-lag, l, between testing with PCR and the onset of clinical disease. Let us consider one approach to characterizing this TPF function. Suppose we model it as a cubic polynomial in l:

$$\text{logit TPF}(l) = \text{logit P}[Y = 1 | \mathcal{L} = l]$$
$$= \beta_0 + \beta_1 l + \beta_2 l^2 + \beta_3 l^3 \, .$$

The parameters in this model can be estimated using the marginal regression methods described in Section 3.5. Subjects that developed CMV contributed records to the analysis until clinical disease developed. There may be multiple records because these subjects were tested with PCR at approximately weekly intervals. For each test, the time of testing defines a time origin and a time-lag l between testing and the onset of disease. Thus, there is one data record in the analysis for each PCR test performed. We refer to Leisenring *et al.* (1997) for details.

The polynomial fit to the data yields the TPF function shown in Fig. 9.3. There is a clear dependence on l. The test appears to be reasonably sensitive for detecting infections that occur clinically within about seven days after testing, but not those occurring later. Frequent testing with PCR is probably necessary in this context.   ∎

Time-dependent ROC incidence curves were defined by Etzioni *et al.* (1999*b*). These are straightforward extensions of the classification probabilities defined above. The controls are again defined as a non-time-dependent group, event free at $\mathcal{L}^\infty$. That is, $D = 0$ if and only if $\mathcal{L} > \mathcal{L}^\infty$. The cases at time l are those

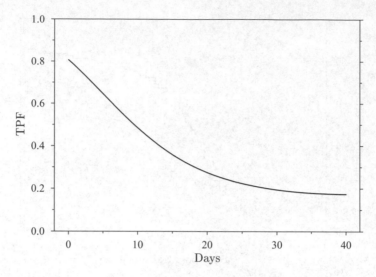

F<small>IG</small>. 9.3. The incidence TPF function calculated for the PCR test for cytomegalovirus infection. The time axis is the number of days between the
PCR test and the subsequent onset of infection

that experience an event at l. The time-dependent ROC curve describes the
separation between cases having an event at l and the controls. At time l and
$\text{FPF} = t$, it is

$$\text{ROC}(l, t) = \text{P}[Y_i > S_{\bar{D}}^{-1}(t)|\mathcal{L}_i = l].$$

We refer back to Example 6.13, where we previously considered these time-
dependent ROC curves in the context of detecting prostate cancer with serum
PSA. These curves were fitted to data using the ROC–GLM regression methodology.

Observe that, in Example 9.3 above, to estimate the time-dependent TPFs
we employed logistic regression using the lag-time l as a covariate. Similarly,
in Example 6.13 we employed ROC regression methods with l, the time-lag
between serum sampling and cancer diagnosis, as a covariate. Although this is a
reasonable strategy, it is not without limitations. It requires that a parametric
functional form be specified for the effect of time on the test accuracy measure of
interest. Nonparametric methods may be more robust. In addition, the regression
methods that are described here require that the event time $\mathcal{L}_i$ is observed for
all cases in the analysis. In prospective studies, event times may be censored for
many subjects, in the sense that their follow-up times are less than $\mathcal{L}^\infty$ and an
event has not yet occurred for them. These observations, censored in $(0, \mathcal{L}^\infty)$, are
omitted from the regression analysis because they cannot be assigned to the case
or control groups. Their partial information is ignored in effect. The approach
we describe in the next section incorporates censored data, but uses somewhat

different notions for defining test accuracy. Extensions of the methods discussed in this section to censored data would be worthwhile.

9.2.3   *Interval cases and controls*

Considering the entire time interval up to l, Heagerty *et al.* (2000) defined a case as

$$D(l) = 1 \quad \text{if and only if} \quad \mathcal{L} \leqslant l.$$

That is, if the subject has an event before l then he is a case. This contrasts with the incident notion of the previous section where a case was defined by an event occurring *at* l. A subject is defined to be a control if

$$D(l) = 0 \quad \text{if and only if} \quad \mathcal{L} > l.$$

Thus, at each time l, all subjects are defined as being cases or controls at l. At $l = 0$, all subjects are controls. Thereafter, the case group accumulates subjects from the control group as they have events. True and false positive fractions for binary tests are then both defined as time-dependent entities based on cumulative events in the interval $(0, l)$:

$$\text{TPF}^C(l) = \text{P}[Y = 1 | \mathcal{L} \leqslant l], \quad \text{FPF}^C(l) = \text{P}[Y = 1 | \mathcal{L} > l]. \qquad (9.6)$$

The notion of a cumulative ROC curve, ROC^C, follows similarly.

It is easy to see that the cumulative entities, TPF^C, FPF^C and ROC^C, can be calculated from the incidence entities described in Section 9.2.2 if the event time distribution is known (Exercise 2). However, Heagerty *et al.* (2000) showed that they can also be calculated directly. Moreover, their approach has the advantages that it accommodates censored data and does not require a parametric model for the time effect. Let us consider a continuous test and the cumulative ROC curve that is defined as a plot of $\text{TPF}^C(l, y)$ versus $\text{FPF}^C(l, y)$ for $y \in (-\infty, \infty)$ and $l \geqslant 0$, where

$$\text{TPF}^C(l, y) = \text{P}[Y > y | \mathcal{L} \leqslant l] = \frac{\text{P}[Y > y, \mathcal{L} \leqslant l]}{\text{P}[\mathcal{L} \leqslant l]}$$

and

$$\text{FPF}^C(l, y) = \frac{\text{P}[Y > y, \mathcal{L} > l]}{\text{P}[\mathcal{L} > l]}.$$

Bivariate and univariate survivor function estimators are used to estimate the numerator and denominator components of the classification probabilities. We refer to Heagerty *et al.* (2000) for details about the estimation procedures.

The next example uses the ROC curve in an interesting non-traditional context. Instead of denoting a diagnostic test result, Y denotes a variable used for determining eligibility for entry into a clinical trial. The event time, $\mathcal{L}$, is the outcome variable in the proposed clinical trial. We will see that the cumulative ROC curve can be used to assist in developing eligibility criteria for the design of a clinical trial.

Example 9.4

Heagerty *et al.* (2000) use the cumulative ROC curve in clinical trial design. They use it to describe the impact on sample size requirements of varying the eligibility criterion associated with a risk factor for the clinical outcome variable. Consider a study population and let $P[\mathcal{L} \leqslant l]$ denote the proportion that experience the clinical outcome of interest when study participants are followed for a time l. The sample size for the study of a relatively rare event is driven by the expected number of clinical events (Collett, 1994). Let Y denote the risk factor and suppose that we impose the eligibility criterion for the trial to be $Y > y$. If this criterion has a high cumulative true positive fraction, $P[Y > y | \mathcal{L} \leqslant l]$, then a trial with this eligibility criterion will include most of those subjects that will have an event. This study, whose sample size is a fraction $P[Y > y]$ of that for a study without the eligibility criterion, will therefore have about the same statistical power. The proportion of essentially uninformative subjects that continue to be included in the trial despite imposing the criterion is $P[Y > y | \mathcal{L} > l]$. A plot of $\mathrm{TPF}^C(l, y) = P[Y > y | \mathcal{L} \leqslant l]$ versus $\mathrm{FPF}^C(l, y) = P[Y > y | \mathcal{L} > l]$ shows the reduction in the expected number of events in the trial by imposing the constraint against the corresponding reduction in the number of uninformative subjects enrolled. If $\mathrm{TPF}^C(l, y)$ is high and $\mathrm{FPF}^C(l, y)$ is low, then this indicates that, by imposing the eligibility criterion $Y > y$, a substantially smaller but almost as powerful study can be performed.

An illustration of these cumulative ROC curves is shown in Fig. 9.4. This illustration concerns a proposed HIV vaccine study where the outcome variable of interest is incidence of HIV infection. The risk factor $Y = $ 'number of male partners in the last six months' may be used for selecting HIV-negative subjects likely to become infected within the follow-up period of the study. The cumulative ROC curves are calculated for follow-up periods l equal to 6, 12 and 18 months. The calculations, derived from the Vaccine Preparedness Study (Koblin *et al.*, 1998), are described in detail in Heagerty *et al.* (2000). It appears that Y is better at distinguishing between subjects likely to have an infection occurring within six months ($l \leqslant 6$) from those infection free at six months ($l > 6$) than it can distinguish between corresponding groups at 12 months or at 18 months. Considering the ROC^C curve for 6 months follow-up, we see that one point on the curve is $(\mathrm{FPF}^C, \mathrm{TPF}^C) = (0.55, 0.90)$. Thus, by imposing an eligibility criterion of the form $Y \geqslant y$, for the corresponding threshold y we can reduce the sample size to about 55% of that required for a trial without that eligibility criterion, while maintaining about 90% of the incident infections.   ■

This example illustrates how the cumulative ROC can be useful for planning enrolment criteria in a clinical trial. This is a setting where the notion of the cumulative ROC curve plays a natural role. However, the incidence ROC curve is a more natural choice in other settings. In the examples of the previous section, we consider biomarkers for conditions that have preclinical states, namely CMV infection and prostate cancer. In such settings, we have discussed that

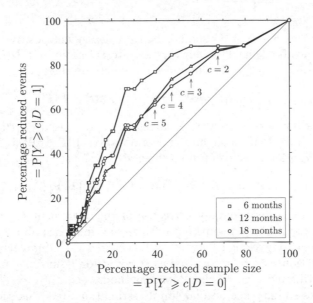

FIG. 9.4. The impact of the eligibility criterion, number of sex partners $\geqslant c$, on the reduction in sample size (horizontal axis) and the power (vertical axis) of a clinical trial with the incidence of HIV infection by 6, 12 or 18 months as outcome measures

the non-time-dependent controls defined by a single large value $\mathcal{L}^\infty$ seem more appropriate because subjects with preclinical disease at l should not be included in the control set at time l. In addition, the incidence ROC curve provides a more detailed description of the effect of the time-lag l between test and event on the detection capacity of the test. It relates the events that occur only at l to Y rather than accumulating all events occurring at or before l. Moreover, the interval notions of sensitivity and specificity can be calculated from the incidence values if the event time distribution is known or can be estimated (Cai *et al.*, 2002).

In cancer research, the notion of non-time-dependent controls is natural. The FPF or specificity may be defined as relating to those not having cancer up to 5 years after the screening test, say. Interestingly, the concept of defining the TPF based on an *interval* after screening is well established. The cases may be defined as those with cancer detected and confirmed at screening or arising clinically within, say, 1 year after screening. There is much debate about how to choose the time interval, of course. In my opinion, the interval concept is attractive mostly because of its computational simplicity (the TPF can be calculated as a simple ratio). The incident TPF function that displays the TPF as a function of the time interval between screening and the onset of clinical disease, however, provides more detailed information.

9.2.4 Predictive values

Suppose that Y is binary. How should the time-dependent positive and negative predictive values be defined? Following the interval notion for $D(l)$ used in the previous section, we define the cumulative predictive values

$$\mathrm{PPV}^C(l) = \mathrm{P}[\mathcal{L} \leqslant l | Y = 1] \quad \text{and} \quad \mathrm{NPV}^C(l) = \mathrm{P}[\mathcal{L} > l | Y = 0].$$

The incidence notions of predictive values could be based on the probability densities, which are, with a slight abuse of notation, $\mathrm{P}[\mathcal{L} = l | Y = 1]$ and $\mathrm{P}[\mathcal{L} = l | Y = 0]$. Alternatively, we can use the hazard functions

$$\lambda[l | Y = 1] = \mathrm{P}[\mathcal{L} = l | Y = 1, \mathcal{L} \geqslant l] \quad \text{and} \quad \lambda[l | Y = 0] = \mathrm{P}[\mathcal{L} = l | Y = 0, \mathcal{L} \geqslant l].$$

We prefer to use hazard functions because of the prominent role they already play in the analysis of event time data. Moreover, inference about these hazard functions is relatively straightforward with censored data. Similarly, the predictive value functions can be recognized as survivor (or 1-survivor) functions that are readily estimated with Kaplan–Meier methods.

Approaches to inference beyond simple estimation are straightforward when each subject contributes a single observation to the analysis. Comparisons between predictive value functions or between hazard functions can proceed using standard methods (Kalbfleisch and Prentice, 1980), as can regression analysis. However, extensions to settings where data are paired, for example where subjects are tested with two tests that are to be compared, have not been discussed in the literature to date. They could proceed using methods analogous to those described in Chapter 3 for analyzing predictive values of non-time-dependent outcomes using paired data. That is, by using regression methods marginal with respect to predictors. However, in-depth discussion or applications have not yet appeared in the literature.

Notions of predictive values when test results are continuous, as opposed to binary, have not received careful attention in the literature either. This is so, not only for event time outcomes, but, as mentioned in Chapter 4, notions of predictive values for continuous tests are not well developed even for simple binary non-time-dependent disease state outcomes. Methodological developments in this direction would obviously be worthwhile.

9.2.5 Longitudinal measurements

In the previous sections we have assumed that the test result is measured at a baseline time, $l = 0$, and that its capacity for 'diagnosing' future events at $l > 0$ is to be explored. If only the time-lag between the measurement of Y and the event time is relevant, then the time-dependent accuracy parameters defined earlier can be estimated using multiple measurements made over time by including them as separate observations in the analysis, each measurement time defining the baseline for that observation. In both Examples 9.3 and 6.13, we employ marginal regression methods in this way, noting that the marginal distributions that relate a single measure Y to $\mathcal{L}$ are the entities of interest in those examples.

There has been much recent interest in joint modeling of the longitudinal biomarker process and event times. A comprehensive joint model for $\{Y(l),\ l > 0;\ \mathcal{L}\}$ yields a lot more information than the simple marginal models we employ. For example, one can calculate the predictive values associated with a sequence of test result measurements made at arbitrary time points. Skates *et al.* (2001) use this to develop the 'risk of cancer' algorithm for ovarian cancer screening. Joint modeling of processes over time is challenging in practice. It requires that one models the evolution of the biomarkers over time in relation to the biological process that terminates in the clinical event at $\mathcal{L}$. With careful and sophisticated work, however, these approaches appear to have met with some success (see Wulfsohn and Tsiatis, 1997; Henderson *et al.*, 2000).

9.3 Combining multiple test results

Most diagnostic tests are not perfect. On the other hand, several such tests may be available. Strategies for combining information from multiple tests are therefore important since a combination may provide a better diagnostic tool than any single test can on its own.

This issue is currently receiving considerable attention in the search for cancer biomarkers. No single biomarker is sufficiently sensitive and specific for the purposes of population screening for ovarian cancer, for example. The hope is, instead, that a panel of serum biomarkers will lead to a composite screening test with adequate operating characteristics (Bast, 1993; Woolas *et al.*, 1995). As a second example, in clinical practice multiple sources of information are often available to a clinician. Signs and symptoms of disease, family and personal medical histories, in addition to results of formal medical tests, can all be used to decide on a diagnosis.

The question we address in this section is how to formally combine multiple such predictors to yield an optimal diagnostic test. As mentioned above, the predictors may include diagnostic tests as well as other sources of information pertinent to the diagnosis. We write the P predictors as $Y = (Y_1, \ldots, Y_P)$ and write $(\mathrm{FPF}_p, \mathrm{TPF}_p)$ for the classification probabilities associated with the pth predictor.

9.3.1 *Boolean combinations*

Let us consider the simplest case where the predictors are binary. For example, each Y_p might be the result of a binary test, the presence or absence of a clinical symptom, say. Boolean operators are often used to combine the Ys. These combinations are defined by the operators 'AND', 'OR' and 'NOT' applied to $(Y_1, \ldots, Y_P)$. When $P = 2$, only four configurations are possible and the decision rules are classified as the 'believe the positive' (BP) and the 'believe the negative' (BN) rules (Marshall, 1989).

Definition (for two binary tests)

- The 'believe the positive' rule means that if Y_1 *OR* Y_2 is positive then the subject is classified as diseased.

- The 'believe the negative' rule means that if Y_1 *AND* Y_2 are positive then the subject is classified as diseased.   ∎

Example 9.5

Consider the CASS data and the cross-tabulation of the EST and CPH tests for subjects with and without coronary artery disease.

	$D = 0$		$D = 1$	
	$Y_{\text{EST}} = 0$	$Y_{\text{EST}} = 1$	$Y_{\text{EST}} = 0$	$Y_{\text{EST}} = 1$
$Y_{\text{CPH}} = 0$	151	46	25	29
$Y_{\text{CPH}} = 1$	176	69	183	786

The BP combination has a TPF = 998/1023 = 97.6% and FPF = 291/442 = 66%, while the BN combination has TPF = 786/1023 = 76.8% and FPF = 69/442 = 15.6%. These contrast with the classification probabilities of the individual tests which are TPF = 815/1023 = 79.7% and FPF = 115/442 = 26% for the EST test, and TPF = 969/1023 = 94.7% and FPF = 245/442 = 55.4% for the CPH test. We see that the BP test is more sensitive but less specific than the component tests, while the BN test is more specific but less sensitive than each test on its own. These observations are true in general.   ∎

Result 9.2

1. The BP rule increases sensitivity relative to the component tests. It also increases the FPF, but by no more than $\text{FPF}_1 + \text{FPF}_2$.

2. The BN rule increases specificity and decreases the sensitivity, but maintains the TPF of the composite test above $\text{TPF}_1 + \text{TPF}_2 - 1$.   ∎

We leave the proof of this result as an exercise. The result is easily generalized to $P > 2$ tests and it has important implications for practice. It implies that, if several highly specific but inadequately sensitive tests are available, then they should be combined with a BP rule. The combination will remain specific, with FPF no larger than $\text{FPF}_1 + \text{FPF}_2$ when $P = 2$ (or no larger than $\sum \text{FPF}_p$ more generally). The sensitivity may be increased by the combination. This depends on whether or not the component tests detect different diseased subjects or the same diseased subjects. The BP combination will only prove to be useful if each component test detects some subjects that are not detected with the others.

On the other hand, if several highly sensitive but non-specific tests are available, then a BN combination should be considered. It might lead to improved specificity while maintaining adequate sensitivity. Improvements in specificity will result if non-diseased subjects testing positive on one test do not test positive on another. The sensitivity is maintained above the lower bound of $\text{TPF}_1 + \text{TPF}_2 - 1$, but will be higher if false negatives on one test are also false negatives on the other.

More complex combinations formed by Boolean operators can be considered when $P > 2$. However, the problem of finding the best decision rule quickly becomes very complex indeed. For example, if 4 tests are available, then $2^4 = 16$ combinations of test results are possible and an enormous number of different decision rules can be based on the 16 possibilities. When the predictors are continuous the problem becomes essentially infinite. A search among all possible rules in order to find the best is not feasible except in very simple settings. In the next sections we show that there is in fact an elegant solution to this apparently enormous problem.

9.3.2   *The likelihood ratio principle*

In Chapter 4 we considered the likelihood ratio function, $\mathcal{L}\text{R}(Y) = \text{P}[Y|D = 1]/\text{P}[Y|D = 0]$, for a single test result, Y. We noted there that the $\mathcal{L}\text{R}$ function of Y has the best ROC curve among all possible functions of Y. Throughout the text we have assumed that Y is such that its $\mathcal{L}\text{R}$ function is monotone increasing. Therefore, further consideration of the $\mathcal{L}\text{R}$ transformation was unnecessary because $\mathcal{L}\text{R}(Y)$ and Y then have the same ROC curve.

The $\mathcal{L}\text{R}$ transformation becomes a very useful tool, however, when considering multiple tests. With $Y = (Y_1, \ldots, Y_P)$ we define it, as before, to be

$$\mathcal{L}\text{R}(Y) = \frac{\text{P}[Y|D = 1]}{\text{P}[Y|D = 0]}. \tag{9.7}$$

Result 4.4, which concerns the optimality of $\mathcal{L}\text{R}(Y)$, is true when Y is multidimensional. We restate the general result here and provide arguments for its validity because of its key role in solving the optimal combination problem.

Result 9.3

The scalar function of $(Y_1, \ldots, Y_P)$, namely $\mathcal{L}\text{R}(Y)$, yields all optimal decision rules based on $(Y_1, \ldots, Y_P)$ in the sense that a criterion of the form

$$\mathcal{L}\text{R}(Y) > c \tag{9.8}$$

 (i) maximizes the TPF among all rules with FPF $= t$, for each $t \in (0, 1)$;

 (ii) minimizes the FPF among all rules with TPF $= r$, for each $r \in (0, 1)$;

 (iii) minimizes the overall misclassification probability, $\rho(1 - \text{TPF}) + (1 - \rho)\text{FPF}$; and

 (iv) minimizes the expected cost, regardless of the costs associated with false negative and false positive errors.

The criterion threshold value c depends on the chosen values for: t in (i); r in (ii); the prevalence in (iii); and both prevalence and costs in (iv).

Proof The result is essentially the Neyman–Pearson lemma that was developed in the context of statistical hypothesis testing (Neyman and Pearson, 1933), but applies equally well to medical diagnostic testing. We refer to Table 9.2 for the analogy between the two classification scenarios. We see that the significance level in hypothesis testing is equivalent to the false positive fraction in diagnostic testing. Statistical power and the true positive fraction are the same entities, but given different names in the two settings. The Neyman–Pearson lemma applies to any decision problem. In statistical hypothesis testing it is stated as follows. Among all decision rules based on W with significance level α, that which maximizes statistical power is of the form $\mathcal{LR}(W) > c$, where the threshold c is chosen so that $\alpha = P[\mathcal{LR}(W) > c|H_0]$. In medical diagnostic testing it is stated in the same way but with different terminology as follows. Among all classification rules based on Y with $\mathrm{FPF} = t$, that which maximizes the TPF is $\mathcal{LR}(Y) > c$, where c is the $1 - t$ quantile of $\mathcal{LR}(Y)$ among non-diseased subjects. That is, part (i) of the result holds.

Part (i) of the result implies that no decision rule based on Y can have an $(\mathrm{FPF}, \mathrm{TPF})$ point that lies anywhere above the ROC curve for $\mathcal{LR}(Y)$. Parts (ii), (iii) and (iv) of the result then follow easily from (i). For example, consider (iv) and let C_{FP} and C_{FN} denote the costs of false positive and false negative errors, respectively. Suppose that the rule R^* minimizes the expected cost and let $(\mathrm{FPF}^*, \mathrm{TPF}^*)$ be the classification probabilities of R^*. Thus

$$C^* = C_{\mathrm{FP}}(1 - \rho)\mathrm{FPF}^* + C_{\mathrm{FN}}\rho(1 - \mathrm{TPF}^*) \qquad (9.9)$$

is the minimum expected cost. Now consider the $\mathcal{LR}$ rule with false positive fraction FPF^*. Its true positive fraction must be at least TPF^*. The above equation therefore indicates that its expected cost can be no more than C^*.

Table 9.2 *The analogy between statistical hypothesis testing and medical diagnostic testing*

	Statistical hypothesis testing	Medical diagnostic testing
Possible states	H_0 versus H_1	$D = 0$ versus $D = 1$
Information	Data for n subjects denoted by W	Test results for a subject denoted by Y
Rule	Classify as H_0 or H_1 using W	Classify as $D = 0$ or 1 using Y
Type 1 error	Significance level $\alpha = P[\text{reject } H_0|H_0]$	False positive fraction $\mathrm{FPF} = P[\text{classify } D = 1|D = 0]$
Type 2 error	Power $1 - \beta = P[\text{reject } H_0|H_1]$	True positive fraction $\mathrm{TPF} = P[\text{classify } D = 1|D = 1]$
$\mathcal{LR}$ function	$\mathcal{LR}(W) = P[W|H_1]/P[W|H_0]$	$\mathcal{LR}(Y) = P[Y|D = 1]/P[Y|D = 0]$

That is, the $\mathcal{LR}$ rule also minimizes the expected cost, and part (iv) is proven. We leave (ii) and (iii) as exercises.   ∎

Example 9.6

McIntosh and Pepe (2002) develop a simulation model for two ovarian cancer biomarkers. Briefly, they assume that the two markers $Y = (Y_1, Y_2)$ have a standard bivariate normal distribution among controls:

$$Y_{\bar{D}} = \begin{pmatrix} Y_{1\bar{D}} \\ Y_{2\bar{D}} \end{pmatrix} \sim \mathrm{N}\left(\begin{pmatrix} 0 \\ 0 \end{pmatrix}, \begin{pmatrix} 1 & 0 \\ 0 & 1 \end{pmatrix}\right).$$

Diseased subjects belong to one of four classes, each class representing a subtype of ovarian cancer, with the probability of being in the kth class being denoted by P_k. Within each class, $Y_D = (Y_{1D}, Y_{2D})$ has a bivariate normal distribution with mean (μ_{1k}, μ_{2k}), variances $(\sigma_{1k}^2, \sigma_{2k}^2)$ and covariance ρ_k. We refer to McIntosh and Pepe (2002) for details and the rationale for using this model to simulate biomarker data for ovarian cancer, as well as choices of parameter values.

The $\mathcal{LR}$ function can be calculated as

$$\mathcal{LR}(Y_1, Y_2) = \frac{\sum_k P_k \mathrm{BVN}_k(Y_1, Y_2)}{\mathrm{BVN}_0(Y_1, Y_2)},$$

where BVN_k denotes the bivariate normal density for the kth class and the 0 subscript denotes the density for $Y_{\bar{D}}$. In Fig. 9.5(a) we show the distribution of $\mathcal{LR}(Y_1, Y_2)$ for the diseased and non-diseased populations. In Fig. 9.5(b) we display the contours of the $\mathcal{LR}$ function in the two-dimensional marker space for (Y_1, Y_2). Suppose that we set the target FPF of a test based on (Y_1, Y_2) at 0.1. We find the 90th percentile of the $\mathcal{LR}$ function among controls and consider the corresponding contour in the marker space. Result 9.3 indicates that, on the basis of only their biomarkers, we should classify subjects as positive for disease if their marker values fall in the region above or to the right of the contour. That is, if $\mathcal{LR}(Y) > c(0.10)$, as shown in Fig. 9.5. This classification rule has the highest TPF among all rules based on (Y_1, Y_2) with FPF $= 0.1$.

The ROC curves associated with the use of each marker on its own are shown in Fig. 9.6. We also calculate the ROC curve associated with the $\mathcal{LR}$ score based on (Y_1, Y_2). No classification rule based on (Y_1, Y_2) can have operating points anywhere above this curve. Although the combination has improved performance compared with the single markers, it certainly does not produce the perfect diagnostic test.   ∎

9.3.3 *Optimality of the risk score*

The $\mathcal{LR}$ function, as written above in (9.7), does not seem to be very useful from a practical point of view. It appears that the multivariate probability distributions for Y in the diseased and non-diseased populations must be known (or estimated)

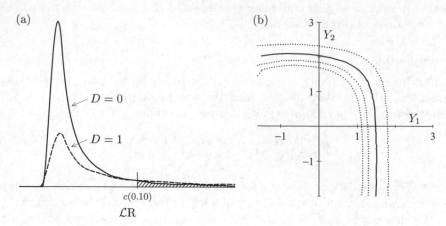

FIG. 9.5. (a) Frequency distributions of $\mathcal{L}$R among diseased and non-diseased populations. Shown is the 90th percentile of $\mathcal{L}$R in the controls, denoted by $c(0.10)$. The distribution for the diseased population is highly skewed and extends well beyond the range shown in the plot. (b) Contours in the marker space that correspond to fixed thresholds for $\mathcal{L}$R(Y_1, Y_2). The highlighted contour corresponds to a false positive fraction of 0.10. That is, classifying values above or to the right of the contour line as positive for disease yields FPF $= 0.10$

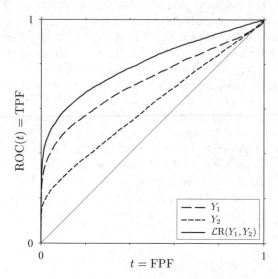

FIG. 9.6. ROC curves for each marker on its own and for the optimal combination $\mathcal{L}$R(Y_1, Y_2), or equivalently RS(Y_1, Y_2)

in order to calculate $\mathcal{L}R(Y)$. The evaluation of multivariate distributions is not an easy task. The next result states that the $\mathcal{L}R$ function is equivalent to a more familiar entity that is commonly estimated with data, namely the risk score. We formally define the risk score function as

$$RS(Y) = P[D = 1|Y]. \tag{9.10}$$

Result 9.4

The risk score $RS(Y)$ has the same ROC curve as $\mathcal{L}R(Y)$. Moreover, it yields the same optimal decision rules as the $\mathcal{L}R$ function, rules that are of the form

$$RS(Y) > c^*,$$

where the threshold chosen, c^*, depends on the optimality criterion.

Proof If we can show that $RS(Y)$ is a monotone increasing function of $\mathcal{L}R(Y)$, then they have the same ROC curve and the result follows. Using Bayes' rule, observe that

$$
\begin{aligned}
RS(Y) &= P[D = 1|Y] \\
&= \frac{P[Y|D = 1]P[D = 1]}{P[Y]} \\
&= \frac{P[Y|D = 1]P[D = 1]}{P[Y|D = 1]P[D = 1] + P[Y|D = 0]P[D = 0]} \\
&= \frac{\mathcal{L}R(Y)P[D = 1]}{\mathcal{L}R(Y)P[D = 1] + P[D = 0]},
\end{aligned}
$$

which is monotone increasing in $\mathcal{L}R(Y)$. ∎

The conclusion to be drawn from this result is that, in order to optimally combine the results of multiple tests, one should ascertain the risk score function $P[D = 1|Y]$. Moreover, any monotone increasing function of the risk score works just as well.

Results 9.3 and 9.4 provide a remarkably simple solution to a problem that seemed at first glance to be very difficult. The results were noted decades ago by Green and Swets (1966) and by Egan (1975), amongst others, in the context of signal detection theory. They were noted more recently by Baker (2000) and by McIntosh and Pepe (2002). However, they do not appear to be well known among statisticians, or at least among statisticians that use frequentist concepts for inference. We emphasize that our discussion here is entirely within the frequentist domain.

Bayesians, on the other hand, have long argued for optimality of the $\mathcal{L}R$ score and have noted the relationship between the $\mathcal{L}R$ and RS functions (see classic Bayesian decision theory as described by McLachlan, 1992 or Ripley, 1996). Their arguments are based on minimizing an expected loss (or cost) function. Indeed, if $P[D = 1]$ is regarded as the prior probability of disease, then the Bayesian arguments yield parts (iii) and (iv) of Result 9.3. However, arguments that derive parts (i) and (ii) of Result 9.3 are not well known in the Bayesian literature either.

9.3.4 *Estimating the risk score*

We now turn to the practical implications of these results. Suppose that a training set of data is available to develop a classification rule. How should we proceed? It seems reasonable to use the data to estimate the risk score function (or some monotone function of it) and to base the classification rule on a suitable threshold for the resulting estimated function, $\hat{RS}(Y)$. Amongst the many approaches to estimating $RS(Y) = P[D = 1|Y]$ are binary regression methods, logic regression (Ruczinski *et al.*, 2003), classification trees (Breiman *et al.*, 1984), neural network techniques, and machine learning techniques including support vector machines (Cristianini and Shawe-Taylor, 2000) and boosting (Schapire *et al.*, 1998; Friedman *et al.*, 2000). These can all yield predicted values given Y, i.e. $\hat{P}[D = 1|Y]$. Bayesian procedures can be used to yield a posterior probability function for D given Y. This too can be interpreted simply as an estimate of the risk score. The most appropriate choice for estimating the risk score function depends on the problem at hand and we do not promote one technique over another here. Several texts describe and contrast techniques (Ripley, 1996).

Classification procedures that do not involve risk score estimates have a long history in statistical practice. Notably, discriminant analysis methods seek to define a score that maximizes the ratio of between-group ($D = 0$ versus $D = 1$) to within-group variance. The rationale for using such a criterion is not compelling in general. If in large samples it does not yield a monotone function of the risk score, then it does not yield classification rules with optimal operating characteristics. Interestingly, it does yield a monotone function of the risk score when Y is multivariate normal in the diseased and non-diseased populations (Su and Liu, 1993; Pepe and Thompson, 2000).

Although we do not promote one technique over another for estimating the risk score, we recognize one important advantage of logistic regression for this problem, namely its ability to handle retrospective study designs. Part (i) of the following result is well known in epidemiologic research (Breslow and Day, 1980) and is the basis of inference from case-control studies in evaluating risk factors for disease. We restate it here because of its applicability to our problem in diagnostic test development.

Result 9.5

Suppose that the population risk score can be written as

$$\text{logit}\, P[D = 1|Y] = \alpha + h(\beta, Y),$$

where h is a specified parametric function. Then

(i) the parameter β can be estimated (from the prospective likelihood) even when a retrospective design is employed in which sampling depends on D; and

(ii) the function $h(\beta, Y)$ is optimal for classification.

Proof We refer to Breslow and Day (1980) for a proof of (i). Part (ii) follows from the fact that $h(\beta, Y)$ is a monotone function of the risk score $P[D = 1|Y]$ under the model. ∎

Most studies in diagnostic test development are retrospective case-control studies. In particular, many studies that seek to combine multiple 'sources of information' to define a prospective classification rule are phase 3 retrospective studies. Therefore, statistical techniques must accommodate such designs. The above result indicates that logistic regression is one technique that does so. The next example uses simple logistic regression to combine two biomarkers.

Example 9.7

The data displayed in Fig. 9.7 are a random sample of 200 cases and 200 controls from the simulation model of McIntosh and Pepe (2002) that we described earlier in Example 9.6. The markers Y_1 and Y_2 are rescaled to have variance 1 and a linear logistic regression model is fitted to the data:

$$\text{logit}\, P[D = 1|Y] = \alpha + \beta_1 Y_1 + \beta_2 Y_2. \tag{9.11}$$

The estimated linear combination of Y_1 and Y_2 is $h(\hat{\beta}, Y) = \hat{\beta}_1 Y_1 + \hat{\beta}_2 Y_2 = 1.17 Y_1 + 0.584 Y_2$, a weighting of 0.50 for Y_2 relative to Y_1. The true ROC curve

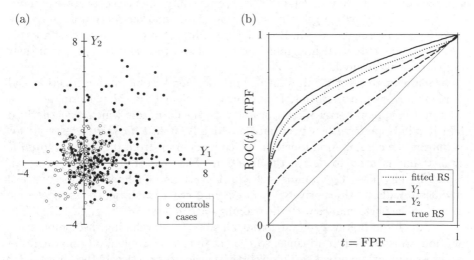

FIG. 9.7. (a) A sample of 200 cases and 200 controls simulated from the bivariate cancer biomarker model. (b) ROC curves for each marker alone, the estimated linear combination $h(\hat{\beta}, Y)$ and for the true risk score $RS(Y_1, Y_2)$

for this linear score function is shown in Fig. 9.7. Also displayed in Fig. 9.7 are the ROC curves shown previously in Fig. 9.6 for Y_1 alone, Y_2 alone and for the optimal biomarker combination $RS(Y_1, Y_2)$. Although the linear combination has improved performance relative to either marker alone, it does not have optimal performance. This is likely to be due to the fact that the linear logistic model (9.11) is not a good model for the risk score. This is evident from the nonlinearity of the contours for the $\mathcal{L}R$ function (or equivalently for $RS(Y_1, Y_2)$) that we observed earlier. We refer to McIntosh and Pepe (2002) for methodology that modifies the logistic regression approach to target better estimation of the $\mathcal{L}R$ contours over subregions of the predictor space that pertain to levels of operating characteristics for the test that may be of practical interest. They show that such an approach leads to an approximately optimal score in this simulated example.

■

9.3.5 *Development and assessment of the combination score*

One simple approach to estimating the risk score function was demonstrated in Example 9.7. Modifications to this procedure are available, as are many alternative approaches mentioned in the previous section. It must be emphasized, however, that they all require some degree of modeling of the risk score function and that misspecification can therefore lead to a non-optimal combination score even in large samples. Flexible approaches are therefore appealing. Baker's nonparametric method, demonstrated with a simple example in Baker (2000), is particularly worth noting and may be worth extending to continuous covariates and/or higher dimensions. Some techniques, e.g. the modified logistic regression approach of McIntosh and Pepe (2002), require only that the risk score is modeled appropriately over a relevant subregion of the marker space and so reduce modeling requirements as well. Boosting and support vector machines share this feature to some extent, although further rigorous statistical investigation of their properties is warranted.

In many analyses one will want to both develop a combination function and to assess how well it performs. It is intuitively clear that the performance of a function will appear better when assessed with the data from which it was derived than it will appear with a new dataset. Ideally, a *test dataset* is reserved for evaluating the combination function, which is different from the original *training dataset* that is used to derive the function. The size of the test dataset can be chosen based on the sample size considerations of Chapter 8 for phase 2 validation studies. Alternatively, by employing cross-validation techniques, one can assess the performance with the training data in a relatively unbiased fashion. Cross-validation, however, requires that all steps for developing the combination function are specified in advance, so that they can be applied automatically in the cross-validation process. This is hard to do in practice if the process for developing $\hat{RS}(Y)$ is complex or involves any subjective judgments.

9.4 Concluding remarks

9.4.1 *Topics we only mention*

There are several additional topics relating to diagnostic test development and evaluation that must at least be mentioned here. Although a full treatment of these subjects cannot be given, we try to provide a few key references.

Establishing the reliability and reproducibility of a new test is often one of the first steps taken in its development. A test that does not yield a reproducible result cannot be informative of disease state. Laboratory assays must be reliable and quality control measures must be taken to ensure that results are reproducible over time and across technicians. When a test is to be disseminated across multiple testing sites, it must be documented that test results are reproducible across sites. In a similar vein, it is usually desirable that subjective assessments made by testers are reproducible, at least as far as recommendations for subsequent medical procedures are concerned. Thus, pathologists should agree on the histologic type of cancer presenting on a biopsy slide if treatment recommendations vary with histology.

When test results are either binary, ordinal or nominal, cross-tabulations along with the Kappa summary statistic are often used to summarize reliability within or between testers. Statistical techniques including log–linear modeling and latent class modeling have also been advocated. We refer to review articles by Landis and Koch (1977) and Nelson and Pepe (2000) for a discussion. For continuous test results, scatterplots along with intraclass correlation coefficients are typically employed. The concordance correlation coefficient (Lin, 1989) is a related measure that is natural for summarizing reproducibility. We are not aware of articles that provide specific guidance on study design for assessing reliability. Such developments would be a useful contribution in this area.

A second topic that must be mentioned has to do with the use of diagnostic tests in the scheme of providing healthcare to a patient. Medical decision making is a field where knowledge about tests, treatments, the patient populations and the costs are synthesized in order to understand the implications of different decisions to the patient. More broadly, the impact of different policies on populations are assessed. Thus the decision to implement a diagnostic test in practice can be assessed given disease prevalence, test accuracy, treatment success rates and costs. These techniques were mentioned in relation to phase 5 of medical test development, but probably should be undertaken much earlier too, in order to determine if the development of a test is even worthwhile. Key references for the techniques of medical decision making are Weinstein and Fineberg (1980) and Gold *et al.* (1996). A recent book by Sackett *et al.* (2000), which is geared towards practicing physicians, may also be of interest.

9.4.2 *New applications and new technologies*

This book concerns the assessment of diagnostic tests and biomarkers for distinguishing subjects with disease from those without. However, as mentioned in Section 1.1.1, the methods apply to a much wider variety of problems. For example, the state to be detected need not be 'disease' *per se*, but might represent prognosis, response to treatment, a change in behavior or indeed any dichotomous variable. The classification problem arises in many fields outside of medicine and, since this book in essence concerns the classification problem, the methods apply to many non-medical fields. Swets (1988) mentions weather forecasting, economic forecasting, criminal investigations and so forth.

The methods actually apply more generally, incorporating problems outside of classification as well. The framework presented fundamentally asks how much a measure, Y, differs between two groups, those denoted by $D = 1$ from those denoted by $D = 0$. From this point of view, we see that the methods can be used to evaluate treatment effects in a two-arm clinical trial (Example 4.2), or to compare health measures in exposed versus unexposed populations, for example. I think that methodologies such as ROC curves are potentially very valuable for these non-traditional applications.

There is a virtual explosion of new technologies emerging recently in medicine, many of which are proposed for the purposes of diagnosis and prediction. These include gene expression arrays, protein mass spectrometry, cell flow cytometry, and imaging modalities such as proton emission tomography. It is hoped that these technologies will provide precise biological information that will lead to better predictions about presence and course of disease than do currently available clinical measures. For example, the gene expression profile of a tumor may predict metastatic potential (van 't Veer *et al.*, 2002). It is critical that these technologies be subjected to rigorous scientific evaluations of their capacities to classify correctly before being disseminated for widespread use. Methods for the design and evaluation of the necessary research studies do exist but are not very well known. As described in Chapter 8, the approaches taken must be quite different from those for evaluating new treatments with which the biotechnology industry is already familiar. I particularly hope that this book will disseminate knowledge to move forward the rigorous evaluation of new technologies for prediction in medicine.

The new technologies also highlight some major gaps that exist in statistical methodology in this field. One is how to best combine the information from huge numbers of predictors. A gene expression array provides expression levels for thousands of genes, each of which can be considered a predictor or diagnostic test in its own right. Protein mass spectrometry similarly provides densities for thousands of protein mass units. Although estimation of the risk score or a monotone function of it seems appropriate (Result 9.4), it is not at all clear how to do this practice when the dimension of Y is very large. I hope that as resources are invested in the development of these emerging technologies, research efforts will also be invested in the development of statistical techniques that will guide their optimal use in practice.

9.5   Exercises

1. Consider the Moses algorithm for calculating the sROC curve. Show that the procedure is symmetric in its handling of the TPF and FPF values in the sense that the same curve will be calculated if 'disease' is considered to be the control state and 'non-disease' is the case state.

2. Show that the cumulative time-dependent classification probabilities, $\text{TPF}^C(l)$ and $\text{FPF}^C(l)$, can be calculated from the incident TPF function and the event time hazard rate function.

3. Prove formally Result 9.2.

4. Using part (i) of Result 9.3, prove parts (ii) and (iii).

BIBLIOGRAPHY

Agresti, A. (1990). *Categorical data analysis.* Wiley, New York.

Agresti, A. and Caffo, B. (2000). Simple and effective confidence intervals for proportions and differences of proportions result from adding two successes and two failures. *The American Statistician*, **54**, 280–8.

AHCPR (1999). *Publication No. 99-E0: Evidence report/technology assessment No. 5, evaluation of cervical cytology.* Agency for Health Care Policy and Research, Rockville, MD.

Alonzo, T. A. (2000). *Assessing accuracy of a continuous medical diagnostic or screening test in the presence of verification bias.* University of Washington, Seattle.

Alonzo, T. A. and Pepe, M. S. (1999). Using a combination of reference tests to assess the accuracy of a new diagnostic test. *Statistics in Medicine*, **18**, 2987–3003.

Alonzo, T. A. and Pepe, M. S. (2002). Distribution-free ROC analysis using binary regression techniques. *Biostatistics*, **3**, 421–32.

Alonzo, T. A., Pepe, M. S. and Lumley, T. (2002*a*). Estimating disease prevalence in two-phase studies. *Biostatistics.* (In press.)

Alonzo, T. A., Pepe, M. S. and Moskowitz, C. S. (2002*b*). Sample size calculations for comparative studies of medical tests for detecting presence of disease. *Statistics in Medicine*, **21**, 835–52.

American College of Radiology (1995). *Breast imaging reporting and data system.* American College of Radiology, Reston, Virginia.

Baker, S. G. (1991). Evaluating a new test using a reference test with estimated sensitivity and specificity. *Communications in Statistics*, **20**, 2739–52.

Baker, S. G. (1995). Evaluating multiple diagnostic tests with partial verification. *Biometrics*, **51**, 330–7.

Baker, S. G. (2000). Identifying combinations of cancer markers for further study as triggers of early intervention. *Biometrics*, **56**, 1082–7.

Baker, S. G. and Pinsky, P. F. (2001). A proposed design and analysis for comparing digital and analog mammography: Special receiver operating characteristic methods for cancer screening. *Journal of the American Statistical Association*, **96**, 421–8.

Balasubramanian, R. and Lagakos, S. W. (2001). Estimation of the timing of perinatal transmission of HIV. *Biometrics*, **57**, 1048–58.

Bamber, D. (1975). The area above the ordinal dominance graph and the area below the receiver operating characteristic graph. *Journal of Mathematical Psychology*, **12**, 387–415.

Barndorff-Nielsen, O. E. and Cox, D. R. (1989). *Asymptotic techniques for use in statistics*. Chapman and Hall, London.

Barratt, A., Irwig, L. M., Glasziou, P. P., Cumming, R. G., Raffle, A., Hicks, N., Gray, J. A. and Guyatt, G.H. (1999). Users' guides to the medical literature: XVII. How to use guidelines and recommendations about screening. Evidence-based medicine working group. *Journal of the American Medical Association*, **281**, 2029–34.

Bast, R. C. (1993). Perspective on the future of cancer markers. *Clinical Chemistry*, **39**, 2444–51.

Begg, C. B. (1987). Biases in the assessment of diagnostic tests. *Statistics in Medicine*, **6**, 411–23.

Begg, C. B. and Gray, R. (1984). Calculation of polychotomous logistic regression parameters using individualized regressions. *Biometrika*, **71**, 11–18.

Begg, C. B. and Greenes, R. A. (1983). Assessment of diagnostic tests when disease verification is subject to selection bias. *Biometrics*, **39**, 207–15.

Begg, C. B. and McNeil, B. J. (1988). Assessment of radiologic tests: Control of bias and other design considerations. *Radiology*, **167**, 565–9.

Begg, C. B. and Metz, C. E. (1990). Consensus diagnoses and 'gold standards'. *Medical Decision Making*, **10**, 29–30.

Begg, C. B., Greenes, R. A. and Iglewicz, B. (1986). The influence of uninterpretability on the assessment of diagnostic tests. *Journal of Chronic Disease*, **39**, 575–84.

Boyd, J. C. (1997). Mathematical tools for demonstrating the clinical usefulness of biochemical markers. *Scandinavian Journal of Clinical and Laboratory Investigation*, **Supplement 227**, 46–63.

Boyko, E. J. (1994). Ruling out or ruling in disease with the most sensitive or specific diagnostic test: Short cut or wrong turn? *Medical Decision Making*, **14**, 175–9.

Breiman, L., Friedman, J. H., Olshen, R. A. and Stone, C. J. (1984). *Classification and regression trees*. Wadsworth, Belmont, CA.

Breslow, N. E. and Day, N. E. (1980). *Statistical methods in cancer research. Volume 1: Analysis of case-control studies*. World Health Organization.

Cai, T. and Pepe, M. S. (2002). Semi-parametric ROC analysis to evaluate biomarkers for disease. *Journal of the American Statistical Association*. (In press.)

Cai, T., Pepe, M. S., Lumley, T., Zheng, Y. and Jenny, N. S. (2002). The sensitivity and specificity of markers for event times. (Unpublished manuscript.)

Campbell, G. (1994). Advances in statistical methodology for the evaluation of diagnostic and laboratory tests. *Statistics in Medicine*, **13**, 499–508.

Carroll, R. J., Ruppert, D. and Stefanski, L. A. (1995). *Measurement error in nonlinear models*. Chapman and Hall, London.

Cheng, H. and Macaluso, M. (1997). Comparison of the accuracy of two tests with a confirmatory procedure limited to positive results. *Epidemiology*, **8**, 104–6.

Cheng, H., Macaluso, M. and Waterbor, J. (1999). Letter to the editor: Estimation of relative and absolute test accuracy. *Epidemiology*, **10**, 566–8.

Cheng, H., Macaluso, M. and Hardin, J. M. (2000). Validity and coverage of estimates of relative accuracy. *Annals of Epidemiology*, **10**, 251–60.

Chock, C., Irwig, L. M., Berry, G. and Glasziou, P. P. (1997). Comparing dichotomous screening tests when individuals negative on both tests are not verified. *Journal of Clinical Epidemiology*, **50**, 1211–17.

Clayton, D., Spiegelhalter, D., Dunn, G. and Pickles, A. (1998). Analysis of longitudinal binary data from multiphase sampling. *Journal of the Royal Statistical Society, Series B*, **60**, 71–87.

Cole, P. and Morrison, A. S. (1980). Basic issues in population screening for cancer. *Journal of the National Cancer Institute*, **64**, 1263–72.

Cole, T. J. (1990). The LMS method for constructing normalized growth standards. *European Journal of Clinical Nutrition*, **44**, 45–60.

Cole, T. J. and Green, P. J. (1992). Smoothing reference centile curves: The LMS method and penalized likelihood. *Statistics in Medicine*, **11**, 1305–19.

Collett, D. (1994). *Modelling survival data in medical research*. Chapman and Hall/CRC, London.

Coughlin, S. S., Trock, B., Criqui, M. H., Pickle, L. W., Browner, D. and Tefft, M. C. (1992). The logistic modeling of sensitivity, specificity and predictive value of a diagnostic test. *Journal of Clinical Epidemiology*, **45**, 1–7.

Cristianini, N. and Shawe-Taylor, J. (2000). *An introduction to support vector machines: And other kernel-based learning methods*. Cambridge University Press.

DeLong, E. R., DeLong, D. M. and Clarke-Pearson, D. L. (1988). Comparing the areas under two or more correlated receiver operating characteristic curves: A nonparametric approach. *Biometrics*, **44**, 837–45.

Dempster, A. P., Laird, N. M. and Rubin, D. B. (1977). Maximum likelihood from incomplete data via the EM algorithm. *Journal of the Royal Statistical Society B*, **39**, 1–38.

Dendukuri, N. and Joseph, L. (2001). Bayesian approaches to modeling the conditional dependence between multiple diagnostic tests. *Biometrics*, **57**, 158–67.

DeSutter, P., Coibion, M., Vosse, M., Hertens, D., Huet, F., Wesling, F., Wayembergh, M., Bourdon, C. and Autier, P. H. (1998). A multicenter study comparing cervicography and cytology in the detection of cervical intraepithelial neoplasia. *British Journal of Obstetrics and Gynaecology*, **105**, 613–20.

Diamond, G. A. (1992). Clinical epistemology of sensitivity and specificity. *Journal of Clinical Epidemiology*, **45**, 9–13.

Diggle, P., Heagerty, P. J., Liang, K. Y. and Zeger, S. L. (2002). *Analysis of longitudinal data*. Oxford University Press.

Dodd, L. E. (2001). *Regression methods for areas and partial areas under the ROC curve*. Ph.D. thesis, University of Washington.

Dorfman, D. D. and Alf, E. (1968). Maximum likelihood estimation of parameters of signal detection theory—a direct solution. *Psychometrika*, **33**, 117–24.

Dorfman, D. D. and Alf, E. (1969). Maximum likelihood estimation of parameters of signal detection theory and determination of confidence intervals–rating method data. *Journal of Mathematical Psychology*, **6**, 487–96.

Dorfman, D. D., Berbaum, K. S. and Metz, C. E. (1992). Receiver operating characteristic rating analysis: Generalization to the population of readers and patients with the jack-knife method. *Investigative Radiology*, **27**, 723–31.

Dorfman, D. D., Berbaum, K. S. and Lenth, R. (1995). Multireader, multicase receiver operating characteristic methodology: A bootstrap analysis. *Academic Radiology*, **2**, 626–33.

Dorfman, D. D., Berbaum, K. S., Metz, C. E., Lenth, R. V., Hanley, J. A. and Dagga, H. A. (1997). Proper ROC analysis: The bigamma model. *Academic Radiology*, **4**, 138–49.

Dujardin, B., van den Ende, J., van Gompel, A., Unger, J. P. and van der Stuyft, P. (1994). Likelihood ratios: A real improvement for clinical decision making? *European Journal of Epidemiology*, **10**, 29–36.

Efron, B. (1991). Regression percentiles using asymmetric squared error loss. *Statistica Sinica*, **1**, 93–125.

Efron, B. and Tibshirani, R. J. (1993). *An introduction to the bootstrap* (1st edn). Chapman and Hall/CRC Press, New York.

Egan, J. P. (1975). *Signal detection theory and ROC analysis*. Academic Press, New York.

Etzioni, E., Cha, R. and Cowen, M. (1999a). Serial prostate specific antigen screening for prostate cancer: A computer model evaluates competing strategies. *Journal of Urology*, **162**, 741–8.

Etzioni, R., Pepe, M., Longton, G., Hu, C. and Goodman, G. (1999*b*). Incorporating the time dimension in receiver operating characteristic curves: A case study of prostate cancer. *Medical Decision Making*, **19**, 242–51.

Fagan, T. J. (1975). Letter: Nomogram for Bayes theorem. *New England Journal of Medicine*, **293**, 257.

Fahey, M. T., Irwig, L. M. and Macaskill, P. (1995). Meta-analysis of Pap test accuracy. *American Journal of Epidemiology*, **141**, 680–9.

Feinstein, A. R. (2002). Misguided efforts and future challenges for research on 'diagnostic tests'. *Journal of Epidemiology and Community Health*, **56**, 330–2.

Ferraz, M. B., Walter, S. D., Heymann, R. and Atra, E. (1995). Sensitivity and specificity of different diagnostic criteria for Behcet's disease according to the latent class approach. *British Journal of Rheumatology*, **34**, 932–5.

Fine, J. P. and Bosch, R. J. (2000). Risk assessment via a robust probit model, with application to toxicology. *Journal of the American Statistical Association*, **95**, 375–82.

Fleischmann, K. E., Hunink, M. G. M., Kuntz, K. M. and Douglas, P. S. (1998). Exercise echocardiography or exercise SPECT imaging? *The Journal of the American Medical Association*, **280**, 913–20.

Fletcher, S. W., Black, W., Harris, R., Rimer, B. K. and Shapiro, S. (1993). Report of the international workshop on screening for breast cancer. *Journal of the National Cancer Institute*, **85**, 1644–56.

Foulkes, A. S. and DeGruttola, V. (2002). Characterizing the relationship between HIV-1 genotype and phenotype: Prediction-based classification. *Biometrics*, **58**, 145–56.

Friedman, J., Hastie, T. and Tibshirani, R. (2000). Additive logistic regression: A statistical view of boosting. *Annals of Statistics*, **28**, 400–7.

Friedman, L. M., Furberg, C. D. and DeMets, D. L. (1996). *Fundamentals of clinical trials.* P. S. G. Publications, Littleton, MA.

Gail, M. H. and Green, S. B. (1976). A generalization of the one-sided two-sample Kolmogorov–Smirnov statistic for evaluating diagnostic tests. *Biometrics*, **32**, 561–70.

Gart, J. J. and Buck, A. A. (1966). Comparison of a screening test and a reference test in epidemiologic studies II: A probabilistic model for the comparison of diagnostic tests. *American Journal of Epidemiology*, **83**, 593–602.

Gatsonis, C. A. (1995). Random-effects models for diagnostic accuracy data. *Academic Radiology*, **2**, S14–21.

Gatsonis, C. A., Begg, C. B. and Wieand, S. (1995). Introduction to advances in statistical methods for diagnostic radiology: A symposium. *Academic Radiology*, **2**, S1–3.

Georgiadis, M. P., Johnson, W. O., Singh, R. and Gardner, I. A. (2003). Correlation-adjusted estimation of sensitivity and specificity of two diagnostic tests. *Applied Statistics*. (In press.)

Giard, R. W. and Hermans, J. (1993). The evaluation and interpretation of cervical cytology: Application of the likelihood ratio concept. *Cytopathology*, **4**, 131–7.

Gold, M. R., Siegel, J. E., Russell, L. and Weinstein, M. C. (1996). *Cost-effectiveness in health and medicine*. Oxford University Press, New York.

Gray, R., Begg, C. and Greenes, R. (1984). Construction of receiver operating characteristic curves when disease verification is subject to selection bias. *Medical Decision Making*, **4**, 151–64.

Green, D. M. and Swets, J. A. (1966). *Signal detection theory and psychophysics*. Wiley, New York.

Green, T. A., Black, C. M. and Johnson, R. E. (1998). Evaluation of bias in diagnostic test sensitivity and specificity estimates computed by discrepant analysis. *Journal of Clinical Microbiology*, **36**, 375–81.

Green, T. A., Black, C. M. and Johnson, R. E. (2001). Letter to the editor: In defense of discrepant analysis. *Journal of Clinical Epidemiology*, **54**, 210–11.

Greenhouse, S. W. and Mantel, N. (1950). The evaluation of diagnostic tests. *Biometrics*, **6**, 399–412.

Guyatt, G. H., Tugwell, P. X., Feeny, D. H., Haynes, R. B. and Drummond, M. (1986). A framework for clinical evaluation of diagnostic technologies. *Canadian Medical Association Journal*, **134**, 587–94.

Hadgu, A. (1996). The discrepancy in discrepant analysis. *The Lancet*, **348**, 592–3.

Hadgu, A. (1997). Bias in the evaluation of DNA-amplification tests for detecting chlamydia trachomatis. *Statistics in Medicine*, **16**, 1391–9.

Hadgu, A. (2001). Letter to the editor: Response. *Journal of Clinical Epidemiology*, **54**, 212–15.

Hajian-Tilaki, K. O., Hanley, J. A., Joseph, L. and Collet, J. P. (1997). Extension of receiver operating characteristic analysis to data concerning multiple signal detection tasks. *Academic Radiology*, **4**, 222–9.

Hamill, P. V., Drizd, T. A., Johnson, C. L., Reed, R. B. and Roche, A. F. (1977). *NCHS growth curves for children birth–18 years*. United States, Vital Health Statistics 11, pp. 1–74. Washington, DC.

Hanley, J. A. (1988). The robustness of the 'binormal' assumptions used in fitting ROC curves. *Medical Decision Making*, **8**, 197–203.

Hanley, J. A. (1989). Receiver operating characteristic (ROC) methodology: The state of the art. *Critical Reviews in Diagnostic Imaging*, **29**, 307–35.

Hanley, J. A. (1996). The use of the 'binormal' model for parametric ROC analysis of quantitative diagnostic tests. *Statistics in Medicine*, **15**, 1575–85.

Hanley, J. A. and Hajian-Tilaki, K. O. (1997). Sampling variability of nonparametric estimates of the areas under receiver operating characteristic curves: An update. *Academic Radiology*, **4**, 49–58.

Hanley, J. A. and McNeil, B. J. (1982). The meaning and use of the area under an ROC curve. *Radiology*, **143**, 29–36.

Hauck, W. W., Hyslop, T. and Anderson, S. (2000). Generalized treatment effects for clinical trials. *Statistics in Medicine*, **15**, 887–99.

He, X. (1997). Quantile curves without crossing. *The American Statistician*, **51**, 186–92.

Heagerty, P. J. and Pepe, M. S. (1999). Semiparametric estimation of regression quantiles with application to standardizing weight for height and age in US children. *Applied Statistics*, **48**, 533–51.

Heagerty, P. J., Lumley, T. and Pepe, M. S. (2000). Time-dependent ROC curves for censored survival data and a diagnostic marker. *Biometrics*, **56**, 337–44.

Henderson, R., Diggle, P. and Dobson, A. (2000). Joint modelling of longitudinal measurements and event time data. *Biostatistics*, **1**, 465–80.

Henkelman, R. M., Kay, I. and Bronskill, M. J. (1990). Receiver operator characteristic (ROC) analysis without truth. *Medical Decision Making*, **10**, 24–9.

Hilgers, R. A. (1991). Distribution-free confidence bounds for ROC curves. *Methods of Information in Medicine*, **30**, 96–101.

Horvitz, D. G. and Thompson, D. J. (1952). A generalization of sampling without replacement from a finite universe. *Journal of the American Statistical Association*, **47**, 663–85.

Hosmer, D. W. and Lemeshow, S. (2000). *Applied logistic regression*. Wiley, New York.

Hsieh, F. and Turnbull, B. W. (1996). Nonparametric and semiparametric estimation of the receiver operating characteristic curve. *Annals of Statistics*, **24**, 25–40.

Hui, S. L. and Zhou, X. H. (1998). Evaluation of diagnostic tests without gold standards. *Statistical Methods in Medical Research*, **7**, 354–70.

Hunink, M. G. M., Richardson, D. K., Doubilet, P. M. and Begg, C. B. (1990). Testing for fetal pulmonary maturity: ROC analysis involving covariates, verification bias, and combination testing. *Medical Decision Making*, **10**, 201–11.

Hunink, M. G. M., Polak, J. F., Barlan, M. M. and O'Leary, D. H. (1993). Detection and quantification of carotid artery stenosis: Efficacy of various Doppler velocity parameters. *American Journal of Roentgenology*, **160**, 619–25.

ICH E9 Expert Working Group (1999). Statistical principles for clinical trials: ICH harmonised triparite guideline. *Statistics in Science*, **18**, 1905–42.

Irwig, L. M., Groeneveld, H. T., Pretorius, J. P. and Hnizdo, E. (1985). Relative observer accuracy for dichotomized variables. *Journal of Chronic Diseases*, **38**, 899–906.

Irwig, L. M., Glasziou, P. P., Berry, G., Chock, C., Mock, P. and Simpson, J. M. (1994a). Efficient study designs to assess the accuracy of screening tests. *American Journal of Epidemiology*, **140**, 759–69.

Irwig, L. M., Tosteson, A., Gatsonis, C. A., Lau, J., Colditz, G., Chalmers, T. and Mosteller, F. (1994b). Guidelines for meta-analyses evaluating diagnostic tests. *Annals of Internal Medicine*, **120**, 667–76.

Irwig, L. M., Macaskill, P., Glasziou, P. P. and Fahey, M. (1995). Meta-analytic methods for diagnostic test accuracy. *Journal of Clinical Epidemiology*, **48**, 119–30.

Irwig, L., Bossuyt, P., Glasziou, P., Gatsonis, C. and Lijmer, J. (2002). Designing studies to ensure that estimates of test accuracy are transferable. *British Medical Journal*, **324**, 669–71.

Ishwaran, H. and Gatsonis, C. A. (2000). A general class of hierarchical ordinal regression models with applications to correlated ROC analysis. *The Canadian Journal of Statistics*, **28**, 731–50.

Jiang, Y., Metz, C. E. and Nishikawa, R. M. (1996). A receiver operating characteristic partial area index for highly sensitive diagnostic tests. *Radiology*, **201**, 745–50.

Joseph, L., Gyorkos, T. W. and Coupal, L. (1995). Bayesian estimation of disease prevalence and the parameters of diagnostic tests in the absence of a gold standard. *American Journal of Epidemiology*, **141**, 263–72.

Kalbfleisch, J. D. and Prentice, R. L. (1980). *The statistical analysis of failure time data*. Wiley, New York.

Kerlikowske, K., Grady, D., Barclay, J., Sickles, E. A. and Ernster, V. (1996). Likelihood ratios for modern screening mammography. Risk of breast cancer based on age and mammographic interpretation. *Journal of the American Medical Association*, **276**, 39–43.

Koblin, B. A., Heagerty, P. J., Sheon, A., Buchbinder, S., Celum, C. and Douglas, J. M. (1998). Readiness of high-risk populations in the HIV Network for Prevention Trials to participate in HIV vaccine efficacy trials in the United States. *AIDS*, **12**, 785–93.

Koenker, R. and Bassett, G. (1978). Regression quantiles. *Econometrica*, **46**, 33–50.

Kosinski, A. S. and Flanders, W. D. (1999). Evaluating the exposure and disease relationship with adjustment for different types of exposure misclassification: A regression approach. *Statistics in Medicine*, **18**, 2795–808.

Kraemer, H. C. (1992). *Evaluating medical tests: Objective and quantitative guidelines.* Sage Publications, Newbury Park, CA.

Kwok, Y., Kim, C., Grady, D., Segal, M. and Redberg, R. (1999). Meta-analysis of exercise testing to detect coronary artery disease in women. *American Journal of Cardiology*, **83**, 660–6.

Lachenbruch, P. A. and Lynch, C. J. (1998). Assessing screening tests: Extensions of McNemar's test. *Statistics in Medicine*, **17**, 2207–17.

Landis, R. J. and Koch, G. G. (1977). The measurement of observer agreement for categorical data. *Biometrika*, **33**, 159–74.

Lee, W. C. (1999). Probabilistic analysis of global performances of diagnostic tests: Interpreting the Lorenz curve-based summary measures. *Statistics in Medicine*, **18**, 455–71.

Lee, W. C. and Hsiao, C. K. (1996). Alternative summary indices for the receiver operating characteristic curve. *Epidemiology*, **7**, 605–11.

Leisenring, W. and Pepe, M. S. (1998). Regression modelling of diagnostic likelihood ratios for the evaluation of medical diagnostic tests. *Biometrics*, **54**, 444–52.

Leisenring, W., Pepe, M. S. and Longton, G. (1997). A marginal regression modelling framework for evaluating medical diagnostic tests. *Statistics in Medicine*, **16**, 1263–81.

Leisenring, W., Alonzo, T. and Pepe, M. S. (2000). Comparisons of predictive values of binary medical diagnostic tests for paired designs. *Biometrics*, **56**, 345–51.

Liang, K. Y. and Zeger, S. L. (1986). Longitudinal data analysis using generalized linear models. *Biometrika*, **73**, 13–22.

Lilienfeld, A. M. (1974). Some limitations and problems of screening for cancer. *Cancer*, **33**, **Supplement**, 1720–4.

Lin, L. (1989). A concordance correlation coefficient to evaluate reproducibility. *Biometrics*, **45**, 255–68.

Little, R. J. A. and Rubin, D. B. (1987). *Statistical analysis with missing data.* Wiley, New York.

Lusted, L. B. (1960). Logical analysis in roentgen diagnosis. *Radiology*, **74**, 178–93.

Ma, G. and Hall, W. J. (1993). Confidence bands for receiver operating characteristic curves. *Medical Decision Making*, **13**, 191–7.

Mahoney, W. J., Szatmari, P., MacLean, J. E., Bryson, S. E., Bartolucci, G., Walter, S. D., Jones, M. B. and Zwaigenbaum, L. (1998). Reliability and accuracy of differentiating pervasive developmental disorder subtypes. *Journal of the American Academy of Child and Adolescent Psychiatry*, **37**, 278–85.

Mantel, N. (1951). Evaluation of a class of diagnostic tests. *Biometrics*, **7**, 240–6.

Marshall, R. J. (1989). The predictive value of simple rules for combining two diagnostic tests. *Biometrics*, **45**, 1213–22.

McClish, D. K. (1989). Analyzing a portion of the ROC curve. *Medical Decision Making*, **9**, 190–5.

McCullagh, P. and Nelder, J. A. (1999). *Generalized linear models*. Chapman and Hall, London.

McIntosh, M. and Pepe, M. S. (2002). Combining several screening tests: Optimality of the risk score. *Biometrics*, **58**, 657–64.

McLachlan, G. J. (1992). *Discriminant analysis and statistical pattern recognition*. Wiley, New York.

Mee, R. W. (1990). Confidence intervals for probabilities and tolerance regions based on a generalization of the Mann–Whitney statistic. *Journal of the American Statistical Association*, **85**, 793–800.

Metz, C. E. (1978). Basic principles of ROC analysis. *Seminars in Nuclear Medicine*, **8**, 283–98.

Metz, C. E. (1989). Some practical issues of experimental design and data analysis in radiologic ROC studies. *Investigative Radiology*, **24**, 234–45.

Metz, C. E. and Kronman, H. B. (1980). Statistical significance tests for binormal ROC curves. *Journal of Mathematical Psychology*, **22**, 218–43.

Metz, C. E. and Pan, X. (1999). 'Proper' binormal ROC curves: Theory and maximum-likelihood estimation. *Journal of Mathematical Psychology*, **43**, 1–33.

Metz, C. E., Herman, B. A. and Roe, C. A. (1998a). Statistical comparison of two ROC curve estimates obtained from partially-paired datasets. *Medical Decision Making*, **18**, 110–21.

Metz, C. E., Herman, B. A. and Shen, J. H. (1998b). Maximum likelihood estimation of receiver operating characteristic (ROC) curves from continuously-distributed data. *Statistics in Medicine*, **17**, 1033–53.

Miller, W. C. (1998a). Bias in discrepant analysis: When two wrongs don't make a right. *Journal of Clinical Epidemiology*, **51**, 219–31.

Miller, W. C. (1998b). Editorial response: Can we do better than discrepant analysis for new diagnostic test evaluation? *Clinical Infectious Diseases*, **27**, 1186–93.

Moses, L. E., Shapiro, D. and Littenberg, B. (1993). Combining independent studies of a diagnostic test into a summary ROC curve: Data-analytic approaches and some additional considerations. *Statistics in Medicine*, **12**, 1293–316.

Muller, C., Wasserman, H. J., Erlank, P., Klopper, J. F., Morkel, H. R. and Ellmann, A. (1989). Optimisation of density and contrast yielded by multi-format photographic imagers used for scintigraphy. *Physics in Medicine and Biology*, **34**, 473–81.

Nelson, J. C. and Pepe, M. S. (2000). Statistical description of interrater variability in ordinal ratings. *Statistical Methods in Medical Research*, **9**, 475–96.

Neyman, J. and Pearson, E. S. (1933). On the problem of the most efficient tests of statistical hypothesis. *Philosophical Transactions of the Royal Society of London, Series A*, **231**, 289–337.

Norton, S. J., Gorga, M. P., Widen, J. E., Folsom, R. C., Sininger, Y., Cone-Wesson, B., Vohr, B. R., Mascher, K. and Fletcher, K. (2000). Identification of neonatal hearing impairment: Evaluation of transient evoked otoacoustic emission, distortion product otoacoustic emission, and auditory brain stem response test performance. *Ear and Hearing*, **21**, 508–28.

Obuchowski, N. A. (1994). Computing sample size for receiver operating characteristic studies. *Investigative Radiology*, **29**, 238–43.

Obuchowski, N. A. (1995). Multireader, multimodality receiver operating characteristic curve studies: Hypothesis testing and sample size estimation using an analysis of variance approach with dependent observations. *Academic Radiology*, **2**, S22–9.

Obuchowski, N. A. (1997a). Nonparametric analysis of clustered ROC curve data. *Biometrics*, **53**, 567–78.

Obuchowski, N. A. (1997b). Testing for equivalence of diagnostic tests. *American Journal of Roentgenology*, **168**, 13–17.

Obuchowski, N. A. (1998). Sample size calculations in studies of test accuracy. *Statistical Methods in Medical Research*, **7**, 371–92.

Obuchowski, N. A. and Lieber, M. L. (1998). Confidence intervals for the receiver operating characteristic area in studies with small samples. *Academic Radiology*, **5**, 561–71.

Obuchowski, N. A. and Lieber, M. L. (2002). Confidence bounds when the estimated ROC area is 1.0. *Academic Radiology*, **9**, 526–30.

Obuchowski, N. A. and McClish, D. K. (1997). Sample size determination for diagnostic accuracy studies involving binormal ROC curve indices. *Statistics in Medicine*, **16**, 1529–42.

Obuchowski, N. A. and Zhou, Z. H. (2002). Prospective studies of diagnostic test accuracy when disease prevalence is low. *Biostatistics*. (In press.)

Obuchowski, N. A., Graham, R. J., Baker, M. E. and Powell, K. A. (2001). Ten criteria for effective screening: Their application to multislice CT screening for pulmonary and colorectal cancers. *American Journal of Roentgenology*, **176**, 1357–62.

Ogilvie, J. C. and Creelman, C. D. (1968). Maximum-likelihood estimation of receiver operating characteristic curve parameters. *Journal of Mathematical Psychology*, **5**, 377–91.

Pan, W. and Louis, T. A. (2000). A note on marginal linear regression with correlated response data. *American Statistician*, **54**, 191–5.

Pepe, M. S. (1997). A regression modelling framework for receiver operating characteristic curves in medical diagnostic testing. *Biometrika*, **84**, 595–608.

Pepe, M. S. (1998). Three approaches to regression analysis of receiver operating characteristic curves for continuous test results. *Biometrics*, **54**, 124–35.

Pepe, M. S. (2000). An interpretation for the ROC curve and inference using GLM procedures. *Biometrics*, **56**, 352–9.

Pepe, M. S. and Alonzo, T. A. (2001a). Author's reply: Using a combination of reference tests to assess the accuracy of a new diagnostic test. *Statistics in Medicine*, **20**, 658–60.

Pepe, M. S. and Alonzo, T. A. (2001b). Comparing disease screening tests when true disease status is ascertained only for screen positives. *Biostatistics*, **2**, 249–60.

Pepe, M. S. and Anderson, G. L. (1994). A cautionary note on inference for marginal regression models with longitudinal data and general correlated response data. *Communications in Statistics*, **23**, 939–51.

Pepe, M. S. and Thompson, M. L. (2000). Combining diagnostic test results to increase accuracy. *Biostatistics*, **1**, 123–40.

Pepe, M. S., Reilly, M. and Fleming, T. R. (1994). Auxiliary outcome data and the mean score method. *Journal of Statistical Planning and Inference*, **42**, 137–60.

Pepe, M. S., Whitaker, R. C. and Seidel, K. (1999). Estimating and comparing univariate associations with application to the prediction of adult obesity. *Statistics in Medicine*, **18**, 163–73.

Pepe, M. S., Etzioni, R., Feng, Z., Potter, J. D., Thompson, M., Thornquist, M., Winget, M. and Yasui, Y. (2001). Phases of biomarker development for early detection of cancer. *Journal of the National Cancer Institute*, **93**, 1054–61.

Pepe, M. S., Longton, G., Anderson, G. and Schummer, M. (2003). Selecting differentially expressed genes from microarray experiments. *Biometrics*. (In press.)

Pocock, S. J. (1982). *Clinical trials: A practical approach*. Wiley, New York.

Qu, Y. and Hadgu, A. (1998). A model for evaluating sensitivity and specificity for correlated diagnostic tests in efficacy studies with an imperfect reference test. *Journal of the American Statistical Association*, **93**, 920–8.

Qu, Y., Tan, M. and Kutner, M. H. (1996). Random effects models in latent class analysis for evaluating accuracy of diagnostic test. *Biometrics*, **52**, 797–810.

Ramsey, B. W., Pepe, M. S., Quan, J. M., Otto, K. L., Montgomery, A. B., Williams-Warren, J., Vasiljev, K. M., Borowitz, D., Bowman, C. M., Marshall, B. C., Marshall, S. and Smith, A. L. (1999). Efficacy and safety of chronic intermittent administration of inhaled tobramycin in patients with cystic fibrosis. *New England Journal of Medicine*, **340**, 23–30.

Reilly, M. and Pepe, M. S. (1995). A mean-score method for missing and auxiliary covariate data in regression models. *Biometrika*, **82**, 299–314.

Ripley, B. D. (1996). *Pattern recognition and neural networks*. Cambridge University Press.

Robins, J. M. and Rotnitzky, A. (1995). Semiparametric efficiency in multivariate regression models with missing data. *Journal of the American Statistical Association*, **90**, 122–9.

Robins, J. M., Rotnitzky, A. and Zhao, L. P. (1994). Estimation of regression coefficients when some regressors are not always observed. *Journal of the American Statistical Association*, **89**, 846–66.

Rodenberg, C. and Zhou, X. H. (2000). ROC curve estimation when covariates affect the verification process. *Biometrics*, **56**, 1256–62.

Roe, C. A. and Metz, C. E. (1997). Variance-component modeling in the analysis of receiver operating characteristic index estimates. *Academic Radiology*, **4**, 587–600.

Ross, K. S., Carter, H. B., Pearson, J. D. and Guess, H. A. (2000). Comparative efficiency of prostate-specific antigen screening strategies for prostate cancer detection. *Journal of the American Medical Association*, **284**, 1399–405.

Ruczinski, I., Kooperberg, C. and LeBlanc, M. L. (2003). Logic regression. *Journal of Computational and Graphical Statistics*. (In press.)

Rutter, C. M. and Gatsonis, C. A. (1995). Regression methods for meta-analysis of diagnostic test data. *Academic Radiology*, **2**, **Supplement 1**, S48–56.

Rutter, C. M. and Gatsonis, C. A. (2001). A hierarchical regression approach to meta-analysis of diagnostic test accuracy evaluators. *Statistics in Medicine*, **20**, 2865–84.

Sackett, D. L., Haynes, R. B. and Tugwell, P. (1985). *Clinical epidemiology: A basic science for clinical medicine*. Little & Brown, Boston.

Sackett, D. L., Strauss, S. E., Richardson, W. S., Rosenberg, W. and Haynes, R. B. (2000). *Evidence-based medicine: How to practice and teach EBM*. Churchill Livingstone, Edinburgh.

Schachter, J. (2001). Letter to the editor: In defense of discrepant analysis. *Journal of Clinical Epidemiology*, **54**, 211–12.

Schapire, R., Freund, Y., Bartlett, P. and Lee, W. (1998). Boosting the margin: A new explanation for the effectiveness of voting methods. *Annals of Statistics*, **26**, 1651–86.

Schatzkin, A., Connor, R. J., Taylor, P. R. and Bunnag, B. (1987). Comparing new and old screening tests when a reference procedure cannot be performed on all screenees. *American Journal of Epidemiology*, **125**, 672–8.

Selby, J. V., Friedman, G. D., Quesenberry, C. P. and Weiss, N. S. (1992). A case-control study of screening sigmoidoscopy and mortality from colorectal cancer. *New England Journal of Medicine*, **326**, 653–7.

Shapiro, D. E. (1999). The interpretation of diagnostic tests. *Statistical Methods in Medical Research*, **8**, 113–34.

Shorack, G. R. and Wellner, J. A. (1986). *Empirical processes with applications to statistics*. Wiley, New York.

Simel, D. L., Samsa, G. P. and Matchar, D. B. (1991). Likelihood ratios with confidence: Sample size estimation for diagnostic test studies. *Journal of Clinical Epidemiology*, **44**, 763–70.

Simonoff, J. S., Hochberg, Y. and Reiser, B. (1986). Alternative estimation procedures for Pr(X less than Y) in categorized data. *Biometrics*, **42**, 895–907.

Simpson, A. J. and Fitter, M. J. (1973). What is the best index of detectability? *Psychological Bulletin*, **80**, 481–8.

Skates, S. J., Pauler, D. K. and Jacobs, I. J. (2001). Screening based on the risk of cancer calculation from Bayesian hierarchical change-point models of longitudinal markers. *Journal of the American Statistical Association*, **96**, 429–39.

Smith, D. S., Bullock, A. D. and Catalona, W. J. (1997). Racial differences in operating characteristics of prostate cancer screening tests. *The Journal of Urology*, **158**, 1861–6.

Smith, P. J. and Hadgu, A. (1992). Sensitivity and specificity for correlated observations. *Statistics in Medicine*, **11**, 1503–9.

Song, H. H. (1997). Analysis of correlated ROC areas in diagnostic testing. *Biometrics*, **53**, 370–82.

Spiegelhalter, D. J., Thomas, A., Best, N. G. and Gilks, W. R. (1996). *BUGS: Bayesian inference using Gibbs sampling*. Software, version 0.5. MRC Biostatistics Unit, Cambridge.

Staquet, M., Rozencweig, M., Lee, Y. J. and Muggia, F. M. (1981). Methodology for the assessment of new dichotomous diagnostic tests. *Journal of Chronic Diseases*, **34**, 599–610.

Sternberg, M. R. and Hadgu, A. (2001). A GEE approach to estimating sensitivity and specificity and coverage properties of the confidence intervals. *Statistics in Medicine*, **20**, 1529–39.

Stover, L., Gorga, M. P., Neely, S. T. and Montoya, D. (1996). Toward optimizing the clinical utility of distortion product otoacoustic emission measurements. *Journal of the Acoustical Society of America*, **100**, 956–67.

Su, J. Q. and Liu, J. S. (1993). Linear combinations of multiple diagnostic markers. *Journal of the American Statistical Association*, **88**, 1350–5.

Swets, J. A. (1986). Indices of discrimination or diagnostic accuracy: Their ROCs and implied models. *Psychological Bulletin*, **99**, 100–17.

Swets, J. A. (1988). Measuring the accuracy of diagnostic systems. *Science*, **240**, 1285–93.

Swets, J. A. and Pickett, R. M. (1982). *Evaluation of diagnostic systems: Methods from signal detection theory*. Academic Press, New York.

Szatmari, P., Volkmar, F. and Walter, S. (1995). Evaluation of diagnostic criteria for autism using latent class models. *Journal of the American Academy of Child and Adolescent Psychiatry*, **34**, 216–22.

Thibodeau, L. A. (1981). Evaluating diagnostic tests. *Biometrics*, **37**, 801–4.

Thompson, M. L. and Zucchini, W. (1989). On the statistical analysis of ROC curves. *Statistics in Medicine*, **8**, 1277–90.

Toledano, A. and Gatsonis, C. A. (1995). Regression analysis of correlated receiver operating characteristic data. *Academic Radiology*, **2**, **Supplement 1**, S30–6.

Torrance-Rynard, V. L. and Walter, S. D. (1997). Effects of dependent errors in the assessment of diagnostic test performance. *Statistics in Medicine*, **16**, 2157–75.

Tosteson, A. A. N. and Begg, C. B. (1988). A general regression methodology for ROC curve estimation. *Medical Decision Making*, **8**, 204–15.

Tsimikas, J. V., Bosch, R. J., Coull, B. A. and Barmi, H. E. (2002). Profile-likelihood inference for highly accurate diagnostic tests. *Biometrics*. (In press.)

Vacek, P. M. (1985). The effect of conditional dependence on the evaluation of diagnostic tests. *Biometrics*, **41**, 959–68.

Vamvakas, E. C. (1998). Meta-analyses of studies of the diagnostic accuracy of laboratory tests: A review of the concepts and methods. *Archives of Pathology and Laboratory Medicine*, **122**, 675–85.

van 't Veer, L. J., Dai, H., van de Vijver, M. J., He, Y. D., Hart, A. A. M. *et al.* (2002). Gene expression profiling predicts clinical outcome of breast cancer. *Nature*, **415**, 530–6.

Venkatraman, E. S. (2000). A permutation test to compare receiver operating characteristic curves. *Biometrics*, **56**, 1134–8.

Venkatraman, E. S. and Begg, C. B. (1996). A distribution-free procedure for comparing receiver operating characteristic curves from a paired experiment. *Biometrika*, **83**, 835–48.

Walter, S. D. (1999). Estimation of test sensitivity and specificity when disease confirmation is limited to positive results. *Epidemiology*, **10**, 67–72.

Walter, S. D. and Irwig, L. M. (1988). Estimation of test error rates, disease prevalences, and relative risk from misclassified data: A review. *Journal of Clinical Epidemiology*, **41**, 923–37.

Walter, S. D., Frommer, D. J. and Cook, R. J. (1991). The estimation of sensitivity and specificity in colorectal cancer screening methods. *Cancer Detection and Prevention*, **15**, 465–9.

Weiner, D. A., Ryan, T. J., McCabe, C. H., Kennedy, J. W., Schloss, M., Tristani, F., Chaitman, B. R. and Fisher, L. D. (1979). Correlations among history of angina, ST-segment response and prevalence of coronary artery disease in the coronary artery surgery study (CASS). *New England Journal of Medicine*, **301**, 230–5.

Weinstein, M. C. and Fineberg, H. V. (1980). *Clinical decision analysis*. Saunders, Philadelphia.

Weiss, N. S. (1996). *Clinical epidemiology: The study of the outcome of illness* (2nd edn). Oxford University Press, New York.

Weiss, N. S. (1997). Case-control studies of the efficacy of screening for cancer: Can we earn them some respect? *Journal of Medical Screening*, **4**, 57–9.

Whitaker, R. C., Wright, J. A., Pepe, M. S., Seidel, K. D. and Dietz, W. H. (1997). Predicting adult obesity from childhood and parent obesity. *New England Journal of Medicine*, **337**, 869–73.

Wieand, S., Gail, M. H., James, B. R. and James, K. L. (1989). A family of nonparametric statistics for comparing diagnostic markers with paired or unpaired data. *Biometrika*, **76**, 585–92.

Wilson, J. M. G. and Jungner, Y. G. (1968). *Principles and practice of screening for disease*. Public Health Papers 34. World Health Organization, Geneva, Switzerland.

Woolas, R. P., Conaway, M. R., Xu, F., Jacobs, I. J. *et al.* (1995). Combinations of multiple serum markers are superior to individual assays for discriminating malignant from benign pelvic masses. *Gynaecologic Oncology*, **59**, 111–16.

Wu, C., Lee, M., Yin, S., Yang, D. and Cheng, S. (1992). Comparison of polymerase chain reaction, monoclonal antibody based enzyme immunoassay, and cell culture for detection of chlamydia trachomatis in genital specimens. *Sexually Transmitted Diseases*, **19**, 193–7.

Wulfsohn, M. S. and Tsiatis, A. A. (1997). A joint model for survival and longitudinal data measured with error. *Biometrics*, **53**, 330–9.

Yang, I. and Becker, M. P. (1997). Latent variable modeling of diagnostic accuracy. *Biometrics*, **53**, 948–58.

Youden, W. J. (1950). Index for rating diagnostic tests. *Cancer*, **3**, 32–5.

Zelen, M. (1976). Theory of early detection of breast cancer in the general population. In *Breast cancer: Trends in research and treatment* (ed. J. C. Heuson, W. H. Mattheim and M. Rozencweig), 287–300. Raven Press, New York.

Zhou, X. H. (1993). Maximum likelihood estimators of sensitivity and specificity corrected for verification bias. *Communication in Statistics–Theory and Methods*, **22**, 3177–98.

Zhou, X. H. (1996). A nonparametric maximum likelihood estimator for the receiver operating characteristic curve area in the presence of verification bias. *Biometrics*, **52**, 299–305.

Zhou, X. H. (1998). Correcting for verification bias in studies of a diagnostic test's accuracy. *Statistical Methods in Medical Research*, **7**, 337–53.

Zhou, X. H., McClish, D. K. and Obuchowski, N. A. (2002). *Statistical methods in diagnostic medicine*. Wiley, New York.

Zou, K. H. and Hall, W. J. (2000). Two transformation models for estimating an ROC curve derived from continuous data. *Journal of Applied Statistics*, **27**, 621–31.

Zweig, M. H. and Campbell, G. (1993). Receiver-operating characteristic (ROC) plots: A fundamental evaluation tool in clinical medicine. *Clinical Chemistry*, **39**, 561–77.

INDEX

agreement, 76, 277
AND rule
  in combining tests, 207, 267–8
area under ROC curve (AUC)
  confidence intervals, 107, 224–5
  definitions, 77, 92
  empirical estimates, 103–7, 110
  for binormal curve, 83
  for comparing ROC curves, 108–10,
    112, 118–19, 126
  in multireader radiology studies, 126,
    166
  in sample size calculations, 224–8,
    234–7
  interpretations, 77–8, 92
  magnitudes, 94
  parametric estimates, 110, 116
  regression modelling, 164, 166
  small sample inference, 107, 126
ascertainment bias, 169
auxiliary variables, 175–7

Bayes factor, 19
Bayes theorem, 16, 170–1
Bayesian methods
  in combining tests, 273–4
  in latent class analysis, 202
  in meta-analysis, 258–9
  software, 259
believe the positive (negative) rules, 207,
  268
bias
  publication, 254
  survey of sources, 6–8
  with imperfect reference, 195–6
  with selected verification, 168–70
bin and smooth, 139
binary regression
  for AUC models, 164
  for classification probabilities, 51–8
  for detection and false referral
    probabilities, 186–7
  for estimating the ROC curve, 121
  for predictive values, 58–60
  for ROC–GLM models, 155
  in meta-analysis, 258
binormal ROC curve
  area under the ROC curve, 83–4
  comparing, 118–19, 124–5, 158–9

covariate effects on, 144–5, 152–3,
  158–60, 162
definition and properties, 81–5
estimation with continuous data, 122–3
estimation with ordinal data, 115–18
in discrete function framework, 91
in latent decision variable model, 87–8
sample size calculations, 223–4, 226–8,
  236
slope, 223
BIRADS, 86
blinding, 5, 36, 217
Boolean combination, 207, 268
boosting, 174–6
Box–Cox power transform, 140
bronze standard, 200
BUGS, 259

case-control
  definition, 3–4
  in phase 5, 246
  in phases of test development, 215–17
  merits relative to cohort, 26–7
  sample sizes, 218–38, 249–51
classification probabilities
  confidence regions, 22–4, 218–20
  definition, 15
  hypothesis tests, 15, 218–19, 230–4
  regression, 51–8
  regression with verification bias, 178–9
  relation to other accuracy measures,
    16–17, 19–21, 61–2
  sample sizes, 218–20, 250
  time-dependent, 260–3
  see also relative classification
    probabilities
classifier, 1
clinical trial
  applications of ROC analysis, 74, 81,
    93, 264, 278
  in comparing tests, 35–7
  in phase 5 development, 217, 245
clustered data, 52, 63–4, 97, 118, 126,
  150–1
  see also paired design
cohort
  definition, 3–4
  in phases of test development, 215–17
  merits relative to case-control, 26–7

297